Indian Plants and Drugs

With their Medicinal Properties and Uses

Indian Plants and Drugs

With their Medicinal Properties and Uses

By

K. M. Nadkarni, F. S. Sc. L. A. (London),

Member of the Paris Chemical Society,

Member of the British Pharmaceutical Conference, England

ASIATIC PUBLISHING HOUSE

B-181/4, J-Extn, Street No-5, Laxmi-Nagar

Delhi-110092 Ph.: (011) 22449904

(India)

Asiatic Publishing House (India)

Third Indian Print : 2010
Price : Rs. 1250/-

ISBN : 81-87067-07-1

Published by Asiatic Publishing House,
B-181/4, J-Extn, Street No-5, Laxmi-Nagar,
New Delhi-110092. Ph. (011) 22449904

Printed By
Ruchika Printers
Shahdara, Delhi-110032

Printed and Bound in India

PREFACE

If the object of my previous publications was mainly to serve my brethren of the Medical Profession by strengthening their hands in their sacred duties of combating disease and alleviating the suffering of the countless millions entrusted to their care, the aim and object of this little volume is to serve not only the professional medical men in India but also the non-professional educated public in general; and this object is sought to be attained by rendering the book useful to both these classes in the following ways:—

(1) *To the Medical Profession*:—

(*a*) By introducing to them the therapeutical properties of the numerous remedial drugs and agents of indigenous origin, and thus awakening an interest for their further study, research and application for helping the poorer classes of their patients by using cheaper and equally, if not more, efficacious native remedies in the treatment of diseases in preference to their costly foreign substitutes.

(*b*) By placing before them the value and composition of several dietetic articles, such as fruits, grains, vegetables, etc., thereby helping them in prescribing diets more accurately and suitably to their patients who are naturally accustomed to native foods rather than foreign ones.

(c) By stimulating in them a desire for keeping ready the pharmacological preparations of important Indian drugs made according to Western preservative methods so that they can be readily employed in emergent cases.

(d) By enabling them, with the help of their knowledge of the Indian drugs as well as of the various Ayurvedic preparations described in the book, to better diagnose and treat the conditions of patients who come under their care after undergoing a previous course of treatment by kavirajees, pundits, vaidyans, and hakims.

(2) *To the Educated Public in general :—*

(a) By initiating them into a knowledge of the medicinal uses and applications of indigenous drugs and remedies procurable at a nominal price in all Indian bazaars, or at the mere cost of collection from the road-sides or gardens in immediate neighbourhood, whereby they can help themselves in cases of very minor complaints, or in cases where efficient medical aid is unattainable, and thus relieve many a pain and suffering and, perhaps even, save a valuable life.

(b) By placing before them the nature, composition and preparation of several select remedies belonging to the Ancient Ayurvedic System whose merits and benefits, in chronic cases, are already well known throughout the country.

(c) By enabling them to find out by themselves the medical and hygienic effect of numerous fruits, foods and vegetables in common use in order to regulate their own diet according to the needs of their conditions.

(*d*) By helping, with all these means and resources, the innumerable individuals, families and establishments, Agricultural, Industrial and Government, such as Public Works, Forests, Railways, Telegraph and other Departments, those engaged in Tea, Coffee, Cotton and other plantations and those employed in commercial pursuits in stations far away from regular medical aid and consequently thrown, at such times, on their own resources.

With these aims and objects I have compiled and condensed the notes embodied in this little volume, with the hope that, to the intelligent Householder it will serve as a safe and reliable Family Medical Aid, and to the Medical Practitioner, a powerful weapon added to his already existing armoury. I have endeavoured to give, within the prescribed limits of this volume, an epitome of the largest possible amount of valuable information, compressed as much as is consistent with clearness, accuracy and practical usefulness. In selecting this mass of facts I have made use of, besides the notes occassionally jotted down during the last fifteen years as a result of personal observation of cases cured with marvellous beneficial results in competition with the Western Allopathic System, several Standard Authorities on Indian products; among these may be named prominently, that of Dr. Watt, a monumental work replete with information about products of Indian origin, containing a vast store of personal investigation by a large army of eminent Physicians, Scientists and Workers in the field of Indian Therapeutics; that of Dr. K. L. Dey, C.I.E., F.C.S., the invaluable product of his forty years' experience and research in the domain of Indian Pharmacology; that of Dr. U. C. Dutt who, in his "Materia Medica of the Hindus" has unravelled the precious knowledge that lay hidden in ancient Sanscrit medical works; and that of Dr. E. J. Waring, already well known and popular in India. Among the rest may be mentioned the works of Dymock, Druary, Khory, Moideeen Sheriff and Sakharam Arjoon. To all these I owe my grateful acknowledgements, as I have availed myself of the valuable information contained in their works.

The Index of Diseases and Remedies given at the end has been prepared with the special purpose of helping the reader to track out at once the particular remedies for the particular ailment; and, under their respective headings, he can readily find out the methods of their application which, when employed with ordinary care and intelligence, will never fail to do good in most cases; and if, through the instrumentality of this little work, the physical suffering of the millions may be, in any degree, alleviated, my highest aim and ambition will be fulfilled and my labours abundantly rewarded.

tonic and aphrodisiac action on the nervous system Dose of the powder is 1 to 3 grains. If administered un-cooked they act as a strong purgative and emetic; when used in large doses they are acrid poïson, giving rise to symptoms like those of cholera. The active principle has been isolated and named *abrin*. The seeds are rubbed down with a small quantity of water into a paste and applied to contusions to reduce pain and swelling. It is also recommended to be applied to the bare skin in alopecia, in sciatica, stiffness of the shoulder joint, paralysis and other nervous diseases. Mixed with the paste made of plumbago root it is applied as a stimulant dressing in white leprosy. When decorticated and finely ground they are used for *pannus cornea* (vascularisation of the cornea, usually due to the irritation of granulations in conjunctivitis; the cornea is normally non-vascular) and granular lids. They cause a true purulent ophthalmia. A three per cent solution prepared by steeping the decorticated and powdered seeds in cold water for 24 hours and brushed over the reversed lids two or three times a day will cause purulent ophthalmia. In bad cases 5 per cent infusion is required, or it may be prepared thus:—Take 32 seeds, pulverise them and steep the powder in 16 ounces of cold water for 24 hours; then add 16 ounces of hot water, and filter when cooled; bathe the eyes with this infusion several times a day until sufficient irritation is set up; after the first application, irritation of the conjunctiva can be noticed; on the following day severe inflammation of the eyelids will set in, lasting from 5 to 15 days, when it gradually ceases and the patient is free from pannus and granulations. Even moderate ulceratïon is not a contra-indication for the use of the remedy ; this ulceration speedily improves.

Native Indian Preparations.—*Gunjabhadrarasa* :—Take of the seeds of *Abrus precatorius* six parts, mercury three parts, sulphur twelve parts, *nim* seeds, *cannabis sativa* leaves and croton seeds each one part. Rub them together and soak for one day in each of the following fluids, *viz.*, lemon juice, juice of the leaves of *cannabis sativa*, of datura leaves and of the leaves of *solanum nigrum*. This medicine is given in doses of 8 grains with rock salt and assafœtida, in paraplegia (Rasendra-sârsangrah).

Gunjâdya tailam.—Take of prepared sesamum oil four seers, juice of the leaves of *Wedelia calendulacea* (*bhringaraja*) sixteen seers, seeds of *Abrus precatorius* reduced to a paste one seer, and boil them together in the usual way. This oil is used as a local application in scurf of the scalp, prurigo and other skin diseases.

---

3. ACACIA ARABICA.

(N. O.—LEGUMINOSÆ.)

Sans.—Vabboola. *Eng.*—Indian gum arabic tree. *Hind.*, *Pers.*, and *Mah.*—Bâbul. *Ben.*—Bâbla. *Duk.*—Kali-kikar. *Guz.*—Kaloabaval. *Tel.*—Nallatumma. *Tam.*—Karuvel. *Can.*—Karijali *Mal.*—Karuvelum. *Kon.*—Shameeruku.

Habitat.—Common all over India ; plentiful in Western Peninsula, the Deccan and Coromandal Coast.

Properties and Uses.—The tender growing tops rubbed into a paste with sugar and water and given morning and evening act as demulcent, useful in coughs. The extract is an astringent and injected to allay irritation

Indian Plants and Drugs.

1. ABIES WEBBIANA.

(*Natural Order.*—CONIFERÆ.)

Sanskrit—Tâlisapatram. *English*—Himalayan Silver Fir. *Hindustani* and *Bengalee*—Tâlispatra. *Telugu, Tamil* and *Canarese*—Tâlispatri. *Malayalum*—Tâleesapatram.

Habitat.—This lofty fir is widely distributed on the higher ranges of the Himalayas.

Properties and Uses.—This drug is used as an astringent, carminative, expectorant and antiperiodic. The dried terebinthinous leaves are useful in coughs, phthisis, asthma, bronchitis and catarrh of the bladder. The juice of the fresh leaves is administered in fevers of infants during dentition and also in affections of the chest, the dose being 5 to 10 drops in water or mother's milk. In Bengal the juice is administered as a tonic in cases of parturition. Powder of the leaves in doses of half to one drachm is given with the juice of *Adhatoda vasica* and honey in cough, asthma and hæmoptysis.

Native Indian Preparations.—A confection called *Tâlisadya Churna* is prepared with *Tâlispatra*, black-pepper, long-pepper, ginger, bamboo-manna, cardamoms, cinnamon and sugar, and is used in cough, asthma and hæmoptysis (Sarangadhara).

2. ABRUS PRECATORIUS.

(*N. O.*—LEGUMINOSÆ.)

Sans.—Gunja. *Eng.*—Jequirity, Indian liquorice. *Pers.*—Gungchi. *Hind.*, *Duk.*, and *Guz.*—Gumchi. *Ben.*—Kunch. *Mah.*—Gunja. *Tel.*—Guriginja. *Tam.*—Gundumani. *Can.*—Gurugunji. *Mal.*—Kunni.

Habitat.—This beautiful climbing plant, remarkable for its small egg-shaped beads of a brilliant scarlet colour with a black scar is found all over India, spreading through the plains from the Himalayas down to Ceylon and Siam.

Properties and Uses.—Its leaves are used to relieve local pain in swellings, rheumatism, etc. The leaves steeped in warm mustard oil are applied over the seat of pain; or they are warmed over the fire and applied after smearing the part with warm castor oil. The juice of fresh leaves mixed with some bland oil and applied to the painful part relieves pain and reduces the swelling. The juice rubbed daily to leucodermatic spots for about a month has been found to remove them. The leaves are chewed and the juice swallowed in cases of hoarseness.

The root is made use of in the same manner as the liquorice root, *i.e.*, as a laxative, and as an adjunct in mixture. The watery extract of the root is useful in relieving obstinate cough.

The seeds contain an albuminous substance of a poisonous nature, similar in its action to the poison extracted from castor oil seeds. Like all albuminous seeds it loses its activity when boiled, and therefore the seeds when cooked may be even used as food. When powdered and boiled with milk they have a powerful copper sulphate (15 grains to the ounce) may be added. The tincture is an excellent application for threatened bed sores, and the decoction is useful for washing sore or cracked nipples.

Kath-bol is a mixture of catechu and myrrh and is given to women after confinement, as a tonic and to promote secretion of milk. Combined with the seeds of *Bonducella* and with ferri sulphas it is useful for strengthening gums.

Native Indian Preparations.—*Svalpakhadiravatika* is a favourite medicine in diseases of the mouth and gums. To prepare it, take of catechu twelve seers and a half, water sixty-four seers, boil down to eight seers, then add nutmeg, camphor, betel-nuts and *kakkola* each half a seer in fine powder, and prepare a mass fit for being made into balls or boluses. They are directed to be kept in the mouth, in affections of the teeth, gums, palate and tongue (Chakradatta).

The following decoction called *Khadirâstaka* is prescribed for internal use in boils, prurigo, measles, and other skin diseases. Take of catechu, the three myrobalans, *nim* bark, leaves of *Trichosanthes dioica* (*patola*) *gulancha* and *adhatoda vasica* equal parts and prepare a decoction in the usual way. Sarangadhara describes a fermented liquor called *Khadirârishta* for use in skin diseases. It is prepared with catechu and the wood of *Pinus Deodara* and some other ingredients in smaller proportions.

5. ACACIA CONCINNA.

(N. O.—LEGUMINOSÆ.)

Sans.—Saptata. *Hind.*—Kochi. *Duk.*—Siki. *Ben.*—Banritha. *Mah.*—Shikâkâi. *Tel.*—Cheekâya. *Tam.*—Sheeyakây. *Can.*—Sheegæ. *Mal.*—Cheeyakâyi. *Kon.*—Shikâyi.

Habitat.—In the tropical jungles throughout India: in Bengal, in East and Central Mysore.

Properties and Uses.—The pods are externally used as detergent; internally they are used as aperient and expectorant. The decoction of the pods and leaves is a useful aperient in bilious affections. The decoction of the pods made by boiling half ounce of the pods in one pint of water is used as hair-wash; it is said to promote growth of the hair and remove dandruff. The tender leaves ground up with salt, tamarind and chillies form an excellent chutney, useful in bilious affections. The infusion thereof is useful in checking malarious fevers; it also prevents flatulence, as it acts as a mild laxative. The pods ground up and formed into an ointment make a good application in skin diseases.

---

6. ACACIA FARNESIANA.

(N. O.—LEGUMINOSÆ.)

Sans.—Arimædah. *Eng.*—The Cassie flower. *Hind.*—Gandbabul. *Ben.*—Guyabâbla. *Duk.*—Gu-kikar. *Guz.*—Gu-baval. *Tel.*—Nugatumma. *Tam.*—Pikkaruvil. *Can.*—Karijali. *Mal.*—Kariveelum. *Kon.*—Kusrijhâd.

Habitat.—It is found everywhere in India and is well known for its bright yellow flowers, which yield a most delicious perfume.

Properties and Uses.—The decoction of the bark together with ginger is an astringent wash for the teeth.

in acute gonorrhœa and leucorrhœa. The tender leaves beaten into a pulp are administered in dysentery and diarrhœa; the decoction is used in the same complaints as an astringent enemata. Bruised tender leaves formed into a poultice and applied to ulcers act as stimulant and astringent. The bark contains a large quantity of tannin and is a powerful astringent; its decoction is largely used as a gargle and mouth-wash in cancerous and syphilitic affections. It is a useful injection in gonorrhœa, cystitis, vaginitis, leucorrhœa, &c. The infusion of the bark (1½ ounces to one pint of water) is given in chronic diarrhœa and diabetes mellitus, in doses of 1½ to 2 ounces twice a day The juice of the bark mixed with milk is dropped into the eye in conjunctivitis. The burnt bark and burnt almond shell both pulverised and mixed with salt make a good tooth-powder. The gum is administered in the form of mucilage in diarrhœa and dysentery and also in diabetes mellitus as the gum is not converted into sugar. The powdered gum mixed with quinine is useful in fever cases complicated with diarrhœa and dysentery. The powdered gum mixed with the white of an egg is applied to burns and scalds. The powdered gum is also used to arrest hæmorrhages. Fried in ghee it is useful as a nutritive tonic and aphrodisiac in cases of sexual debility.

4. ACACIA CATECHU.

(*N. O.*—LEGUMINOSÆ.)

Sans., *Mah.* and *Can.*—Khadira. *Eng.*—Catechu. *Hind.*—Kathâ. *Ben.*—Khair. *Guz.*—Kher. *Duk.*—Kath-khair. *Tel.*—Poogamu. *Tam.*—Voadalam. *Mal.*—Khadiram. *Kon.*—Kâthu.

Habitat.—This tree is common in the forests of many parts of India and Burma.

Properties and Uses.—Catechu is an extract prepared from the wood of *Acacia Catechu* by boiling it in water and inspissating the decoction. Its chief use in India is as an ingredient of the packet of betel leaves chewed by the people. It is a valuable astringent in passive diarrhœas and hæmorrhages, either in powder or as tincture, combined with other astringents; especially useful for children. Take powdered catechu and powdered cinnamon bark each 10 or 15 grains, mix them together in sufficient honey or syrup and make into four pills; or take of catechu powder three drachms and cinnamon bark powder one drachm; infuse both in half-pint of boiling water for 2 hours; filter and administer in doses of 1½ to 2 ounces three times a day. For adults 5 drops of laudanum may be added to each dose during administration, but not for young children. A small piece held in the mouth and allowed slowly to dissolve acts like an astringent lozenge, and is of great service in hoarseness, relaxed sore throat, loss of voice, etc.; also in cases of mercurial salivation, bleeding, ulcerations and sponginess of the gums. In toothache it is employed to stuff the hollow of the aching tooth. When mixed with lard or simple ointment it makes a useful application to chronic ulcerations with fœtid discharges; in obstinate cases a little of powdered of spirit of wine in a closed jar for seven days, occasionally agitating the same, strain, press, filter and add sufficient spirits of ether to make one pint; dose is from 20 to 60 minims frequently repeated during the day in honey. Hakims treat cases of acute mania in early stages by the following mode: Take of one ounce of fresh juice of the leaves and dissolve in it six grains of common salt; drop a little of this mixture in both nostrils every morning and then place the patient under cold shower baths for three mornings regularly; this causes a quantity of mucus and other matter to escape from the nostrils.

---

9. ACHYRANTHES ASPERA.

(*N. O.*—AMARANTACEÆ.)

Sans.—Apâmârga. *Eng.*—Prickly chaff-flower. *Ben.*—Apâng. *Duk.*—Agari. *Guz.*—Aghedo. *Mah.*—Aghada. *Tel.*—Uttarœni. *Tam.*—Shiru-kadalâdi. *Mal.*—Kadalâdi. *Can.*—Uttaranee.

Habitat.—A small plant three or four feet in height, found all over India.

Properties and Uses.—The decoction of the plant made with 2 oz. of the plant in 1½ pints of water is a good diuretic which acts mildly on the kidneys and tends to increase their secretions; found efficacious in renal dropsies; the juice is also useful in such complaints as piles, boils, skin eruptions, &c.; in large doses it produces abortion or labour pains. Fresh leaves ground into a paste and mixed with black-pepper and garlic and made into pills are used as antiperiodic; leaves rubbed into a paste with water are applied with much benefit to bites of poisonous insects, wasps, bees, &c. Fresh juice of the leaves thickened into an extract by exposure to the sun and mixed with a little opium is an efficacious application to primary syphilitic sores. An infusion of the root is given as a mild astringent in bowel complaints. The spike with the seeds is often used as an expectorant.

Native Indian Preparations.—*Apámárga taila:* Take of sesamum oil four seers, the alkaline water prepared from the ashes of *Achyranthes aspera* sixteen seers, the ashes of the plant one seer and boil them together in the usual way. This oil is poured into the meatus in cases of noise in the ears and in deafness.

---

10. ACONITUM FEROX.

(*N. O.*—RANUNCULACEÆ.)

Sans.—Visha. *Eng.*—Indian aconite. *Hind.* and *Arab.*—Bish, *Pers.*—Bishnâg. *Ben.*—Katbish or Mitha. *Guz.*—Vuchnag. *Mah.*—Bachanâg. *Tel.*—Vasanubhi. *Tam.*—Vishna nuir. *Can.*—Vatsanâbhi.

Habitat.—It grows plentifully in the temperate and sub-Alpine regions of the Himalayas.

Properties and Uses.—This root is distinctly more powerful than that of *Aconitum napellus*, and therefore more suited for the external applications or the manufacture of *aconitine*. The root yields a comparatively larger quantity of *pseudo-aconitine* or *nepaline* and a smaller quantity of aconitine than other species of aconite, the former being the more powerful physiologically of the two alkaloids. It is therefore not to be given in the same doses as the true aconite. It is a narcotic and powerful sedative. In large doses it acts as a virulent poison. In the form of liniment it is useful in cases of neuralgia and muscular rheumatism. It is used in very small doses and so it is useful in the bleeding of the gums, etc. A gum exudes from the bark of the tree which is a good substitute for gum arabic, but yields a gelatinous fluid on treatment with water. The tender leaves are bruised with a little water and swallowed in gonorrhœa. The pods or the round yellow heads constitute the Cassia flowers, which when distilled yield a delicious perfume. They contain a balsamic liquid which is employed as an adjunct to aphrodisiacs in spermatorrhœa.

---

7. ACACIA SPECIOSA.

(*N. O.*—LEGUMINOSÆ.)

Sans.—Sahasraki, Pruthushrangi. *Eng.*—Sirissa tree. *Hind.*—Siris. *Ben.*—Siriz. *Guz.*—Pitosarshio. *Mah.*—Siras. *Tel.*—Girishamu. *Tam.*—Chireedam. *Can.*—Shireesha-mara. *Mal.*—Nannæni.

Habitat.—Sub-Himalayan tract, Bengal, Central and South India.

Properties and Uses.—The seeds are astringent and given in bleeding piles, diarrhœa, gonorrhœa &c., in the form of powder. In doses of 1½ drachms the powder has been successfully administered in cases of scrofulous enlargement of the glands; locally a paste made of the powder and water is also applied. The oil extracted from the seeds is given in leprosy. The leaves are applied to any eye-complaints as in ophthalmia; the flowers form a cooling application to boils, eruptions and swellings.

---

8. ACALYPHA INDICA.

(*N. O.*—EUPHORBIACEÆ.)

Sans.—Arittamanjaric. *Eng.*—Indian acalypha. *Hind.*—Kupi. *Ben.*—Muktajhuri. *Guz.*—Vanchi Kânto. *Mah*—Khokali. *Tel.*—Kuppichettu. *Tam.*—Kuppivæni. *Can.*—Kuppigida. *Mal.*—Kuppamæni. *Kon.*—Kunkmiphal.

Habitat.—This plant is a common annual in Indian gardens.

Properties and Uses.—The leaves possess laxative properties used in the form of powder or decoction; mixed with garlic they are used as anthelmintic. Mixed with common salt the leaves are applied to scabies; and their juice mixed with oil forms a useful application in rheumatic arthritis. The expressed juice of the leaves is a safe, certain and speedy emetic for children in one tea-spoonful doses, found useful in cases of croup; in smaller doses it is expectorant, and in bronchitis and asthma. The decoction is employed in ear-ache as instillation and also as fomentation round the aching ear; and a cataplasm of the bruised leaves is applied to syphilitic ulcers, to maggot-eaten sores, and also to relieve the pain of snake bites. The powder of dry leaves is used in bed sores. In congestive head-aches a piece of cotton saturated with the expressed juice of the plant or leaves and inserted into each nostril is said to relieve by causing hæmorrhage from the nose. In cases of obstinate constipation of children the leaves ground into a paste and made into a ball and introduced into the rectum, relieves the contraction of the sphincter ani and produces free motions. The root bruised in water acts as a cathartic.

Native Indian Preparations.—Macerate three ounces of the fresh leaves, stalks and flowers with a pint the watery portion is evaporated. This oil is said to be useful in boils, prurigo, psoriasis, leucoderma and other skin diseases.

11. ACONITUM HETEROPHYLLUM.

(N. O.—RANUNCULACEÆ.)

Sans.—Ativisha. *Eng.*—Indian atees. *Hind.* and *Ben.*—Atis. *Pers.*—Vuggi-turki. *Mah.*—Ativisha. *Tel.*—Ativasu. *Tam.*—Ativudayam.

Properties and Uses.—The tuberous roots of this plant are considered tonic, astringent, stomachic and aphrodisiac. The drug is chiefly used in the form of powder. The active principle is *atisine*, an amorphous alkaloid of intensely bitter taste but non-poisonous. Aconitine is absent in the true *Atis*. It is a valuable febrifuge and antiperiodic, and for combating debility after fevers it is an excellent tonic, and very efficacious in diarrhœa and dysentery.

Native Indian Preparations.—In fever with diarrhœa the following decoction is recommended in Sarangadhara:—Take of *atis*, ginger, *kurchi* bark, tubers of *Cyperus rotundus* (*mustaka*) and root of *Tinospora cordifolia* (*gulancha*) equal parts, in all two tolas, water thirty-two tolas. Boil till the water is reduced to eight tolas. This quantity is given in two or three divided doses during the course of the day. Chakradatta recommends the following called *Hriveradi* in similar cases:—Take of *atis*, dried *bela*, root of *pavonia odorata* and *Cyperus rotundus* (*mustaka*) and the horny excrescence of *Rhus succedanea* equal parts, powder and mix. This compound powder is given in suitable doses with the addition of honey. Sometimes, long-pepper is added to the above ingredients, when the powder is called *Bâla-chatur bhadraka* from its being composed of four ingredients.

---

12. ACONITUM NAPELLUS.

(*N. O.*—RANUNCULACEÆ.)

Sans.—Visha. *Eng.*—Monkshood, aconite. *Hind.*—Mithazahar. *Ben.*—Katbish. *Mah.*—Nagpuri bachanâg.

Habitat.—Indigenous to the temperate Himalayan region, where it grows in abundance.

Properties and Uses.—The dried root is extensively used in Indian medicine. It yields several chemical principles, the principal of which being the alkaloid *aconitine*. The uses of this root have already been indicated under *Aconitum Ferox*. Most of the preparations are made from the root, but an extract is made from the fresh leaves and flowering tops.

---

13. ACORUS CALAMUS.

(*N. O.*—AROIDEÆ.)

Sans.—Vacha. *Eng.*—Sweetflag. *Hind.* and *Ben.*—Bach. *Pers.*—Agri-turki. *Duk.*—Vach. *Guz.*—Godavâj. *Mah.*—Vekhand. *Tel.*—Vasa. *Tam.*—Vashambu. *Can.*—Baje. *Mal.*—Vayampu. *Kon.*—Ekhanda.

Habitat.—A semi-aquatic perennial growing in damp marshy places and indigenous to India and Burma.

Properties and Uses.—The dried rhizome of this plant is stimulant and aromatic, yielding a glucocide *acorin* and a volatile oil. Given in the form of infusion it is tonic and stomachic, useful in dyspepsia, flatulence, loss of appetite, etc., and also in atonic and choleraic diarrhœa of children; as antiperiodic it is given in

(½ to ¼ grain) as an antiperiodic and alterative and as a nervine tonic in cases of paralysis; for internal administration it must be used with great caution on account of the virulent character of the drug.

Native Indian Preparations.—Aconite is purified by being cut in small slices and steeped in cow's urine for three days before being used.

Mrityunjaya Rasa—is a favourite medicine, which is prepared as follows:—Take of purified aconite, sulphur, black-pepper, long-pepper, and borax each one part, cinnaber two parts, powder and beat them into a mass with water and make into two-grain pills. These pills are given in ordinary remittent fever and in that of typhoid type (Rasaratnakara). A composition very similar to the above is recommended by Sarangadhara under the name of *Ananda Bhairavarasa*. If there is much constipation along with the fever, croton seeds are added to the above ingredients, as in the preparations called *Jvara Murari Rasa* (Bhasajyaratnavali).

Panchavaktra Rasa.—Take of purified mercury, aconite, sulphur, black-pepper and borax, rub them together with the juice of datura leaves for twelve hours and make into four-grain pills; these pills are administered in fever complicated with cerebral symptoms. Along with these pills a decoction of the root of *Calotropis gigentia* (arka) with the addition of long-pepper, black-pepper and ginger is recommended to be taken.

Saubhâgya Vatika—described in *Bhaishajya-ratnavali* is prepared thus:—Take of aconite, borax, cumin seeds, the five salts, *viz.*, rock, sea, *sonchal*, *vit*, and *sambar* salts, the three myrobalans, ginger, long-pepper and black-pepper prepared talc, mercury and sulphur in equal parts. First rub the mercury and sulphur together, then mix them with the other ingredients, soak the mixture seven times successively in the juice of the following leaves, *viz.*, of *vitex negundo*, *nyctanthes arbor-tristis*, *eclipta prostrata*, *adhatoda vasica*, and *achyranthes aspera*, and make into four-grain pills.

Ramabana Rasa.—Take of mercury, aconite, cloves and sulphur, each one part, black-pepper two parts, nutmeg half a part, rub them together with tamarind juice and make into two-grain pills; these pills are used in dyspepsia with loss of appetite; they are given with the addition of powdered black-pepper. (Rasendrachintamani.)

Kaphaketu Rasa.—Take of aconite, borax, long-pepper and conch-shell lime, equal parts; powder, mix, and soak the mixture three times successively in fresh ginger juice. Dose: two grains to be given with ginger juice. This is useful in catarrh, sore-throat, cough, asthma, discharges from the ears and nose, etc. (Rasendrasârsangrah.)

Visha taila.—Take of sesamum oil four seers, aconite root eight tolas, seeds of *pongamia glabra*, turmeric, wood of *Berberis Asiatica*, root of *Calotropis gigentia*, of *Nerium odorum*, flowers of *Tabernæmontana coronaria* (*tagara*), *Acorus calamus*, *Aplotaxis auriculata*, *Vallaris dichotoma*, red sandalwood, flowers of *Aganosma Caryophyllata*, bark of *Alstonia scholaris*, madder and leaves of *Vitex negundo* each four tolas, cow's urine sixteen seers. The solid ingredients should be beaten into a paste with water and then boiled with the oil and cow's urine till tertian fevers. With the addition of a little liquorice root it is administered in cases of cough, fever, colic, etc., especially in children. In cases of irritation of the throat and cough the root simply chewed produces copious salivation and an agreeable sensation of warmth; in large doses, 30 grains and upwards, it is nauseant and emetic; in small doses it is carminative and nervine. It is eaten freely during the prevalence of any epidemic, as it is supposed to be an antidote for several poisons. Externally it is used in chronic rheumatism, the root being powdered and rubbed up with cachew spirit; the powder is a very effective insecticide, keeps moths from woollen goods and fleas from rooms. The root burnt to cinder, mixed with cocoanut or castor oil and smeared over the abdomen relieves flatulent colic.

Native Indian Preparations.—Take of *Acorus calamus* root, assafœtida, *atis*, long-pepper, black-pepper, ginger, chebulic myrobalan and sonchal salt equal parts; powder and mix. Dose is about half a drachm. This is prescribed in dyspepsia; in combination with other medicines it is used as a stimulant in low fevers, epilepsy, and insanity.

---

14. ADANSONIA DIGITATA.

(*N. O.*—BOMBACEÆ).

Eng.—Boabab, or monkey bread-tree. *Hind.* and *Guz.*—Gorakhamli. *Duk.*—Hathi-khatiyan. *Mah.*—Gorakh-chinch. *Tam.*—Papperappuli. *Can.*—Brahmamlika.

Habitat.—One of the largest and long-lived trees in the world, met with chiefly in Bombay, Guzarat and Coromandel Coast.

Properties and Uses.—The fruit is somewhat acid and makes a cooling and refrigerent drink in fevers. The pulp of the seed is refrigerent and diuretic. Externally it is applied in skin diseases. The fresh juice of the leaves mixed with powdered ginger together with the expressed juice of the fresh root of *Salvadora Indica* is applied with considerable benefit to painful joints, indolent syphilitic ulcers, and chancres. The leaves are used as fomentations and poultices for rheumatic affections of the limbs and irritable inflammatory ulcers. The bark is used as an antiperiodic. It contains a principle called *adansonia*. The bark yields a gum which has an acid reaction insoluble in water, and which appears to be allied to gum tragacanth.

15. ADHATODA VASIKA.

(*N. O.*—ACANTHACEÆ)

Sans.—Vàsaka. *Eng.*—Malabar nut. *Hind.*—Arusha. *Ben.*—Bákash. *Pers.*—Bànsa. *Duk.*—Adarsa. *Tel.*—Addasaram. *Tam.*—Adatodai. *Can.*—Adusogae. *Mal.*—Ataloetakam.

Habitat.—This plant grows wild all over Bengal, and also in most other parts of India.

Properties and Uses.—The root, bark, leaves and flowers are all used medicinally, mostly in the form of powder or infusion of the root and extract of the leaves in cough, asthma, ague and phthisis. The fresh juice two drachms with honey or with one drachm of ginger juice or a decoction of the leaves and root with pepper is an excellent cough mixture useful in chronic bronchitis, asthma and consumption. The juice of the leaves is considered useful for diarrhœa and dysentery, especially in hæmoptysis and in the bleeding of dysentery. The strong decoction is an efficacious fomentation to rheumatic and painful swellings and neuralgias. The dried leaves are smoked as cigarettes with much benefit in asthma. The fresh flowers are bound over the eyes in ophthalmia.

Native Indian Preparations.—Sarangdara describes a compound decoction of the root of *Adhatoda vasica*, much used in fever with cough, and which is as follows:—Take of *vâsaka* root, *gulancha* and the root of *Solarium Jacquinii* (*Kantakâri*) in equal parts, two tolas in all, and prepare a decoction in the usual way. This is given with the addition of honey. A *ghrita* is prepared with clarified butter, a decoction of the plant and a paste of the root taken in the usual proportions, and is used in phthisis. *Vâsâvaleha* or electuary of *Vâsaka* is prepared thus:—Take of the juice of vâsaka leaves four seers, white sugar one seer, long-pepper sixteen tolas, clarified butter sixteen tolas, boil them together till reduced to the consistence of an extract. When cool add honey one seer and stir with a ladle till intimately mixed. Dose is one to two tolas in phthisis, cough with pain in the sides, hæmoptysis and asthma (Bhâvaprakash).

Vâsachandanâdi taila:—Take of *vasaka* root twelve seers and a-half, water sixty-four seers; boil till reduced to one-fourth. Take of lac eight seers, water sixty-four seers; boil down to sixteen seers. Take of red sandalwood, *guluncha*, root of *Clerodendron Siphonanthus*, the ten drugs called *dasamula* and *Solanum Jacquinii*, each two seers and a-half, water sixty-four seers; boil down to sixteen seers. To these decoctions add of whey and prepared sesamum oil sixteen seers each, and the following substances in the form of a paste, *viz.*, red sandalwood, liquorice, wood of *Berberis Asiatica*, long-pepper, black-pepper, ginger, termuric, *pâchak* root, embelic myrobalans, *tejapatra* leaves, wood of *Cedrus Deodâra*, cinnamon and cardamom, seeds called *renuka*, pouch of civet cat, root of *Withania somnifera (asvaganda) Pæderia fœtida, Vanda Roxburghii, saileya* (a sort of lichen), Zedoary root, and the fruit of *Aglaia Roxburghiana* each eight tolas ; and boil them together in the usual way. This oil is rubbed on the body in affections of the chest and especially in phthisis (Bhaishajyaratnavali).

---

16. AEGLE MARMELOS.

(*N. O.*—RUTACEÆ.)

Sans.—Bilva, Sriphal. *Eng.*—Bæl fruit, Bengal quince. *Hind.*—Bel. *Guz.*—Bilivaphal. *Pers.*—Shul. *Mah.*—Bæla. *Tel.*--Bilvamu. *Tam.*—Vilvam. *Can.*—Belapatre. *Mal.*—Koovalam, vilvam.

Habitat.—Found in cultivation all over India, wild in sub-Himalayan forests, in Central and South India, and Burma.

Properties and Uses.—The fruit is alterative and nutritive, acts as a laxative in health ; very valuable in habitual constipation and dyspepsia. The unripe or half ripe fruit cut up and sun-dried is astringent, digestive and stomachic, and is prescribed in diarrhœa and dysentery, with debility of the mucous membrane. It is specially useful in chronic diarrhœa and dysentery of children. It contains a small quantity of tannin, pectin and some astringent acids. The ripe fruit is sweet, aromatic and cooling when made into morning sherbat, which is made by mixing two ounces of pulp in three or four ounces of water or syrup. It is pleasantly laxative and a good simple cure for dyspepsia. Bæl-marmalade or aromotised confection is useful at the breakfast during convalescence from chronic dysentery or diarrhœa.

The decoction of the root and sometimes the stem bark is useful in intermittent fever, also in hypochondriasis and palpitation of the heart. The decoction is given with sugar and fried rice for checking diarrhœa and gastric irritability in children. A poultice made of the leaves is useful in ophthalmia. The fresh juice is given with the addition of black-pepper in anasarca with costiveness and jaundice, and when diluted with water or honey it is a highly-praised remedy in catarrh and feverishness; it is largely used in Bengal as antibilious and febrifuge. The astringent rind of the ripe fruit is employed in acute dysentery; its usefulness is enhanced by the combination of opium. Powder of the dried pulp is given with treacle in recent dysentery with griping pain in the loins and costiveness. Dose, as tonic, is from 12 to 15 grains of the powdered pulp; as a febrifuge and antiscorbutic it is from 16 to 20 grains; and as nauseant and antidysenteric it is from 20 grains to 2 drachms. For a child the following is an excellent prescription in cases of chronic diarrhoea :—Powder of unripe fruit six grains, compound powder of kino one grain, and pure white sugar in fine powder one grain; mix together; this dose is to be given two or three times a day. The pulp of the fresh fruit is mixed with milk and administered with cubeb powder in chronic gonorrhœa.

Native Indian Preparations.—Chakradatta mentions a compound powder which is prepared with equal parts of dried *baela*, tubers of *Cyperus Rotundus*, flowers of *Woodfordia floribunda*, root of *Stephania hernandifolia*, ginger and *mocharasa*. It is given in doses of 22 to 44 grains with buttermilk and treacle, in recent dysentery with griping pain in the loins and costiveness. In the dysentery of children a decoction and an electuary of the following drugs is used, *viz.*, dried *baela*, fruits of *Pothos officinalis*, root of *Pavonia odorata*, flowers of *Woodfordia floribunda* and bark of *Symplocos racemosa* in equal parts.

Vilva taila is thus prepared:—Take of dried *baela* fruits twelve seers and a half and boil in 64 seers of water till reduced to one-fourth. To the strained decoction, add 4 seers of prepared sesamum oil and 6 tolas each of the following substances in the form of paste, *viz.*, *Vanda Roxburghii*, *Boerhavia diffusa*, *Aplotaxis auriculata*, ginger, dried *baela*, flowers of *Woodfordia floribunda*, wood of *Pinus deodâra*, bark of *Symplocos racemosa*, tubers of *Cyperus rotundus*, *Acorus Calamus* and gum of *Bombax Malabaricum*, and prepare an oil in the usual way. This oil is used externally in chronic bowel complaints.

---

17. AGATI GRANDIFLORA.

(*N. O.*—LEGUMINOSÆ.)

Sans.—Agastya. *Ben.*—Buko. *Mah.*—Agasti. *Tel.*—Avisi. *Tam.*—Akatti. *Can.*—Agase. *Mal.*—Agatti.

Properties and Uses.—The bark is very astringent and is given as infusion in the first stages of small-pox and other eruptive fevers. The root of the red-flowered variety rubbed into a paste with water is applied to rheumatic swellings. The leaves are aperient. The juice of the leaves and flowers is a popular remedy for nasal catarrh and headache when it is sniffed up the nostrils. The juice of the flowers is squeezed into the eyes to relieve dimness of vision.

---

18. AGAVE AMERICANA.

(*N. O.*—AMARYLLIDEÆ.)

Sans.—Kantala. *Eng.*—American aloe, Carata. *Hind.* and *Duk.*—Rakaspattah. *Ben.*—Jangli-ânanash. *Guz.*—Jangli-kanvâr. *Mah.*—Jangli-anânas. *Tel.*—Râkâshimatalu. *Tam.*—Anekatalai. *Can.*—Anekatali. *Mal.*—Erœppakaita.

Habitat.—The century plant naturalised in many parts of India.

Properties and Uses.—Its roots have diuretic and antisyphilitic properties, used with sarsaparilla in the form of decoction (4 ounces to 1 pint of water); the juice which yields on cutting the leaves and the root is specially useful in syphilis. The sap is laxative, diuretic and emmenagogue; the dose is two fluid ounces. It is found very useful in scurvy. The fresh juice is a good external application to bruises and contusions. The gum exuding from the leaves and root is used as a cure for toothache. The pulp of the leaves mixed with sugar is a popular remedy for gonorrhœa.

---

19. AILANTHUS EXCELSA.

(*N. O.*—SIMARUBEÆ).

Sans.—Mâdala. *Hind.*, *Ben.*, and *Mah.*—Maharukha. *Tel.*—Peddamânu. *Tam.*—Perumaruttu. *Can.*—Doddamani or hiremara.

Habitat.—Common in many parts of India.

Properties and Uses.—The bark is intensely bitter, resembling quassia. It yields an important bitter principle which has been named *ailantic acid.* The bark and the leaves are reputed as tonic, especially in debility after child-birth. They also possess febrifuge properties and are useful in dyspeptic complaints.

20. AILANTHUS MALABARICA.

(*N. O.*—XANTHOXYLACEÆ).

Sans.—Mahânimba, Pishâchavraksha. *Mah.*—Guggula-dhup. *Tel.*—Maddipalu. *Tam.* and *Mal.*—Perumaram. *Can.*—Hemmara.

Habitat.—Malabar Coast and Travancore.

Properties and Uses.—The bark is bitter and is given in dyspepsia. The fresh juice of the bark (one ounce) with equal quantity of curd given morning and evening proves beneficial in dysentery. The resin or gum has a strong balsamic odour, useful in dysentery in the form of powder. Milk mixed with the powder and strained is given in dysentery; it is also a good stimulant in bronchitic affection.

21. ALANGIUM DECAPETALUM.

(*N. O.*—CORNACEÆ.)

Sans.—Shoedhanam, Ankoela, Ankoeda. *Eng.*—Sage-leaved alangium. *Hind.*—Akola. *Ben.*—Akar-kanta, Baghankurâ. *Guz.*—Onkla. *Mah.*—Ankol *Tel.*—Ankoelamu. *Tam*—Ankolum, atikoevam. *Can.*—Ankoelaemara. *Mal.*—Ankolam, Chemmaram.

Habitat.—Common in tropical forests of South India and Burma; occasionally found in gardens.

Properties and Uses.—The root-bark is an efficient and safe emetic in doses of 50 grains; in smaller doses, *i.e.*, 10 grains, it is nauseant and febrifuge. It has a reputation in leprosy and syphilitic and other skin diseases: it is also diaphoretic and antipyretic, therefore used in simple-continued fevers. The root is laxative and anthelmintic, useful in worms, colic, inflammations and poisonous bites, including snake-bites. The oil of the root-bark is said to be a useful external application in acute rheumatism. The fruit is said to be cooling, tonic, nutritive, useful in burning of the body, consumption and hæmorrhages. Dose of the root-bark as an alterative tonic is from two to five grains in powder.

---

22. ALEURITES MOLUCCANA.

(*N. O.*—EUPHORBIACEÆ).

Sans.—Askhota. *Eng.*—Indian walnut. *Hind.*—Akhrot. *Ben.*—Jangli akrot.

Habitat.—This plant, which is a native of the Malay Archipelago is found wild in many parts of South India.

Properties and Uses.—The kernels of the nuts, which taste like English walnuts, yield by expression a very agreeable fixed oil, which has a mild aperient action like castor oil. The kernels are supposed to possess aphrodisiac properties.

---

23. ALLIUM CEPA.

(*N. O.*—LILIACEÆ.)

San.—Palându. *Eng.*—Onion. *Hind.* and *Ben.*—Pyaj. *Guz.*—Dungari.' *Mah.*—Kândâ. *Tel.* and *Can.*—Neerulli. *Tam.*—and *Mal.*—Eerulli.

Habitat.—Cultivated all over India.

Properties and Uses.—The onions are largely used as an article of food and condiment. The bulbs contain an acrid volatile oil which possesses stimulant, diuretic and expectorant properties; are useful in fever, dropsy, catarrh and chronic bronchitis; mixed with common salt the onions are a domestic remedy in colic and scurvy;

eaten raw they are diuretic and emmenagogue. Roasted they are applied as poultice to indolent boils for their rubefacient action. The juice is used like smelling salts in faintness and hysterical fits; it is dropped into the ear to relieve earache; it is applied to allay irritation of insect bites, scorpion stings and also in skin diseases. Mixed with mustard oil in equal proportions it is a good application to rheumatic pains; onions are used to mitigate cough in phthisis; mixed with vinegar they are useful in cases of sorethroat. Cooked with vinegar they are very useful in jaundice, splenic enlargement and dyspepsia. In malarial fevers they are eaten twice a day with two or three black-peppers with remarkable relief. A decoction of the onions is found to benefit much the cases of strangury.

---

24. ALLIUM SATIVUM.

(*N. O.*—LILIACEÆ).

Sans.—Lashuna. *Eng.*—Garlic. *Hind.* and *Ben.*—Lasun. *Pers.*—Sir. *Guz.*—Lasan, shunam. *Mah.*—Lasoona. *Tel., Tam.,* and *Mal.*—Vellulli. *Can.*— Bellulli.

Habitat.—Cultivated all over India.

Properties and Uses.—The seeds yield an aromatic oil of a stimulant nature, prescribed internally to prevent recurrence of the cold fits of intermittent fever; externally it is used in paralytic and rheumatic affections. As resolvent the garlic is applied to indolent tumours; internally it is stomachic and carminative, tonic and alterative; useful in affections of the nervous system, flatulence, hysteria, etc. In the form of confection it is given in rheumatism. Used as a liniment it acts very beneficially in infantile convulsions and other nervous and spasmodic affections, relaxed sorethroat, in asthma, general paralysis, facial paralysis, gout, and sciatica. When eaten in the cold season it is said to ward off attacks of rheumatism and neuralgia. Mustard or cocoanut oil in which garlic has been fried is an excellent application for scabies and maggots infesting ulcers. Its juice mixed with salt is applied to bruises and sprains and also to relieve neuralgia and earache. Garlic oil is stimulant and rubefacient. A clove or two of garlic boiled in half ounce of gingili oil is useful as ear-drops in atonic deafness and to allay the pain in otorrhœa. Expressed juice is applied in case of elongated uvula with some good effect, like that of silver nitrate.

Native Indian Preparations.—Decoction of garlic described by Chakradatta:—Take of garlic 32 tolas, water 4 seers, milk 4 seers; boil together till the water is evaporated, and strain. This decoction in milk is given in small doses in hysteria, flatulence, sciatica and heart disease.

Svalparasuna pinda:—Take of garlic 12 tolas, assafœtida, cumin seeds, rock salt, *sonchal* salt, ginger, long-pepper and black-pepper each one-eighth of a tola; powder them finely and mix. Dose is about 22 grains every morning with a decoction of the root of the castor-oil plant, in facial paralysis, hemiplegia, sciatica, paraplegia and convulsive affections. This medicine should be continued for a month.

25. ALOE BARBADENSIS.

(*N. O.*—LILIACEÆ.)

Sans.—Kumâree. *Eng.*—Indian aloes. *Hind.*—Ghikanvâr. *Ben.*—Ghirta-Kumari. *Guz.*—Kunvár. *Mah.*—Pivalâboel. *Tel.*—Kalabanda. *Tam.*—Kattalai. *Can.*—Kathaligida. *Mal.*—Kattavâla.

Habitat.—Cultivated throughout India in many varieties, some of which run wild as on the coasts of South India.

Properties and Uses.—In small doses it is a stomachic tonic; in large doses it is purgative and indirectly emmenagogue. It is a favourite remedy for intestinal worms in children. Dissolved in attar of roses it is used externally in various affections of the eye, as in catarrhal and purulent ophthalmia. Dissolved in spirit it is used as a hair-dye to stimulate hair-growth. A sweet confection prepared from the pulp of the leaves is given in piles. To correct its griping effect confection of roses and mastich is added. In colic and pneumonia of infants its inspissated juice with a little gum assafœtida is given internally in doses of 1 grain; it may also be given in mothers' milk with the addition of a little borax. The juice of the leaves is applied to inflammations. The pulp washed in cold water and then mixed with a little burnt alum is a good remedy to persons predisposed to apoplexy.

26. ALOE LITORALIS.

(*N. O.*—LILIACEÆ).

Sans.—Ikshuramallika, Kanyâ, Kumari. *Eng.*—Small aloe. *Hind.*—Chhota kanvâr. *Ben.*—Ananash. *Guz.*—Nahani kanvar. *Mah.*—Lahani kumari, Kâlâboel. *Tel.*—Chinikalabanda. *Tam.*—Chirukattâlai. *Can.*—Lolisara. *Mal.*—Kattavâla.

Habitat.—This has become quite naturalised on the southern coast of the Madras Presidency.

Properties and Uses.—Much the same as those of the above. It is a laxative tonic useful in diseases of the spleen; the decoction of the root is prescribed as a febrifuge; very largely used in Mysore as an aperient and an emmenagogue. The tender leaves mixed with the powder of cummin seeds and sugar-candy is said to be an excellent remedy in dysentery characterised by bloody stools. The juice of the leaves mixed with a little opium and applied to the forehead relieves headache; mixed with gingili oil and boiled it makes a fine hair-oil; useful in cases of sleeplessness. The pulp of the leaves well washed in cold water is prescribed as a refrigerent medicine in conjunctivitis, with a small quantity of sugar-candy; the same pulp so purified and with the addition of a little burnt alum is considered a valuable application in cases of ophthalmia. The freshly-expressed juice is in almost universal use as an external refrigerent application to all external or local inflammations. In glandular enlargements and spleen disease the juice of the leaves is given with the addition of powdered turmuric. The following is a useful prescription, generally employed in Indian households:—Aloe leaves sliced, three ounces, common salt, 3 drachms; heat them to boiling point, strain, and add pure white sugar, one ounce; this is for one dose, to be taken cold, early in the morning.

27. ALSTONIA SCHOLARIS.

(*N. O.*—APOCYNACEÆ).

Sans.—Saptaparna. *Eng.*—Dita Bark. *Hind.*—Chatiun. *Ben*—Chhatin. *Mah.*—Satveena. *Tel.*—Aedakularitichettu. *Tam.*—Aelilaippâlai. *Can.*—Hâle. *Mal.*—Daivapâl, aerilampâl. *Kon.*—Sânthni-rooku.

Habitat.—This tree is common throughout India.

Properties and Uses.—The bark is astringent tonic and febrifuge, valuable in debility and after-effects of fever, also valuable in chronic diarrhœa and dysentery, also in catarrhal fever. The milky juice is applied to ulcers and to rheumatic pains; mixed with oil and dropped into ear it relieves earache.

Ditanin is the active principle of the bark, possessing powerful febrifuge and antiperiodic properties, equal to the best sulphate of quinine without its disagreeable secondary symptoms.

Preparations and their doses:—Of the infusion, 1 to 2 ounces; of the tincure, 1 to 2 drachms diluted in water, and of ditanin 5 to 10 grains given two or three times a day

Native Indian Preparations:—*Amritashtakapachana.*—Take of the bark of *alstonia scholaris*, *gulancha*, leaves of *adhatoda vasica* and *Trichosanthes dioica* (*patola*), tubers of *cyperus rotundas*, *calamus rotung*, catechu and *nim* leaves, and prepare a decoction in the usual way.

28. ALTINGIA EXCELSA.

(*N. O.*—HAMAMELIDEÆ).

San.—Sillhaka. *Hind.*, *Mah.*, and *Can.*—Silâras. *Mal.*—Rasamala. *Bur.*—Nan-ta-yok.

Habitat.—This is a magnificent tree of the Indian Archipelago, common also in Burma and Assam.

Properties and Uses.—It yields a fragrant resin which is regarded as a stimulant expectorant, useful in affections of the throat and skin diseases; it is smeared over the abdomen of children to relieve colicky pains.

29. ALUMEN.

Sans.—Sphatikari. *Eng.*—Alum. *Hind.*—Phitkari. *Pers.*—Zak-safed. *Arab.*—Shib. *Ben.*—Phatkiri. *Mah.*—Phatkee. *Tel.*—Patikuram. *Tam.*—Patikâram. *Can.*—Patikâra.

Origin.—It is extensively manufactured in India, chiefly in the Punjaub, Behar and Cutch States. It is manufactured from alum schist or shale.

Properties and Uses.—It is usually darker in colour than the imported article, due to iron which it contains; it is much cheaper than the imported article. It is a valuable astringent, used as a gargle in relaxed and inflamed throat and as a lotion in leucorrhœa and ophthalmia. Mixed with the white of eggs it is extensively used as an application to contusions, sprains and ecchymosis; when burnt it is a mild caustic and is generally sprinkled as powder on indolent and foul ulcers to stimulate healthy action.

30. ANACARDIUM OCCIDENTALE.

(*N. O.*—ANACARDIACEÆ).

San.—Shœphaharâ. *Eng.*—Cachew nut. *Hind.*, *Duk.*, *Guz.*, and *Mah.*—Kâju. *Ben.*—Hijlibadam, *Tel.*—Jædimâmidi. *Tam.* —Mundirikai. *Can.*—Gærumara. *Mal.*—Kappa-mavu. *Kon.* —Kâjju-rooku.

Habitat.—Established in the coast forests of India and all over South India.

Properties and Uses.—Two distinct oils are obtained from this:—(1) The kernel when pressed yields a light yellow bland oil which is very nutritious and emollient, equal to almond oil and superior to olive oil. (2) Cardole or cashew apple oil prepared from the pericarp or shell of the nut; it is black acrid and powerfully rubefacient and vesicant; it is used to colour and preserve fishing nets. It is an effective preventive against white ants, etc., and therefore applied to floors and wooden rafters of houses, also used by book-binders. It is useful as an anæsthetic in leprosy and psoriasis, and as a blister in warts, corns and ulcers. It is also a good application for cracks of the feet; it contains an active principle, *i. e.*, anacardic acid. The spirit distilled from the fruit is stimulant. The fruit is eaten and is a remedy for scurvy; the juice of the nut is used as a substitute for iodine locally.

---

31. ANACYCLUS PYRETHRUM.

(*N. O.*—COMPOSITÆ).

Sans.—Akarakarava. *Eng.*—Pellitory. *Hind* and *Ben.*—Akarakara. *Tam.*—Akarakaram.

Properties and Uses.—The root is a valuable sialagogue. It is powerfully irritant and has been found successful in toothache. It is frequently employed in gargles. An infusion of this drug is useful in cases of rheumatism.

32. ANANAS SATIVUS.

(*N. O.*—BROMELIACEÆ.)

Eng.—Pineapple. *Hind.*, *Guz.*, and *Mah.*—Anânas. *Arab.*—Aainunnâsa. *Ben.*—Anâras. *Tel.*—Anânash-pandu. *Tam.*—Parangithâlai. *Can.*—Anâsu. *Mal.*—Ananas.

Habitat.—Cultivated throughout India.

Properties and Uses.—Fresh juice of the leaves is a powerful anthelmintic; given with sugar it relieves hiccup; also acts as a purgative. The juice of the ripe fruit is antiscorbutic; also allays gastric irritability in fevers; it is useful in jaundice. It acts also as diuretic, diaphoretic and refrigerent. The juice of the unripe fruits is emmenagogue, and in large quantities causes uterine contractions and ought to be rigorously avoided by pregnant women. The oil or essence of pineapple is used for flavouring purposes in confectionery; it is a solution of ethyl-butyrate in alcohol. This is used to give flavour to Jamaica rum.

33. ANDROGRAPHIS PANICULATA.

(*N. O.*—ACANTHACEÆ.)

Sans.—Mahâteeta. *Eng.*—The Creat. *Hind.*—Kiryât. *Ben.*—Kâlmegh. *Pers.*—Nainehavandi. *Guz.*—Kiryâta. *Duk.*—Kalafnath *Mah.*—Olenkirayet. *Tel.*—Naelavemu. *Tam.*—Nilavaembu. *Can.*—Nelabaevu. *Mal.*—Nilavaepu.

Habitat.—This annual is common in hedge-rows throughout the plains of India, cultivated in gardens in some parts.

Properties and Uses.—The whole plant is intensely bitter and yields its properties readily to water or spirit. The root has stomachic, tonic and alterative properties. Its tincture is said to be stimulant and gently aperient. The expressed juice of the leaves is a domestic remedy in flatulence and diarrhœa of children; is also anthelmintic, useful in dyspepsia, in general debility, in convalescence after fevers and in advanced stages of dysentery. During the last epidemic of influenza a tincture of the plant was found highly efficacious in arresting the progress of the disease.

---

34. ANDROPOGON CITRATIS.

(*N. O.*—GRAMINACEÆ.)

Sans.—Takratrani. *Eng.*—Lemon grass. *Hind.*—Gandhatrana or Hareechâhâ. *Ben.*—Gandha-Benâ. *Guz.*—Lilicha. *Mah.*—Gavatichâhâ. *Tel.*—Nimmagaddi. *Tam.*—Karpoorpul. *Can.*—Majjige-hullu. *Mal.*—Châyapul.

Habitat.—Grows wild in gardens throughout India.

Properties and Uses.—This grass is generally used in the form of infusion (4 ounces of the grass to 1 pint of boiling water). It is an excellent stomachic to children; of much use in typhoid fevers; given with black-pepper it is useful in disordered menstruation and in the congestive and neuralgic forms of dysmenorrhoea. It is carminative and tonic to the intestinal mucous membrane, useful in vomiting and diarrhœa. The grass yields a fragrant volatile oil known as verbena oil or Indian *molissa* oil; it is stimulant, carminative, antispasmodic and diaphoretic; useful in flatulent and spasmodic affections of the bowels, gastric irritability, and is of great value in cholera, as it allays and arrests vomiting and aids the process of reaction. The dose is from 2 to 5 minims on a piece of loaf-sugar. Externally it is rubefacient. Mixed with an equal quantity of pure cocoanut oil it makes an excellent liniment for lumbago, chronic rheumatism, neuralgia, sprains, and other painful affections; it is also a good application for ringworm.

35. ANDROPOGON MURICATUS.

(*N. O.*—GRAMINACEÆ.)

Sans.—Usheera, Veeranam. *Eng.*—Cuscus grass, Koosa. *Hind.*—Khas bena. *Ben.*—Vâlâ, khaskhas. *Guz.*—Vâlo. *Mah.*—Vâla. *Tel.*—Kuruvaeru, Vatevaeru. *Tam.*—Vettivær. *Can.*—Mudivâla, Kuruvælu. *Mal.*—Ramachham.

Habitat.—This perennial tufted grass is common in Coromondel Coast, Mysore, Bengal and Burma, cultivated in Rajputana and Chota-Nagpur.

Properties and Uses.—The long fibrous root of this plant is mostly used for making fans, door-screens or *tatties* or aromatic scented mats; they are kept constantly wet for cooling and perfuming the atmosphere during the hot weather. Medicinally the powdered root is cooling, refrigerent, diuretic, stimulant and tonic. The dose is 20 grains and of the infusion which is made by putting 2 drachms of the grass to ten ounces of water, the dose is from 1 to 2 ounces. Being a cooling medicine it is a grateful drink in fevers, inflammation and irritability of the stomach. Externally a paste of the root is rubbed on the skin to remove oppressive heat or burning of the body. By mixing it with red sandalwood and a fragrant wood called *padma kastha* (all in powder) to a tub of water an aromatic bath is prepared. Its essence or oil or otto is useful as tonic; it is given in two *minim* doses to check the vomiting of cholera. The grass used in the form of cigarettes and smoked with benzoin relieves headache.

Chemical Composition:—It contains:—(1) A resin with odour like that of myrrh; (2) a soluble colouring matter; (3) a free acid; (4) a salt of lime; (5) a considerable quantity of oxide of iron; and (6) a large quantity of woody matter.

36. ANDROPOGON NARDUS.

(*N. O.*—GRAMINACEÆ.)

Eng.—Citronella. *Hind.*—Ganjni. *Ben.*—Kamâkher. *Mah.*—Ooshadhâna. *Sing.*—Maana.

Habitat.—This grass is quite common in the United Provinces and the Punjaub and very largely cultivated in Ceylon and Singapore for the valuable oil it yields.

Properties and Uses.—The citronella oil is a very important product in perfumery. It is little used medicinally, but it has properties similar to those of *A. citratus*, especially in rheumatism. The leaves are occasionally used in the form of infusion.

37. ANDROPOGON SCHŒNANTHUS.

(*N. O.*—GRAMINACEÆ.)

Eng.—The geranium grass. *Hind.*—Ruâghâs. *Ben.*—Agyâghas, Roshel.

Habitat.—This is another of the fragrant grasses which is indigenous to Central India, the United Provinces and the Punjaub.

Properties and Uses.—The oil distilled from the leaves is known in commerce as "rusa" oil, "nimar" oil.

and oil of ginger grass. It is very extensively employed in soap-making and perfumery. Medicinally it is stimulant, carminative, anti-spasmodic and diaphoretic found useful in flatulence and spasmodic affections of the bowels. Externally it is used like the oil of lemon grass in conjunction with or as cajeput oil.

---

38. ANISOCHILUS CARNOSUS.

(*N. O.*—LAMINACEÆ.)

Sans.—Ajapâda, Induparni. *Eng.*—Thick-leaved lavender. *Hind.*—Panjiri. *Guz.*—Ajamanupâtree. *Mah.*—Kâpurli. *Tel.*, *Tam.*, and *Mal.*—Karpooravalli. *Can.*—Doddapatri.

Habitat.—Found in Northern Circars, Mysore, and Malabar.

Properties and Uses.—It has stimulant, diaphoretic and expectorant properties. Fresh juice of the leaves mixed with sugar-candy is given to children in coughs; mixed with sugar and gingelly oil it forms a cooling liniment for the head. The leaves and stems in infusion are useful in coughs and colds. The plant yields a volatile oil which has stimulant, expectorant and diaphoretic properties.

---

39. ANISOMELES MALABARICA.

(*N. O.*—LAMIACEÆ.)

Sans.—Alamoola. *Eng.*—Malabar catmint. *Mah.*—Chodharâ. *Tel.*—Mogbeerâku. *Tam.*—Pæyemaruti. *Can.*—Karithumbi. *Mal.* —Karitumpa.

Habitat.—This plant is met with in Travancore and Malabar Coast.

Properties and Uses.—Infusion of the aromatic bitter plant is useful in affections of the stomach and bowels, in catarrh and intermittent fevers; the juice of the leaves is administered to children in colic, dyspepsia, and fever caused by teething. Vapour of the hot infusion inhaled induces copious diaphoresis (perspiration). The decoction of the plant is an excellent fomentation for rheumatic joints. The essential oil distilled from the leaves is used externally as an embrocation in rheumatic arthritis.

---

40. ANONA SQUAMOSA.

(*N. O.*—ANONACEÆ.)

Sans.—Shubhâ, Suda. *Eng.*—Custard apple. *Hind.*—Sharifah. *Ben.*, *Guz.*, *Duk.*, *Mah.*, and *Can.*—Sitâphal. *Tel.*—Seetâpandu. *Tam.*—Sitaphalam.

Habitat.—Cultivated in gardens all over India for its fruit.

Properties and Uses.—The bark is a powerful astringent and as a tonic is much used in medicine. The rip fruit externally applied is a maturant, and when bruised and mixed with salt it is applied to malignant tumours to hasten suppuration. The seeds, leaves and unripe fruit contain an acid principle fatal to vermin and insects. The leaves made into a paste without adding water are applied to unhealthy ulcers. Leaves are anthelmintic. Seeds applied to os uteri cause abortion. Leaves are applied for extraction of guinea-worm. The seeds yield an oil and resin; the latter is an acrid principle. The seeds are detergent and therefore their powder mixed with gram is a good hair-wash. The root is a violent purgative.

---

41. ANTHEMIS NOBILIS.

(*N. O.*—COMPOSITÆ.)

Eng.—Chamomile. *Hind.*—Bábunkephul. *Pers.*—Bâbunâh. *Arab.*—Bábunaj. *Ben.* Bàbunaphul.

Habitat.—It is a native of Europe and Persia, but cultivated in India chiefly in the Punjaub. The dried flowers are available in all the bazaars.

Properties and Uses.—Chamomile is stomachic, antispasmodic, carminative and tonic useful in dyspepsia and general debility. The warm infusion in large doses is sometimes used to promote the action of emetic; it is useful in hysteria and suppression of menses. Chamomile also acts as a vermifuge. Externally an infusion or decoction or cataplasm of the flowers is used to relieve pain. The essential oil obtained by distillation possesses antispasmodic properties.

---

42. ARACHIS HYPOGEÆ.

(*N. O.*—LEGUMINOSÆ.)

Sans.—Buchanaka. *Eng.*—Earthnut, groundnut. *Hind.*—Mungphali. *Ben.*—Chiner-badâm. *Duk.*—Velaiti-mung. *Mah.*—Bhuichanà. *Tel.*—Værushanagalu. *Tam.*—Vaerkadalai. *Can.*—Nelakadale. *Mal.*—Nelakadalaka.

Habitat.—Cultivated chiefly in South India and Bombay, also in some parts of Bengal.

Properties and Uses.—The ground nuts are said to be very bilious. The roasted seeds are used as a substitute for chocolate. They abound with starch as well as oil and a large proportion of albuminous matter. The oil of the groundnut is, in Pharmacy, a good substitute for olive or almond oil, the latter of which it is said to adulterate. The oil is regarded as an excellent aperient and emollient and is used in catarrh of the bladder. The ground-nut meal as food is superior (rich in all important constituents) to any other vegetable product of a similar nature. Its chemical composition is as follows:—

Moisture	9·6 per cent.
Fatty matter	11·8 ,,
Nitrogenous matter	31·9 ,,
Sugar, starch, etc.	37·8 ,,
Fibre	4·3 ,,
Ash	4·6 ,,

43. ARECA CATECHU.

(*N. O.*—PALMACEÆ.)

Sans.—Kramuka, Pooga. *Eng.*—Areca, or betel-nut palm. *Hind., Guz.* and *Mah.*—Supári. *Ben.*—Supàri, gua. *Tel.*—Kramukamu. *Tam.*—Kamuku, Kiramukam. *Can.*—Adike.

Habitat.—Cultivated throughout tropical India. It flourishes in dry plateau of Mysore, Canara and Malabar.

Properties and Uses.—The kernel of the fruit is one of the constituents of the universal masticatory the "betel" of the East. The arecanut contains tannic properties, fatty and coloring matters and several alkaloids chiefly *arcoline*. The young nut is astringent and carminative useful in bowel complaints. The powder of the dried nuts in 10 to 15 grain doses will check diarrhœa due to debility; is also useful in urinary disorders. It is also said to possess anthelmintic properties when given with milk or butter; or one-fourth tola of the powder rubbed into a paste with two tolas of fresh lemon juice makes an excellent vermifuge. The dried nuts when chewed produce stimulant and exhilarant effect, 4 to 6 drachms of the powder stirred up with 2 or 3 ounces of milk is the dose generally administered for the expulsion of the tape-worm. The tincture forms an astringent gargle when freely diluted with water (1 drachm to 4 ounces of water) useful for bleeding gums and may be used as an injection for stopping watery discharges from the vagina. The nut burnt to charcoal and powdered forms an excellent tooth-powder.

44. ARGEMONE MEXICANA.

(*N. O.*—PAPAVERACEÆ.)

Sans.—Brahmadandi. *Eng.*—Yellow thistle ; Prickly or Maxican poppy. *Hind.*—Pila dhaturâ, Bherband. *Ben.*—Sialkanta. *Guz.* ·Dârudi. *Duk.*—Feringee datura. *Mah.*—Dâruri. *Tel.*—Brahmadandi. *Tam.*—Kudiyœtti. *Can.*—Arasina-ummatta-gida. *Mal.*—Ponnummattam.

Habitat.—This spiny herbacious annual is common everywhere in India on road sides and waste places, self-sown and appearing in the cold season.

Properties and Uses.—The whole plant abounds in a yellow juice resembling gamboge which is diuretic in effect and therefore used in dropsy, jaundice and cutaneous affections. It is administered in conjunction with ghee in gonorrhœa, etc. Externally it relieves blisters and heals excoriations and indolent ulcers acting as anodyne and hypnotic. Care should be taken that it may not come in contact with eyes. The seeds are laxative and stomachic, emetic, expectorant and demulcent and the oil obtained from them is aperient and sedative in colic; a thirty-minim dose acts as cathartic, it is best given in sugar; the oil is applied externally to skin diseases, also in headache; it is a valuable application in herpetic eruptions. The seeds and oil have a beneficent effect in asthma which they control; the largest dose of the seeds is 2½ drachms always used in emulsion which can be sweetened if necessary; of the oil thirty minims is the biggest dose. The fresh root bruised and applied to the part stung by scorpions is said to give relief as it is said to have an anodyne property.

---

45. ARISTOLOCHIA INDICA.

(*N. O.*—ARISTOLOCHIACEÆ.)

Sans.—Ahiganda. *Eng.*—Indian birthwort. *Hind.*, *Ben.*, and *Duk.*—Isharmul, Arkamula, Ruhimula. *Mah.*—Sâpsanda. *Tel.*—Eeshvaraværu. *Tam.*—Eesburvær. *Can.*—Eeshvarabæru. *Mal.*—Eeshvaramulla. *Kon.*—Sapsikaddula.

Habitat.—This twining perennial is found all over India.

Properties and Uses.—The root of this as well as of other species of *Aristolochia* possesses a nauseous bitter taste and a powerful emmenagogue and antiarthritic virtues; it is a valuable antidote to snake-bite and to bites of poisonous insects as scorpion, etc., being used both externally and internally. The dose is 1 to 2 drachms. Mixed with honey it is given in white leprosy, it is also considered useful in dropsy. Macerated with black-pepper corns it is given in cases of cholera and diarrhœa with much benefit. The juice of the leaves has stimulant tonic and antiperiodic properties; so also the bark, chiefly used in the bowel-complaints of children and in intermittent fevers. The dose of the expressed juice is half to two drachms.

46. ARTOCARPUS INTEGRIFOLIA.

(*N. O.*—ARTOCARPACEÆ.)

Sans.—Panasa, Skandaphala. *Eng.*—Indian Jack tree. *Hind.*, *Duk.* and *Mah.*—Phanas. *Ben.*—Kânthâl. *Tel.*—Panasa. *Tam.*—Palachu. *Can.*—Halasu. *Mal.*—Pilâv, Kandakiphala. *Kon.*—Pansau.

Habitat.—A large tree cultivated all over India for its fruit.

Properties and Uses.—The fruit of this tree is one of the most popular fruits in India and is very delicious to taste. It is demulcent, nutritious and laxative in action; if eaten in large quantities it produces diarrhœa, being rather difficult to digest. It is best eaten in empty stomach especially in the mornings. The unripe fruit is astringent and is generally used in the preparation of pickles; when cooked it makes a nice curry. The seed when roasted is good food and resembles chestnuts; it contains a large percentage of starch and as such can be utilised in various forms. The milk juice of the plant mixed with vinegar and applied to glandular swellings and abscesses promotes absorption or suppuration. The tender leaves are useful in skin diseases and the root is administered internally in diarrhœa.

---

47. ARUM COLOCASIA.

(*N. O.*—ARACEÆ.)

San.—Katchu. *Eng.*—Çocco. *Hind.*—Kachu. *Ben.*—Guri, Kachu. *Mah.*—Alu. *Tel.*—Sheemagadda. *Tam.*—Sheemai Kilangu. *Can.*—Kaesave. *Mal.*—Chaemp.

Habitat.—Wild over the greater part of tropical India and also cultivated throughout India on account of its corms.

Properties and Uses.—The pressed juice of petioles is highly styptic and rubefacient useful in arterial hæmorrhages, wounds &c., which are said to heal by first intention after its application. It is sometimes dropped in ear-ache and otorrhœa. It forms a good application to the stings of wasps and other insects. The juice of the leaf stalks of the black species is used with salt as an absorbant in cases of inflamed glands, buboes, &c. Internally it is laxative and is useful in piles, congestion of the portal system.

---

48. ASCLEPIAS ASTHMATICA.

(*N. O.*—ASCLEPIACEÆ.)

Sans.—Moolinee. *Eng.*—Vomiting swallow-wort. *Hind.*—Jangli-pikvân. *Ben.*—Antamool. *Tel.*—Kurinja. *Tam.*—Nalpalai. *Can.*—Kirumanji. *Mal.*—Vallipal.

Habitat.—Bengal and South India.

Properties and Uses.—The root and the leaves which possess a strong emetic property are regarded as a substitute for ipecacuanha, the effect of the dried leaves in half-drachm doses being the same as that of ipecac powder of British Pharmacopœa, in small doses, i.e., 3 to 5 grains their action is expectorant and diaphoretic. The roots are superior to leaves in action. They have an additional laxative property; a good remedy in doses of 15 grains. A liniment prepared with the root is applied in cases of dysentery generally administered in powder and in combination with a little gum acacia and a grain of opium. A liniment prepared with the root is applied to the head in cephalalgia and neuralgia.

---

49. ASPARAGUS RACEMOSUS.

(*N. O.*—LILIACEÆ.)

Sans.—Shatâvari, Shatamoolee. *Ben.* and *Can.*--Satmuli. *Hin.*, *Guz.*, *Mah.*, *Tel.*, and *Mal.*—Satâvare. *Tam.*—Paniyanâku.

Habitat.—This climber is found all over India.

Properties and Uses.—The root of the plant is a refrigerent, demulcent, diuretic, aphrodisiac, antispasmodic and alterative tonic. As it is said to have also antidiarrhœtic proporties it is employed in diarrhœa as well as in cases of colic and dysentery. The root is boiled in milk and the milk is administered to relieve bilious dyspepsia and diarrhœa and to promote appetite. The tubers are candied and taken as a sweetmeat. The fresh root juice is given with honey as a demulcent the bark is poisonous. The boiled leaves smeared with ghee are applied to boils, small-pox, &c., in order to prevent their confluence.

Native Indian Preparations.—*Shatävari ghrita.*—Take of clarified butter four seers, juice of *Asparagus Racemosus* four seers, milk forty seers, boil them together and prepare a *ghrita*. This is given with the addition of sugar, honey and long-pepper as an aphrodisiac tonic.

Phalaghrita :—This is prepared with four seers of clarified butter, and sixteen seers each of the juice of *Asparagus Racemosus* and cow's milk with the addition of a number of other medicines in small quantities in the form of a paste. Its use is said to increase the secretion of semen, to cure barrenness in women and to remove disorders of the female genitals. The juice of this drug taken with milk is useful in gonorrhoea. The chief use of the drug, however, consists in the preparation of several popular, cooling and emollient medicated oils, as for instance, *Narayana taila* used by native physicians in rheumatism, diseases of the joints, sti' neck hemiplegia and other diseases of the nervous system.

Vishnu taila :—This is an oil much used in nervous diseases. It is prepared with sesamum oil, cow's or goat's milk and the juice of *Asparagus Racemosus* with the addition of a number of substances in small quantities in the form of a paste.

Prameha Mihira taila.—This oil is prepared with the juice of *asparagus racemosus*, sesamum oil, decoction of lac, whey and milk with the addition of a number of substances in the form of a paste. It is rubbed on the body and more particularly on the pubic region in chronic gonorrhœa, stricture of the urethra and other diseases of the urinary organs.

50. ASTRAGALAS VIRUS.

(*N. O.*—LEGUMINOSÆ.)

Eng.—Gum Tragacanth. *Hind.*—Angirâ. *Ben.*—Katila.

Habitat.—Himalayan regions.

Properties and Uses.—This gum which exudes during the hot season through the bark of the tree in slender threads gradually increases, hardens and forms tears or worm-like pieces. This gum which is found in the bazaars forms the basis of some medicinal lozenges and styptic powder and is extensively used as an emollient and demulcent. It is very useful in the irritation of the mucous membranes of the pulmonary and genito-urinary organs. It is chiefly used as a vehicle for more active medicines.

51. ATALANTIA MONOPHYLLA.

(*N. O.*—AURANTIACEÆ.)

Sans.—Âtavi-jambira. *Eng.*—Wild lime. *Mah.*—Mâkad-limbu. *Tel.*—Adavi-nimma. *Tam.*—Kâttelumichhai. *Can.*—Kadu-limbe. *Mal.*—Malenârakam.

Habitat.—A small tree of East Bengal, South India and Ceylon.

Properties and Uses.—The berries are made into a nice pickle which forms a useful curry-diet in fevers and ailments attended with loss of taste and appetite. The juice is acid and generally employed in the manufacture of dyes and colors. The berries yield a warm oil which is considered to be a valuable application in chronic rheumatism.

52. AVERRHOA BILIMBA.

(*N. O.*—OXALIDACEÆ.)

Hind.—Tamarang. *Ben.*—Bilimbi. *Guz.*—Blimbu. *Mah.*—Bilambi. *Tam.*—Pilimbi. *Can.*—Bilimbi. *Mal.*—Vilimbi. *Kon.*—Bimbula.

Habitat.—Cultivated in gardens on the plains of India.

Properties and Uses.—The fruits which are acid in taste are generally employed in cookery along with other vegetables and grains to render them more palatable and digestible not only to increase the taste but also to promote the digestion and assimilation of the cooked grains. The fruits are also used in pickles. The juice of the fruit made into a syrup will form a cooling drink in fevers. The fruit is rubbed on clothes to remove any strains.

53. AVERRHOA CARAMBOLA.

(*N. O.*—OXALIDACEÆ.)

Sans. and *Hind.*—Karmaranga. *Ben.*—Kamarak. *Duk.*—Karmal, Meeta-kamarunga. *Guz.* and *Mah.*—Kamarakha. *Tel.*—Tamaratamu. *Tam.*—Tamarattai. *Can.*—Dârehuli. *Mal.*—Tamaratta. *Kon.*—Karmbala.

Habitat.—Cultivated in India as far north as Lahore,

Properties and Uses.—The five angled fruit of this plant contains an acid watery pulp and is eaten raw as well as used in curries and pickles. When cooked with other vegetables and grains it renders them more palatable and easy of digestion. The ripe fruit is antiscorbutic and highly cooling. The fruit juice made into a syrup will form an excellent cooling drink; the fruit juice employed in washing clothes renders them clean, removing any spots or stains found thereon.

---

54. BALSAMODENDRON MUKUL.

(*N. O.* BURSERACEÆ.)

Sans. and *Can.*—Guggula. *Eng.*—Gum gugul. *Hind.*—Gugul. *Ben.*—Gugul, Mukul.

Habitat.—This tree is a native of Sind, Rajputana, Eastern Bengal and Assam.

Properties and Uses.—This yields the guggul gum which is collected in the cold season by making incisions in the tree. It is a gum resin and sometimes used in place of myrrh being much cheaper. It is largely used as incense in religious ceremonies. Medicinally it is demulcent, aperient, alterative and carminative, useful in rheumatism, nervous diseases, scrofulous affections, urinary disorders and skin diseases. This gum mixed with lime juice or cocoanut oil is applied as a plaster to ulcers and bad wounds.

Native Indian Preparations.—In rheumatism it is used by native physicians in a great variety of forms of which a preparation called *Yogaraja guggula* is a favourite one and it is composed of several ingredients. Another preparation similar in composition is *Trayodasanga guggula* which is made with 13 aromatic adjuncts and is recommended for use in rheumatism affecting the loins and the sacrum. In rheumatism affecting the joints and bones a preparation called *Adityapâka guggula* is used. Other preparations are *Vatari rasa, Kaisara guggula* and *Sadanga guggula*. For composition &c., of these, refer to U. C. Dutt's Materia Medica of the Hindus.

55. BALSAMODENDRON MYRRHA.

(*N. O.*—BURSERACEÆ.)

Sans.—Vola. *Eng.*—Myrrh. *Hind.* and *Pers.*—Bol. *Ben.*—Hirabol.

Properties and Uses.—Myrrh is the solid gum obtained from the bark of this tree. It exudes in a soft oily state but soon hardens by exposure to air. It has an aromatic and balsamic odour and a bitter aromatic taste. It has been used from time immemorial as an incense. Medicinally it is stimulant, expectorant and emmenagogue useful in dyspepsia and in amenorrhœa, chlorosis and other atonic uterine affections. It is also useful as an expectorant in chest affections, especially in asthma. Externally it is used as an astringent and stimulating application in ulcerated conditions and a valued wash for the mouth and gums, and a gargle in ulcerated sore-throat.

56. BAMBUSA ARUNDINACEÆ.

(*N. O.*—GRAMINACEÆ.)

Sans.—Vansa. *Eng.*—Bamboo. *Hind.* and *Duk.*—Bhâns. *Ben.*—Bâns. *Guz.*—Wâns. *Mah.*—Bâmboo. *Tel.*—Veduru. *Tam.* and *Mal.*—Moongil. *Can.*— Bedru. *Kon.*—Vâso.

Habitat.—Common in Central and South India, cultivated in many places in Bengal and North-West India.

Properties and Uses.—The young shoots of the bamboo made into a poultice is a most efficacious application for dislodgment of worms from ulcers. The juice is poured in the vermin and the liquid mass applied and secured by a bondage. The leaf-bud is emmenagogue administered in decoction to encourage the free discharge of the menses or lochia after delivery when it is scanty. It is also used in leprosy, fevers and hæmophysia. They also act as anthelmintic and therefore useful in cases of children suffering from thread worms. Pickles or curry prepared out of the tender shoots gives much benefit to persons suffering from lack of digestion, it is said to promote appetite and digestion. The silicious concretion found in the joints of the female bamboo is largely used as a sweet, cooling tonic and aphrodisiac, useful in cough, consumption, asthma, &c.

57. BARLERIA PRIONITIS.

(*N. O.*—ACANTHACEÆ.)

Sans.—Koranta. *Hind.*—Katseriya. *Ben.*—Kântajâti. *Guz.*—Kânta shelio. *Mah.*—Pivala koranta or koreta. *Tel.* and *Can.*—Mullu goranta. *Tam.* and *Mal.*—Chemmulli. *Kon.*—Gorti.

Habitat.—This small spiny bush with buff-colored flowers is met with in tropical India, abundant in Bombay, Madras, Ceylon, Assam and Sylhet.

Properties and Uses.—The juice of this leaf administered in a little honey or sugar and water is a favourite medicine in the catarrhal affections of children accompanied with fever and much phlegm; the dose is two tablespoonfuls twice a day. The juice of the leaves applied to feet in the rainy season prevents their cracking or laceration.

---

58. BASELLA ALBA,—RUBRA,—LUCIDA,—CORDIFOLIA.

(*N. O.*—BASELLACEÆ.)

Sans.—Apœdika. *Eng.*—Indian Spinach or Malabar Nightshade. *Hind.*—Poyi. *Ben.*—Rukhto-puri. *Tel.*—Bachhâli. *Tam.*—Pachalai. *Can.*—Basale. *Mal.*—Pachala. *Kon.*—Vâli.

Habitat.—Cultivated in almost every part of India especially in Lower Bengal and Assam.

Properties and Uses.—It contains a good deal of mucilage and is used as a substitute for spinach. It makes a wholesome spinage. The leaves are reduced to pulp and applied to boils and abscesses to hasten suppuration. The juice of the leaves together with sugar-candy is useful in the catarrhal affections of children. It is demulcent and diuretic and therefore administered with much benefit in gonorrhœa and balanitis. The leaf-juice thoroughly rubbed and mixed with butter is a soothing and cooling application for burns and scalds. The decoction of the root of the red variety (*Basella rubra*) relieves bilious vomiting. The infusion of the dried leaves of *Basella lucida* makes a nice drink. The mucilaginous liquid obtained from the leaves and tender stalks of this plant is a popular remedy for habitual headaches; it is applied to the head about half an hour before bathing; it will produce a cooling sensation and bring on sound refreshing sleep.

---

59. BASSIA LATIFOLIA.

(*N. O.*—SAPOTACEÆ.)

Sans.—Madhookah. *Eng.*—The Indian Butter tree, Mahwah tree. *Hind.*—Jangli mohwâ. *Guz.*—Mahurâ. *Mah.*—Mowdâ. *Tel.*—Ippachettu, Madhookamu. *Tam.* and *Mal.*—Madhookam. *Can.*—Ippe-mara.

Habitat.—In Bombay Presidency, Bengal and South Indian forests.

Properties and Uses.—The seeds yield a thick concrete oil which is useful for application in skin diseases and to the head in cephalalgia. It is also used for adulterating ghee, and for burning and for candle and soap-making. The spirit distilled from the flowers is a powerful diffusible stimulant and is an astringent tonic and appetiser; when matured by age it acts like brandy. The leaves boiled in water form a good stimulant embrocation. The bark is a remedy for rheumatic affections, rubbed on the body it cures itch. The residue cake after the extraction of oil is used to poison fish. The smoke produced in burning the cake is reputed to kill insects and rats. The flowers mixed with milk are useful in impotence due to general debility as they have, at once, a cooling, demulcent, tonic, nutritive and stimulant properties; one ounce with eight ounces of fresh milk is the dose. The dried flowers are used as a fomentation in orchitis.

Native Indian Preparations.—Take of the flowers of *Bassia latifolia*, bark of *Gemelina arborea*, red sandalwood, root of *Andropogon muricatum*, coriander and raisins equal parts and prepare an infusion. This infusion is given with the addition of sugar for the relief of thirst, burning of the body and giddiness.

---

60. BAUHINIA TOMENTOSA.

(*N. O.*—LEGUMINOSÆ.)

Sans.—Phalgu. *Hind.* and *Ben.*—Kachnar. *Guz.*—Asundro. *Mah.*—Pivalâ kunchan. *Tel.*—Adavimandâramu. *Tam.* and *Mal.*—Kâttâtti. *Can.*—Kadatti.

Habitat.—United Provinces and throughout India to Ceylon.

Properties and Uses.—The plant is anti-dysenteric and anthelmintic. The decoction of the root-bark is useful in inflammation of the liver. The infusion is a useful gargle in aphthæ. The dried leaves, buds and young flowers are prescribed in dysentery. The seeds may be eaten, they have a tonic and aphrodisiac action. The seeds made into a paste with vinegar is an efficacious application to wounds inflicted by poisonous animals.

---

61. BAUHINIA VARIEGATA.

(*N. O.*—LEGUMINOSÆ).

Sans.—Kanchanâra, Kovidâra. *Hind.*—Kachnâr. *Ben.* and *Mah.*—Rakta-Kânchan. *Guz.*—Kovidara. *Tel.*—Daevakânchanamu. *Tam.*—Shemmandârai. *Can.*—Kempu mandâra. *Mal.*—Chuvanna-mandâram.

Habitat.—Found in sub-Himalayan tract and throughout the forests of India.

Properties and Uses.—The bark is astringent, tonic and alterative ; it yields a brown-colored gum. The root is carminative and flowers are laxative. The bark rubbed into an emulsion with rice-water and administered with the addition of ginger in scrofulous enlargement of the glands of the neck. The decoction of the bark is a useful wash in ulcers and skin-diseases and a remedy in diarrhœa. The dried buds also are useful in diarrhœa and in worms. The decoction of the root is an anti-fat remedy and therefore valuable for corpulent persons.

Native Indian Preparations.—*Kanchanâra guggula.* —Take of the bark of *Bauhinia Variegata* eighty tolas, the three myrobalans sixty tolas, ginger, black-pepper, long-pepper and the bark of Cratæva religiosa eighty tolas each, cardamoms, cinnamon and *tejapatra* leaves each two tolas; powder them all and rub together with *guggula* equal in weight to all the other ingredients. *Dose.*—Half a tola to be taken every morning with a decoction of Sphæranthus Mollis or of Catechu. This medicine is said to be useful in scrofulous enlargements of glands, tumours, ulcers, skin diseases &c.

---

62. BENINKASA CERIFERA.

(*N. O.*—CUCURBITACEÆ.)

Sans.—Kooshmânda. *Eng.*—White Gourd Melon. *Hind.*—Golkaddu. *Ben.*—Kumra. *Guz.*—Kohwla. *Mah.*—Kohala. *Tel.*—Boodigummadi. *Tam.*—Kalyanapoochuni. *Mal.*—Kumbalam. *Can.*—Bile Kumbala. *Kon.*—Kuvâle.

Habitat.—Cultivated in gardens throughout India; resembles the pumpkin in appearance.

Properties and Uses.—The seeds possess anthelmintic properties and are useful in tænea. The fruit is alterative and styptic and is a valuable anti-malarial, cooling, laxative and nutritious tonic. Its juice (*fresh*) is administered as a specific in hæmoptysis and other hæmorrhages from internal organs, while a slice is applied to the temple. The juice is particularly beneficial in phthisis; it is also useful in insanity, epilepsy and other nervous diseases. It is a good antidote for many kinds of vegetable poisons. In diabetes the juice of the cortical portion 4 ounces with powdered saffron and red rice bran 100 grains each is given morning and evening with strict diet. The fruit is cooked in curries and also made into sweetmeats or confections.

Native Indian Preparations.—*Khanda Kooshmândaka* or confection of squash:—In preparing this old ripe gourds at least a year old are selected; the pulp is scraped out in thin flakes by an iron scratcher. The watery juice that oozes out is preserved; the seeds are rejected and in the juice the pulp is boiled till the whole becomes a soft mass. It is then tied up tightly in a cloth and the fluid portion allowed to strain through it. The softened and drained pulp is dried in the sun and the watery portion is preserved for future use. Fifty tolas of the prepared pulp are fried in 16 tolas of clarified butter and again boiled in the juice till it is reduced to the consistence of honey. To this 50 tolas of refined sugar is added and the whole is heated over a *gentle* fire till the mass assumes such a consistence as to adhere to the ladle. Then the pot is removed from the fire and a number of flavouring demulcents, *viz.*, long-pepper and ginger each two tolas, cummin seeds, cardamoms, cinnamon, *tejapatra* leaves, black-pepper and coriander each half a tola in fine powder are added and the mixture is stirred until cooled; eight tolas of honey are now added to the confection and it is preserved in a new earthen pot. Dose of this confection is from 1 to 2 tolas according to age and strength. It is useful in hæmoptysis, phthisis, marasmus, cough, asthma, ulceration of the lungs, hoarseness, &c.

Vâsâ Kushmânda khanda:—Take of the root of *Justicia adhatoda (Vâsaka)* one seer, water eight seers, boil together till reduced to one-fourth and strain. Then take of the pulp of *Benincasa cerifera* prepared as above fifty tolas, fry it in thirty-two tolas of clarified butter and boil in the decoction of *vâsaka* till the whole is reduced to the consistence of honey. Add to it sugar 100 tolas and apply heat till the mass thickens to the proper consistence. Remove from the fire and add the following substances in fine powder, *viz.*, tubers of *Cyperus rotandus*, dried emblic myrobalan, bamboo manna, root of *Clerodendron siphonanthus*, a fragrant substance called *Elabâluka*, cinnamon, cardamom, *tejapatra* each quarter of a tola, ginger, coriander and black-pepper each one tola, long-pepper 4 tolas, stir well till the confection cools and lastly add 8 tolas of honey. This preparation is used in cough, asthma, phthisis, hæmoptysis, heart disease and catarrh.

Kushmanda ghrita:—Take of the juice of *Benincasa cerifera* 18 seers, clarified butter, 1 seer, liquorice root beaten into a paste with water ¼ seer. Boil them together and prepare a *ghrita* in the usual way. Dose is 1 to 2 tolas. This is given in insanity, epilepsy and other nervous diseases.

63. BERBERIS ARISTATA AND B. LYCIUM.

(*N. O.*—BERBERIDEÆ.)

Sans.—**Dâruharidra.** *Eng.*—**Indian Barberry.** *Hind.*—**Rasaut, Chitra.** *Pers.*—**Filzahrah.** *Ben.*—**Dârhaldi.** *Mah.*—Dâruhalad.

Habitat.—The barberry bushes grow on the Nilgiris and all over the Himalaya whence the root and the root-bark could be obtained in large quantities.

Properties and Uses.—The root occurs in pieces varying in thickness from 2 or 3 to 6 or 8 inches and in length from 10 to 12 inches. It is yellow externally and bitter in taste. The active principle is the alkaloid *Berberine*. The official tincture of the root bark is antipyretic, antiperiodic, diaphoretic and tonic. It is greatly used in cases of remittent fever. As a diaphoretic and antipyretic it is considered equal to quinine and Warburg's tincture and as a diaphoretic may be used in place of James' powder. As an antiperiodic it has some advantage over quinine and cinchona inasmuch as frequently repeated doses do not produce depression of the system or deafness and it may be used during the attack of fever. It is used as a febrifuge in doses of half a drachm. A crude extract known as *Rasaut* and prepared from the root bark is used as a local application in affections of the eyelids as in chronic ophthalmia in which it is painted over the eyelids occasionally combined with opium and alum.

64. BERGERA KOENIGII.

(*N. O.*—AURANTIACEÆ.)

Sans.—Krishnanimba. *Eng.*—Curry-leaf tree. *Hind.*—Karaypâk. *Ben.*—Bursunga. *Mah.*—Kadheenimba. *Tel.*—Karivæpamu. *Tam.*—Karuveppilai. *Can* and *Kon.*—Karibævu. *Mal.*—Karivæpu.

Properties and Uses.—The leaves, bark and root are tonic and stomachic. The root-bark is stimulant and laxative. The infusion of the root-bark or of the leaves is useful in vomiting. The green tender leaves are eaten raw for the cure of dysentery. When boiled in milk and ground they form a good application to poisonous bites and also to eruptions. The decoction of the leaves is given with bitters as a febrifuge in fevers. The leaves are popularly used for flavouring curries and condiments. The seeds yield an oil the properties of which are not yet ascertained.

---

65. BOERHAVIA DIFFUSA.

(*N. O.*—NYCTAGINEÆ.)

Sans.—Punarnava, Sotagni. *Eng.*—Spreading hogweed. *Hind.* Sânt. *Ben.*—Gâdhapurna, Swhetapoorna. *Guz.*—Vakha-khaparo. Motosatado. *Tel.*—Atatamamid. *Tam.*—Mookkirattai. Kadiyirattam. *Can.*—Sanâdika. *Mal.*—Tamilâma, Talutâma.

Habitat.—This weed is found all over India; it is of two kinds, one with white and the other with red flowers. The former is used in medicine.

Properties and Uses.—The root is laxative, diuretic and anthelmintic; it is used in powder, decoction or infusion. As diuretic it is useful in gonorrhœa, in moderate doses it is a good expectorant and antispasmodic, successful in asthma; in large doses it will produce vomiting on account of its emetic properties. In dropsy the decoction of the root is administered together with powdered chiretta and ginger also with about 15 grains of nitrate of potash; it is also applied externally. In mild cases a dish of the fresh herb boiled, salted and eaten with bread (*chappaties*) with any other treatment does give much relief.

Native Indian Preparations.—*Punarnavâstaka.*—Take of *punarnavâ* root, *nim* bark, leaves of *Trichosanthus dioica*, ginger, *Picrorrhiza kurroa*, chebulic myrobalan, *gulancha* and the wood of *Berberis Asiatica* quarter of a tola each, water 32 tolas; boil together till reduced to one-fourth. This decoction is given in general anasarca with ascites, cough, jaundice, difficulty of breathing &c., (Chakradatta). An oil prepared from the root and a number of useful aromatics in the form of a paste is rubbed on the body in general anasarca complicated with jaundice. It is called *Punarnava taila* (Sârkaumudee). Bhavaprakasa gives an electuary under the name of *Punarnava leha*. It is prepared with a decoction of the root and a number of other ingredients and is used in strangury or scanty urine.

---

66. BOMBAX MALABARICUM.

(*N. O.*—MALVACEÆ.)

Sans.—Shalmali, Mocha. *Eng.*—Silk Cotton tree. *Hind.*—Huttian, Shimal. *Ben.*—Simul, Rukta-simal. *Tel.*—Poor. *Tam.*—Elavam. *Can.*—Boorugada-mara. *Mal.*—Poola. *Kon.*—Sâvari-kâppusu.

Properties and Uses.—The gum obtained from this tree is called *Mocharas* and is usually met with in Indian bazaars in roundish tears of a dirty brown color somewhat resembling galls. It contains a large proportion of tannic and gallic acids and is employed in cases where an astringent is indicated. It has been found useful in diarrhœa, dysentery and menorrhagia and as an aphrodisiac; it has also been employed as a styptic. The roots known as *Musla* or *Semul musla* have stimulant and tonic properties attributed to them.

Native Indian Preparations.—In the dysentery of children the following is used:—Take of *mocharasa* flowers of *Woodfordia floribunda*, root of *Mimosa pudica* and the filaments of the lotus equal parts, in all one tola, powdered rice one tola, water 11 tolas and boil together to the consistence of a gruel (Bhavaprakasa). In the dysentery of adults a decoction of *bela* fruit in goat's milk is given with the addition of powdered *mocharasa* and *Indrajava* seeds. (Chakradatta).

67. BORASSUS FLABELLIFORMIS.

(*N. O.*—PALMACEÆ).

Sans.—Tâla, Tranarâja. *Eng.*—Palmyra palm, Brab tree. *Hind.* and *Guz.*—Tâd. *Ben.*—Tâl. *Mah.* and *Kon.*—Talatmâd. *Tel.*—Tati. *Tam.*—Panaimaram. *Can.*—Tâlimara. *Mal.*—Tâlam, Pâna.

Habitat.—This noble and useful palm inhabits dry soils throughout tropical India.

Properties and Uses.—It is from this tree that toddy, jaggery and country sugar have been prepared in large quantities in Southern India. The sugar-candy produced in the manufacture of sugar from the palm is used in cough and pulmonary affections. The fresh saccharine juice obtained by excision of the spadis early in the morning is cooling, stimulant and antiphlogistic; also acts as a laxative taken regularly for several mornings;

it is useful for inflammatory affections and dropsy: also in gastric catarrh and to check hiccup; as diuretic it is useful in gonorrhœa. Slightly fermented juice called *Târi* (toddy) is given in diabetes. With aromatics it is a good tonic in emaciation. The milky fluid from the immature seeds is sweet and cooling and prevents hiccup and sickness. The root is cooling and restorative. The toddy poultice prepared by adding fresh drawn toddy to rice flour and subjected to a gentle fire till fermentation takes place, then spread on a cloth forms a valuable stimulant application to gangrenous and indolent ulcers, carbuncles, &c. The terminal buds of the tree are regarded as nutritive, diuretic and tonic. The yellow pulp surrounding the ripe nuts is sweet, heavy and indigestible. It is made into cakes with flour and other ingredients. The ashes of the following stalk are said to be useful in enlarged spleen. The bark of the tree burnt, reduced to charcoal and pulverised makes a good dentifrice; the decoction of the bark with a little salt added to it is a good astringent gargle for strengthening gums and teeth.

---

68. BOSWELLIA GLABRA & B. THURIFERA.

(*N. O.*—BURSERACEÆ.)

Sans.—Konkanadhoopam, Sâlashi. *Eng.*—Indian olibanam or Frankincense. *Hind.*—Lobhân. *Ben.*—Lubân, Salai, Kundro. *Guz.*—Dhup-gugali. *Mah.*—Pahadi-dhup, Vishesh-dhup. *Tel.*—Parangi sâmbrâni. *Tam.*—Kundrikam. *Mal.*—Sâmbrâni. *Can.*—Guggula, Vishæsha dhoop.

Habitat.—This tree is a native of the mountainous tracts of Central India and very common in Shahabad.

Properties and Uses.—The fragrant resin is a bitter aromatic. It is largely consumed as an incense in religious ceremonies; it is regarded by ancient writers as demulcent, aperient, alterative and a purifier of the blood. It is now used as refrigerent, diuretic, emmenagogue and ecbolic; as astringent in the form of ointment it is useful in chronic ulcers, diseased bones, buboes, &c., in which it promotes absorption. The resin rubbed in cocoanut oil or lemon juice is an application to foul ulcerations. The gum is used in rheumatic and nervous diseases, scrofulous affections, urinary disorders and in skin diseases generally combined with aromatics; mixed with ghee it is prescribed in gonorrhœa and in syphilitic cases; with cocoanut oil it is applied to sores and as a stimulant in pulmonary diseases, in bronchitis, chronic laryngitis and bronchorrhœa. Mixed with gum acacia it is used as a corrective for foul breath. If taken for a length of time in one ounce doses it is said to reduce obesity. The oil in 10 to 20 minim doses is useful in gonorrhœa taken in demulcent drinks. Dose of the gum resin is from 5 to 40 grains used in aphthæ, placenta previa, amenorrhœa, dysmenorrhœa, sore nipples, gonorrhœa and ringworm.

---

69. BRASSICA ALBA.

(*N. O.*—CRUCIFERÆ.)

Sans.—Siddhartha. *Eng.*—White mustard. *Hind.*—Sufed-rai. *Pers.*—Sipandane-sufaid. *Ben.*—Dhop-rai.

Habitat.—These mustard plants are extensively cultivated in many parts of India.

Properties and Uses.—White mustard when triturated with water does not yield the characteristic essential oil of mustard. Mustard-flour made into a paste with water is applied to the skin as a stimulant cataplasm or sinapism to the epigastrium in obstinate vomiting, cholera, &c., to the chest in spasmodic whooping cough with difficulty of breathing and to the calf of the leg in cases of delirium, apoplexy, &c. The interval of keeping the mustard plaster or poultice should not exceed 20 to 30 minutes. In cases of delicate women and children, thin muslin cloth should be laid between the skin and the poultice. The plaster and poultice is prepared in cold water. Mustard seeds are generally added to the foot-bath usually employed in cases of high fevers.

70. BRASSICA JUNCEA.

(*N. O.*—CRUCIFERÆ.)

Sans.—Râjika. *Eng.*—Indian mustard. *Hind.*—Rai. *Ben.*—Raisarisha. *Tel.*—Avâlu. *Tam.*—Kadugu. *Can.*—Sàsive, *Mal.*—Kaduka.

Habitat.—Cultivated throughout India forming an important crop in many districts.

Properties and Uses.—The seed contains about 20 to 25 percent of oil. An essential oil is also produced by the action of water as in *B. Nigra.* Mustard oil is used as an external stimulant application in chest affections especially of children. It is also used for culinary purposes. The whole plant is considered to possess bitter, aperient and tonic properties.

71. BRASSICA NIGRA.

(*N. O.*—CRUCIFERÆ.)

Sans.—Sarshapah. *Eng.*—Black mustard. *Hind.*—Makra-rai. *Pers.*—Sar-shaf. *Ben.*—Rai-sarisha. *Tel.*—Avâlu. *Tam.*—Kadugu. *Can.*—Sasive. *Mal.*—Kaduka.

Habitat.—This is also largely cultivated in India for the fixed oil which it yields.

Properties and Uses.—The seeds yield on distillation the essential oil of mustard produced in the presence of water by the *myrosin* of the black mustard. The powdered seeds combined with that of white mustard in the form of mustard flour is used as a simple vesicant and rubefacient. Mustard plasters are used in gout, sciatica, urticaria, &c. Mustard poultices are useful in febrile cases and in inflammatory swellings, such as parotitis. Mustard is often administered as a simple and effective emetic. It is largely used as a digestive condiment. The leaves of the mustard plant are used as a pot-herb and considered pungent and stomachic.

Native Indian Preparations.—Sarangadhara recommends the following application in urticaria:—Take of mustard seed, turmuric, *patchuk* root, sesamum and the seeds of *Cassia tora* equal parts and rub them together into a paste with mustard oil. In inflammatory affections the following poultice is prescribed by Sarangadhara:—Take of the root of *Boerhavia diffusa*. wood of *Berberis Asiatica*, root of *Moringa pterygosperma*, ginger and mustard seeds equal parts and rub them into a paste with fermented rice water.

72. BRYONIA EPIGŒA.

(*N. O.*—CUCURBITACEÆ.)

Sans.—Kadamba. *Ben.* and *Hind.*—Rakas-gaddâh. *Duk.*—Garajphal. *Pers.*—Lufa. *Tel.*—Akâshagadda. *Tam.*—Akâshakaru-dan. *Can.*—Akâshagaruda-balli. *Mal.*—Kollan-kova-kizhauna.

Habitat.—A herbaceous climber met with in Punjaub, Sindh, Guzarat and south along the Deccan Peninsula to Belgaum and distributed to Ceylon.

Properties and Uses.—This root is of special value among Indians as an alterative tonic, useful in syphilitic cases, old venereal complaints and also in the later stages of dysentery. It is usually administered in powder in one drachm doses. It is an effective remedy for rheumatism and snakebites. For rheumatic complaints it is applied mixed with onion, cummin seeds and castor oil in the form of an embrocation.

---

73. BUTEA FRONDOSA.

(*N. O.*—LEGUMINOSÆ).

Sans, *Hind.* and *Ben.*—Palâsh. *Eng.*—Bastard Teak. *Guz.*—Khâkarâ. *Mah.*—Palas. *Tel.*—Mœduga. *Tam.*—Palâshu. *Can.*—Muttaga-mara. *Mal.*—Pilâcham.

Habitat.—This tree is a native of the mountainous districts of India and Burma and common all over Bengal.

Properties and Uses.—The bark of this tree furnishes a very important exudation which is generally known as butea-gum or Bengal kino; it is very rich in tannic and gallic acids and is an excellent astringent well adapted to children and delicate females, useful in diarrhœa and dysentery; the dose is from 5 to 30 grains with a few grains of cinnamon, the addition of a little opium ($\frac{1}{4}$ to 1 grain) increases the efficacy. In moderately large doses the gum is useful in cases of hæmorrhage from the stomach and bladder. The solution of the gum is applied to bruises and erysipelatous inflammations, ringworms, &c., as an astringent application. The seeds act as laxative and anthelmintic and are given in powder, 10 to 20 grains thrice daily for three successive days, especially for round worms. Externally the powder is a remedy for ringworm, it may be applied better in the form of a paste. The leaves are astringent, tonic and aphrodisiac; externally they are used to disperse boils, pimples, buboes, tumourous hæmorrhoids, &c., and internally in flatulent colic, worms and piles. The flowers also are astringent and aphrodisiac, depurative and diuretic. Applied as poultice they disperse swellings and promote diuresis and menstrual flow; they are applied in orchitis. The bark is given with ginger in snake-bites. A weak decoction of the bark is useful in catarrh, cold and cough. The bark in pieces mixed with sugar-candy and chewed relieves abnormal thirsts. The gum and flower-juice are used in the making of dyes and colors and the root-fibre is used for making good, strong ropes. The charcoal of the wood of this plant possesses decolorising properties which enable it to be used as a substitute for animal charcoal in the purification of alkaloids on account of its comparative freedom from saline matter.

Native Indian Preparations.—Sarangadhara gives the following recipe for worms:—Take of the seeds of *Butea frondosa*, root of *Ipomœ turpethum*, seeds of *Hyoscyamus niger*, *kamala* powder, *baberang* seeds and treacle equal parts; beat them together into a paste with water and administer with butter-milk.

The gum of Butea frondosa was employed by ancient Hindus in the following preparation:—Take of red sandal-wood one part, rock salt two parts, chebulic myrobalans three parts and the gum of *Butea frondosa* four parts, powder and mix. This powder is recommended to be applied to pterygium and opacties on the cornea.

---

74. CÆSALPINIA BONDUC.

(*N. O.*—Leguminosæ.)

Sans.—Kubherâkshi. *Eng.*—Molucca Bean, Bonduc seed, Physic nut, Fever nut. *Hind.*—Kâlkaranj. *Ben.*—Nâtakaranja, Natar-phal. *Duk.*—Gutchka. *Tel.*—Gatchà, Yalakshi. *Tam.*—Kalarkodi, Mulal, Kalangu. *Can.*—Gajike-kayi. Mal.—Kalanchi. *Kon.*—Gajago.

Habitat.—A climbing shrub common all over Bengal, Bombay, Travancore and the Coromandal Coast.

Properties and Uses.—The seeds or nuts and the root-bark are noted as antiperiodic, antispasmodic, anthelmintic and febrifuge, valuable in simple, continued and intermittent fevers, in asthma, colic, &c. Dose is 10 to 30 grains of the powdered seed or kernel with an equal quantity of powdered black pepper; of the root-bark the dose is 10 to 15 grains. The active principle occurs more in the bark of the root. The powdered seed smoked in a *hucca* is said to cure colic; mixed with warm butter-milk and asafœtida it acts as tonic in dyspepsia. The burnt seeds with alum and burnt arecanut is a good dentifrice useful in spongy gums, gum-boils, &c. A cake made of 30 grains of powdered kernel, the contents of an egg and fried in ghee is said to be a valuable remedy taken twice a day in cases of acute orchitis, ovaritis and scrofula. The ointment made from the seeds with castor oil forms an excellent application to hydrocele, acute orchitis and glandular swellings. The seeds contain an oil which is useful as an embrocation. The tender leaves are efficacious in disorders of the liver and are reckoned as deobstruent and emmenagogue and the oil expressed from them is useful in convulsions, palsy and similar nervous complaints. The tender leaves boiled with castor oil or ghee and thickly applied on painful and swollen testicles are found to be very efficacious.

---

75. CÆSALPINIA SAPPAN.

(*N. O.*—LEGUMINOSÆ.)

Sans.—Ruktamukta, Patanga. *Eng.*—Sappan wood, Brasiletto. *Pers* and *Ben.*—Bakam. *Hind.*, *Duk.*, *Guz.*, and *Mah.*—Patang. *Tel.*—Bukkapuchettu, Bakâruchakka. *Tam.*—Parthangi. *Can.*—Sappanga. *Mal.*—Chappanam.

Habitat.—A small thorny tree cultivated in Central India, but found throughout the Eastern and Western Peninsula.

Properties and Uses.—This tree supplies the well-known sappan of Bengal commerce. The solid, heavy, hard and compact wood *Bakam* constitutes a very important article of trade in Calcutta; before the advent of the aniline dyes it was chiefly used as a red dye stuff for cotton fabrics. Medicinally the wood is a powerful astringent containing a principle resembling *Hæmatein*. Its active principle is said to be identical with *Brasilin*. It is recommended as a substitute for logwood. It is used as infusion or decoction in cases of diarrhœa, dysentery, &c., also employed in some forms of skin disease—especially lichen. It has also the property of a powerful emmenagogue. The resinous extract of sappan contains a crystalline principle which, if distilled and fused with potash, yields resorcin.

---

76. CAJANUS INDICUS.

(*N. O.*—LEGUMINOSÆ.)

Sans.—Adhaki, Tuvari, Soopyah. *Eng.*—Pigeon Pea, Dal, Cadjan Pea, Congo Pea. *Hind.*—Arhar dâl. *Ben.*—Arhar, *Guz.*—Dangri. *Mah.*—Turi. *Tel.*—Kandulu. *Tam.*—Adagi, Tuvarai. *Can.*—Togari.—*Mal.*—Adhaki, Tuvara.

Habitat.—Extensively cultivated throughout India.

Properties and Uses.—This pulse is easily digested and therefore suitable for invalids; but it is regarded as hot and dry as it produces costiveness. It is largely used by Indians in preparing a soup which is widely appreciated by all classes. The leaves are used in diseases of the mouth. The pulse and leaves ground into a paste, warmed and applied over the mamma has the effect of checking the secretion of milk. The tender leaves are chewed in cases of aphthæ and spongy gums. A poultice made with the seeds will reduce swelling.

Chemical Composition:—According to Professor Church, 1 lb. of the pulse would contain:—water 1 ounce and 361 grains; albuminoids 3 ounces and 208 grains, and starch 9 ounces and 11 grains.

Percentage Composition:—

Nitrogenous matter.—19·83 to 20·38.

Starch or Carbo-hydrates—61·9 to 64·3.

Oil or fatty matter—1·10 to 1·12.

Nutritive salts—About 3·11.

Water ... „ 10·63.

The nutrient ratio of dal is 1 : 3; the nutrient value is 80.

---

77. CALOPHYLLUM APETALUM AND C. INOPHYLLUM.

(*N. O.*—GUTTIFERÆ.)

Sans.—Punnagam, Namæruká, Panchakæshera. *Eng.*—Alexandrian Laurel. *Hind.*—Undi, Surpan, Sultan Champa. *Duk.*—Oondi. *Mah.*—Undag, Pumag. *Tel.*—Pumagamu, Ponnavittulu. *Tam.*—Punnagam, Punnaivirai. *Can.*—Surahonnæ, Namæru. *Mal.*—Cherupunna, Ponnakam. *Kon.*—Undee-phal.

Habitat.—Cultivated especially near the sea coast throughout India as an ornamental tree.

Properties and Uses.—The oil expressed from the seeds (60 per cent.) is known in Europe as the Domba oil. It is a highly exteemed external application in rheumatism; it is also applied to scabies (itch). The gum exuding from the wounded bark is a remedy for wounds and ulcers; internally it is emetic and purgative. The bark is astringent and is used in decoction in internal haemorrhages. The juice of the bark is a purgative. The leaves soaked in water are applied to inflamed eyes. The gum mixed with strips of the bark and leaves is steeped in water and the oil which rises to the surface is an application to sore eyes. The oil expressed from the seeds is generally used in India as lamp oil.

78. CALOTROPIS GIGENTIA.

(*N. O.*—ASCLEPIADEÆ.)

Sans.—Arkâ, Alark, Mandârah. *Eng.*—Gigantic Swallow wort, Mudar. *Hind.*—Madâr. *Ben.*—Akanda. *Pers.*—Khark. *Mah.*—Ruvi. *Tel.*—Arkamu, Mandaramu. *Tam.*—Badâbadam, Erukku. *Can.*—Ekkemâle. *Mal.*—Erikka.

Habitat.—This perennial shrub is found chiefly and frequently in waste lands throughout India.

Properties and Uses.—The root-bark and inspissated juice are used medicinally. They are alterative, tonic, diaphoretic and, in large doses, emetic. Doses,—as alterative 3 to 10 grains and as emetic 30 to 60 grains. The drug is used in leprosy, constitutional syphilis, mercurial cachexia, syphilitic and idiopathic ulcerations, dysentery, diarrhœa and chronic rheumatism. The root-bark promotes secretions; it is useful in skin diseases, elephantiasis, enlargement of the abdominal viscera, ascites and anasarca. Reduced to a paste with sour conjee it is applied to elephantiasis of the legs and scrotum. The milky juice is recommended for ringworm of the scalp and to destroy piles; mixed with honey it is used in aphthæ of the mouth and with a piece of cotton wool it is inserted into hollow tooth to cure tooth-ache. The dried juice is insoluble in water; it may be administered in the form of pills. The drug is an efficient antispasmodic, alterative and nervine tonic. For medicinal purposes the root-bark should be selected from as old plants as possible in the hot or dry weather and the bark should not be removed as soon as the root is dug out, but twenty-four hours afterwards; the thick, rough, corky epidermis of the bark should be scraped off before the root-bark is reduced to powder

This powder as an emetic and expectorant is a substitute for ipecacuanha in dysentery; in doses of 5 to 10 grains it may be safely substituted for ipecac, though double that quantity is generally required; with opium it forms a good representative of the officinal Dovers' powder; in chronic rheumatism it is given suspended in mucilage and water; with black pepper twice a day in jaundice; given in half a seer of whey of milk with half a drachm of sodium carbonate jaundice is said to be cured within a week. The powdered root-bark is smoked like tobacco in syphilis. The leaves of the plant are also useful in ascites and enlargement of the abdominal viscera; they are mixed with rock salt, roasted in closed vessels and the ash thus produced are given with whey. A fluid extract of the leaves given in doses of one to five drops in intermittent fever during intermission is said to cut off the paroxysm more effectually than quinine. A powder of the dried leaves is dusted on ulcers to promote healthy action or mixed with oil it is applied with a liquid paste to old sores and ulcers.

This drug is employed to cure all kinds of fits—epilepsy, hysteria, lock-jaw, convulsions in children—paralytic complaints, cold sweats, poisonous bites and venereal complaints. The flowers are digestive, tonic and stomachic in action; they are used in cough, catarrh, asthma and loss of appetite. The dried flowers in 1 to 2 grain-doses mixed with sugar are given in leprosy, secondary syphilis and in gonorrhœa with milk diet.

---

79. CAMELLIA THEIFERA.

(*N. O.*—TERNSTRÆMIACEÆ.)

Eng.—Tea plant. *Ver.*—Chhâ, Chai.

Habitat.—This plant which is a native of China is grown in the hill districts of India.

Properties and Uses.—The dried leaves of the plant are the source of the crystalline principle—*Caffeine* also called *Theine* and *Guaranine* obtained by sublimation of an extract made by aqueous infusion and evaporation, astringent and coloring matters having been previously removed. The average yield is 3 to 4 per cent. It might be very profitably manufactured in India from tea dust. An infusion of tea seeds was once used as a remedy for insect blights. The seeds contain about 30 per cent. of fixed oil somewhat resembling olive oil. Tea is seldom used medicinally except as a stimulant in strong infusion or as an astringent lotion on account of the tannin it contains, and which it renders useful as a gargle or injection. In moderate quantities it stimulates the mental faculties, clears the mind and facilitates its working; many, too, have experienced its baneful effect in preventing sleep and occasioning mental irritability. At times, however, the disorder of the faculties of the mind under the influence of strong tea amounts nearly to insanity. In some it is highly stimulating and exhilarating; in others its effects are depression and lowness of spirits. Notwithstanding all this, yet its regular and moderate use will in the great majority of cases, prove beneficial, supplying the necessary stimulus to the flagging powers and reviving and refreshing all the mental powers. But then this, be it remembered, is its moderate use, not its immoderate abuse; like all other stimulants it requires to be taken with due caution. Very strong tea, like alcoholic drink, is mischievous, although not in such a high degree as *Spirits*, *Beer*, &c. Not more than two cups, only moderately strong, should be taken at the morning and evening meals. This quantity is enough for the health.

---

80. CAMPHORA OFFICINARUM.

(*N. O.*—LAURACEÆ.)

Eng.—Camphor. *Hind.* and *Mah.*—Kapur. *Tel.* and *Mal.*—Karpooram. *Tam.*—Karuppooram. *Can.*—Karpoora.

Properties and Uses.—Camphor is a stearoptene or volatile oil in translucent white crystalline masses obtained from the wood of *Cinnamomum camphora* (Camphora officinarum) purified by sublimation in England. It is of a very peculiar, fragrant and penetrating odour, bitter, pungent and aromatic taste. It is extremely volatile and inflammable burning with a bright light and much smoke. In its medical properties it is diaphoretic, antiseptic, stimulant, antispasmodic, narcotic and externally anodyne used in the form of liniments. It is good in typhus, confluent small-pox and all fevers and eruptions of the typhoid class; also in measles, febrile delirium, hiccup, asthma, hysteria, epilepsy, atonic gout, mania, melancholy, acute rheumatism, &c. It exhilarates in moderate doses and raises the pulse without producing febrile symptoms; it also promotes perspiration and in certain states of the body it induces sleep when opium fails to do so; but its effects are transient and therefore it requires frequent administration. It is given in doses of

3 to 10 grains in pills, powder and in emulsion. Sniffed up the nostrils it relieves cold in the head; the vapours inhaled by means of a tube like a cigar are useful in affections of the chest; a piece held in the mouth is said to be a protective against fevers and other infectious diseases; finally its strong odour protects animal substances from the ravages of insects.

In cases of spermatorrhœa, pills of camphor and opium in the proportions of 3 grains of the former to half-grain of the latter taken at bed time are found to be very efficacious. In uterine pains 6 to 8 grain pills are administered and the liniment of camphor is rubbed on the abdomen. In apoplexy fomentations of hot water with liniment of camphor added are applied to feet and calfs of legs with much benefit; so also in cases of delirium. An ounce of camphor liniment added to 15 ounces of conjee water will make an injection usefully employed in cases of apoplexy, convulsions (puerperal), hysteria and similar other affections. Three or four grains of camphor with an equal quantity of asafœtida and made into a pill and administered in asthma has been found to give much relief. Its chief officinal preparations are:—(1) Camphor mixture made by simply immersing in cold water a lump of camphor tied in muslin for a few hours (half ounce of camphor to one gallon of water). Dose is 1 to 2 ounces. (2) Compound tincture of camphor known as *Paregoric Elixir*. Dose 15 to 60 minims. (3) Camphor liniments, simple and compound prepared by dissolving camphor in olive oil or rectified spirits and which are used externally as stimulants and counter-irritants. (4) Spirits of camphor prepared by dissolving 1 ounce of camphor in 9 ounces of rectified spirit. Dose is 10 to 30 minims in emulsion.

---

81. CANARIUM COMMUNE.

(*N. O.*—AMYRIDACEÆ.)

Eng.—Java Almond tree. East Indian Elemi. *Hind.* and *Ben.*—Jangli bâdam. *Can.*—Sâmbrâni. *Mal.*—Kanâri.

Habitat.—This plant of the Malay Archipelago has been cultivated in Southern India.

Properties and Uses.—The resin imported under the name of Manilla Elemi is supposed to be a product of this plant. It is used principally in the manufacture of varnishes; the gum is stimulant and rubefacient and used in the form of ointment for indolent and sluggish ulcers. The nut yields a semi-liquid oil on expression similar in appearance to cocoanut oil. It is used for culinary purposes and is regarded as palatable and demulcent as almond oil. It is also burnt in lamps. The bark of the tree yields an abundance of limpid oil with a pungent turpentine smell congealing to a buttery camphoraceous mass; it is stated to possess the same properties as copaiba applied in the form of an ointment to indolent ulcers. The kernels in emulsion form a substitute for almond mixture.

82. CANNA INDICA.

(*N. O.*—MARANTACEÆ.)

Sans. and *Ben.*—Sarvajaya. *Eng.*—Indian shot. *Hind.*—Sabjaya. *Mah.*—Devakeli. *Tel.*—Krishnatâmara. *Tam.*—Poovalai. *Can.*—Kælahoo. *Mal.*—Katuvarâ. *Kon.*—Kælâphool.

Habitat.—Several varieties are common all over India grown in gardens as ornamental and flowering plants.

Properties and Uses.—The root is diuretic, diaphoretic and demulcent used in fevers and dropsy. The seed is cordial and vulnerary. The seed juice warmed and instilled into ears as ear-drops is said to relieve earaches. When cattle have eaten any poisonous grass which is generally discovered by the swelling of the abdomen the root-bulb of this plant is administered as a remedy :— The root bulb is broken up in small pieces boiled in rice water together with pepper and given to the cattle suffering from poisonous symptoms to drink.

---

83. CANNABIS SATIVA.

(*N. O.*—CANNABINACEÆ.)

Sans.—Vijayâ, Siddhapatri. *Eng.*—Indian Hemp. *Hind.*—Gânjâ. *Ben.*—Bhâng, Sidhi, Ganja. *Arab.*—Kinnab. *Pers.*—Darakte-bang. *Guz.*—Ganja. *Mah.*—Bhanga. *Tel.*—Ganjayi, Jadaganja. *Tam.*—Pangi, Kanja, madamattagam. *Can.*—Bhangi.

Habitat.—The hemp plant is a native of Western and Central Asia, now largely cultivated all over India and is found wild on the western Himalayas and Kashmir and is acclimatised on the plains of India generally.

Properties and Uses.—The hemp plant is sacred to the Hindus. It is chiefly cultivated in India for the various forms of narcotics which it yields and which have been used so largely by Indians from very ancient times. The three principal forms in which the *Cannabis Sativa* is used in India are:—(1) The Ganja consisting of the unfertilized resinous flowering shoots of the female plant grown on the plains; the narcotic principle which is only developed in the *Ganja* in the unfertilized flowers entirely disappears after fertilization has taken place. On the other hand the plant grown on the lower hills of Punjaub and which yields (2) *Bhang* does not develop the narcotic property until the fruits are mature, the dried leaves and fruiting shoots constituting the *Bhang* or *Siddhi* so largely used by Indians in making the intoxicating liquor *Hashish* or the narcotic conserve or confection called *Majum.* (3) The *Charas* is the cannabis resin which exudes naturally on the leaves, stems and fruits, but only on plants growing on the mountain tracts at an altitude of 6000 to 8000 feet. It is powerfully narcotic and is smoked with tobacco. *Ganja* contains about 20 per cent. *Bhang* 10 per cent. and *Charas* 40 per cent. of resin. This contains the active principle besides fatty matters and chlorophyll. A brown syrupy alkaloid—*Cannabine*—has been isolated and a purified resin called *Cannabinone* is now prepared. Both are employed as sedatives. *Cannabine Tannate* is a yellowish brown powder which is said to be free of some of the toxic properties of *Cannabis Indica.*

Siddhi, Subjie and *Bhang* are synonymous with each other and are used with water as a drink which is thus prepared:—About three tolas weight are well washed with cold water, then rubbed to powder, mixed with black pepper, cucumber and melon seeds, sugar, half a pint of milk and equal quantity of water. This is considered sufficient to intoxicate an habituated person. Half the quantity is enough for a novice. This composition is chiefly used by Mahomedans of the better classes.

Another recipe is as follows:—The same quantity of *Siddhi* is washed and ground, mixed with black pepper and a quart of cold water added. This is taken at one sitting. This is the favourite beverage of the Hindus who are accustomed to it, especially the Brijobassies and many of the Rajputana soldiery.

The intoxication caused by either of these beverages is of the most cheerful kind causing the person to sing and dance, to eat food with great relish and to seek aphrodisiac enjoyments. The intoxication lasts about 3 hours when sleep supervenes. No nausea or sickness of stomach follows, nor are the bowels at all affected; next day there is slight giddiness and vascularity of the eyes, but no other symptom worth recording.

Gánja is used for smoking alone:—One rupee weight and a little dried tobacco are rubbed together in the palm of the hand with a few drops of water. A little tobacco is placed in the pipe, then a layer of the prepared *ganja*, then more tobacco and above all, the fire. Four or five persons usually join in the use of this. The *hookah* is passed round and each person takes a single draught. Intoxication ensues almost instantly and within half an hour to the novice and after four or five inspirations to those that are accustomed to it. The effects differ from those occasioned by *siddhi*. Heaviness, laziness and agreeable reveries ensue, but the person can be readily roused and made to discharge his routine duties, such as pulling the punkah, waiting at table, &c.

The *Majoom* or hemp confection is a compound of sugar, butter, flour, milk and *siddhi* or *bhang*. Four ounces of *siddhi* and an equal quantity of ghee are placed in an earthen or well-tinned vessel, a pint of water added, and the whole warmed over a charcoal fire. The mixture is constantly stirred until the water all boils away, which is known by the crackling noise of the melted butter on the sides of the vessel. The mixture is then removed from the fire, squeezed through cloth while hot, by which an oleaginous solution of the active principles and coloring matter of the hemp is obtained; and the leaves, fibres, &c., remaining on the cloth are thrown away. The green oily solution soon concretes into a buttery mass and is then well washed by the hand with soft water, so long as the water becomes coloured. The colouring matter and an extractive substance are thus removed and a very pale green mass of the consistence of simple ointment remains. The washings are thrown away as these are intoxicating and producing constriction of the throat, great pain and very disagreeable and dangerous symptoms.

The operator then takes two pounds of sugar and adding a little water, places it in a pipkin over the fire. When the sugar dissolves and froths, two ounces of milk are added; a thick scum rises and is removed; more milk and a little water are added from time to time and the boiling continued about an hour, the solution being carefully stirred until it becomes an adhesive clear syrup, ready to solidify on a cold surface; four ounces of *tyre* (new milk dried before the sun) in fine powder are now stirred in and lastly, the prepared butter of hemp is introduced, brisk stirring being continued for a few minutes. A few drops of *attar* of roses are then quickly sprinkled in and the mixture poured from the pipkin on a flat, cold dish or slab. The mass concretes immediately into a thick cake which is divided into small lozenge-shaped pieces. A seer thus prepared sells for from four to five rupees. One drachm by weight will intoxicate a beginner; three drachms will be required to one that is accustomed to its use. The taste is sweet and the odour very agreeable. Sometimes, if the customers require, stramonium seeds are introduced, but never nucis vomica. It is most fascinating in its effects, producing extatic happiness, a persuasion of high rank, a sensation of flying, voracious appetite and intense aphrodisiac desire (Bengal Dispensary).

The leaves of *Cannabis Sativa* are purified by being boiled in milk before use. They are regarded as heating, digestive, astringent and narcotic. The intoxication produced by *bhang* is said to be of a pleasant description and to promote talkativeness.

Bhang and *Ganja* are prescribed by native doctors in bowel complaints and recommended as appetisers, valuable as nervous stimulants and as a source of great staying-power under severe exertion or fatigue. Indian hemp is primarily stimulant, secondarily anodyne, antispasmodic and anæsthetic.

The leaves make a good snuff for deterging the brain; their juice applied to the head removes dandruff and vermin; dropped into the ear it allays pain and destroys worms; it checks the discharge in diarrhœa and gonorrhœa and is diuretic. The powder of the leaves applied to fresh wounds promotes granulation; a poultice of the plant is applied to local inflammations, erysipelas, neuralgia, &c., as an anodyne or sedative. The dose of the leaves is 40 grains internally. Externally in the form of poultice it relieves hæmorrhoids; a poultice of the fresh bruised leaves is useful in affections of the eye with photophobia; also applied to relieve pain and swelling in orchitis. The resin extracted from the leaves and flowers and which is known as *nasha* or *charas* is narcotic and is used to produce sleep in cases of sleeplessness, in which opium is contra-indicated; it does not cause nausea, constipation or headache as opium does; it is valuable in preventing and curing sick headaches, malarial and periodical headaches, valuable in acute mania, whooping cough, asthma, dysuria and in relieving pain in dysmenorrhœa; it increases appetite; it is aphrodisiac. For asthma and tetanus the dose of the extract is from ¼ to 2 grains; the leaves mixed with sugar and well-fried in ghee and with black pepper added are administered in chronic diarrhœa; with poppy seeds the extract is given in dysentery; with asafœtida it is given in hysteria. In cases of chronic colic, wonderful effect is produced by the administration of 1 grain of the extract in combination with ¼ grain of ipecacuanha. In dysentery about half a drachm of dried tender leaves mixed with a little sugar and black pepper powder is a well-known and successful remedy; the tincture of the British Pharmacopæa is also used in 15 to 20 minim doses three times a day especially in acute dysentery. The oil extracted from the seeds is used for rubbing in rheumatism.

Native Indian Preparations.—*Jatuphaladya Churna* :—Take of nutmeg, cloves, cinnamon, cardamom, *tejapatra* leaves, flowers of *Mesua ferra (Nagakesara)*, camphor, sandlewood, sesamum seeds, bamboo manna, flowers of *Tabernaemontana coronaria (Tagara)*, chebulic and emblic myrobalans, long pepper, black pepper, ginger, leaves of *Pinus Webiana (Talisa)*, plumbago root, cumin seeds and the seeds of *Embelia ribes (Viranga)*, equal parts, purified *bhang* equal in weight to all the above ingredients, and sugar twice as much as the *bhang*. Powder and mix. Dose—about 20 to 40 grains. This preparation is given in diarrhœa, indigestion and loss of appetite. (Sarangadara.)

Jvalanala rasa:—Take of *Yavakshara* and *Sarjikakshara* (Carbonates of potash and soda), borax, mercury, sulphur, long pepper, black pepper, *Piper chaba (Chavya)* and ginger equal parts, fried leaves of *Cannabis sativa* equal to all the above ingredients, root of *Moringa pterygosperma* half the weight of *bhang* ; powder the ingredients, mix and soak the mixed powder for three days in each of the following fluids, namely, a decoction or fresh juice of the leaves of *Cannabis Indica*, the roots of *Moringa pterygosperma* and *Plumbago rosea* and dry in the sun. Then roast the mass lightly and make into a pill mass with the juice of the leaves of *Wedelia calendulacea* (*Bhringaraja*). Dose, about half a drachm with honey. This medicine is given in indigestion and loss of appetite with nausea and vomiting. (Bhavaprakash.)

Madana modaka :—Take of the three myrobalans, ginger, long pepper, black peper, *Rhus succedanea* (*Sringi*), *pachak* root, coriander, rock salt, zedoary root, leaves of

Pinus webbiana (*Talisa*), bark of *Myrica sapida* (*Katphala*), flowers of *Mesua ferrea* (*Nagakesara*), *ajowan*, seeds of *Sesili Indicum* (*Vanayamani*), liquorice root, seeds of *Trigonella faenum graecum* (*Methi*), cumin and nigella seeds equal parts; hemp leaves with flowers and seeds fried in clarified butter, equal in weight to all the other ingredients; sugar equal in weight to the hemp. Prepare a syrup with the sugar, then add the other substances in fine powder and make into a confection. Lastly add clarified butter, honey, powdered sesamum seeds, cardamoms, cinnamon, *tejapatra* leaves and camphor, each two tolas and make into boluses of about 80 grains each. This confection is used in cough, chronic bowel complaints and impotence.

Numerous confections of *bhang* are described in books. They are, as their names imply, considered aphrodisiac and are used in chronic bowel complaints and nervous debility. Most of them are prepared with equal parts of a number of supposed tonic and aphrodisiac substances in small quantities and *bhang* equal in weight to all the other ingredients, together with sugar, honey and the usual aromatics; and of this, the above is an illustration. *Majoom* the preparation of which has been already described would be a neater substitute for these complicated preparations.

---

84. CANSCORA DECUSSATA.

(*N. O.*—GENTIANACEAE).

Sans.—Sankhapushpi. *Hind.*—Sankhahuli. *Ben.*—Dânkuni.

Habitat.—This little plant grows plentifully from the Himalyas to Burma.

Properties and Uses.—It is regarded as laxative, alterative and tonic and is much praised as a nervine. It is used in insanity, epilepsy and nervous debility.

Native Indian Remedies.—According to Chakradatta the fresh juice of the plant in doses of about an ounce is given with the addition of honey and *pachak* root in all sorts of insanity. A paste made of the entire plant including roots and flowers is recommended to be taken with milk as a nervine and alterative tonic. The following compound powder is used in similar cases, Take of *gulancha*, *Achyranthes aspera*, *baberang*, *pachak* root, root of *Asparagus racemosus*, *Acorus calamus*, chebulic myrobalan and *Canscora decussata* in equal parts ; powder and mix. It is said that the use of this powder for three days will enable a student to learn by rote a thousand couplets of poetry.

---

85. CANTHIUM PARVIFLORUM.

(*N. O.*—Rubiaceae.)

Tel.—Balusu *Tam.*—Karai. *Can*— Kâke-gida. *Mal.*—Kandangâri, Neroori. *Kon.*—Kâyili.

Habitat.—A shrubby plant met with from the Konkan southwards to Ceylon.

Properties and Uses.—A decoction of the edible leaves as well as the root of this plant is prescribed in certain stages of flux and the last is supposed to have anthelmintic properties.

86. CAPSICUM ANNUM AND C. FRUTESCENS.

(*N.O.*—SOLANACEAE.)

Sans.—Marichiphalam. *Eng.*—Spanish pepper, Red pepper, Cayenne pepper. *Hind.*—Lal or Gach-marichi. *Ben* and *Guz.*—Lal-marich. *Mah.*—Mirsinga. *Tel.*—Mirapakaya. *Tam.*—Malagay. *Can.*—Kempu menasu. *Mal.*—Uppaeri-paranki, Parangimulak.

Habitat.—This plant is very largely cultivated for its fruit throughout the plains of India and in the hills in some districts.

Properties and Uses.—Capsicum fruits are universally employed in India as a principal ingredient in the preparation of various curries and *chutneys*. Capsicum owes its pungency and acridity to an oleo-resin called *capsicin*. Capsicum is stomachic and stimulant and externally employed as a rubefacient liniment. Made into a lozenge with sugar and tragacanth it is a favourite remedy for hoarseness with professional singers and public speakers. It is often employed in the form of tincture as an adjunct to bitters, tonics and other stimulants; it is useful in dyspepsia and flatulence; pills made of equal parts of capsicum, rhubarb and ginger are used; with cinchona it is useful in intermittent and lithargic affections and also in atonic gout and in advanced stages of rheumatism; with asafœtida and sweet-flag root or camphor it is used in the form of pills in cases of cholera; also the decoction of the fruit with the addition of opium and fried asafœtida is given with equal success in cholera. Capsicum has a powerful action on the mucous membrane and in sore throat and putrid throat a gargle made of chillies (4 drachms in 1 bottle of boiling water) is found particularly beneficial. By pouring hot vinegar upon the fruits all the essential qualities are preserved. This chilly vinegar is an excellent stomachic imparting a fine flavour to fish and meats. The whole plant steeped in milk is successfully applied to reduce swellings and hardened tumours.

---

87. CAREYA ARBOREA.

(*N. O.*—MYRTACEÆ.

Hind. and *Ben.*—Kumbi. *Mah.*--Vakumbha. *Tel.*—Dudippi. *Tam.*—Pailacputatammi. *Can.*—Daddâla, Guddada-ippæ. *Mal.*—Peelam, Paer, Alam, Ukamaram.

Habitat.—Frequent in sub-Himalayan tract from the Jamna eastward.

Properties and Uses.—The bark is astringent; when moistened it gives out mucilage and is therefore prescribed for emollient embrocations; the flowers are given in sherbat or in infusion after child-birth to heal ruptures caused by child-birth. The juice of the fresh bark as well as flowers is administered with honey as demulcent in coughs and colds. Boils, abscesses and ulcers cleaned and washed with the decoction of the barks are said to heal rapidly; for the same purpose the decoction is employed in cases of dysentery and also internally on account of its astringent action.

---

88. CARICA PAPAYA.

(*N. O.*—PASSIFLOREÆ.)

Eng.—Papaw tree. *Hind.*—Popaiyah. *Pers.* and *Arab.*—Amba-hindi. *Ben.*—Papeya. *Guz.*—Papâyi. *Mah*—Popaya. *Tel.*—Boppayi. *Tam.*—Poppayi. *Can.* —Pappangay. *Mal.*—Kappalam, pappayam.

Habitat.—This valuable tree is commonly cultivated in gardens throughout India.

Properties and Uses.—The milky juice of this fruit contains a ferment which has an extraordinarily energetic action upon albuminous substances and like pepsin curdles milk; it differs from pepsin in being active without the addition of free acid; probably it contains a little quantity of it; it operates at a higher temperature about 60 to 65° C. and in a shorter time 5 minutes at most. The filtered juice unlike pepsin gives no precipitate on boiling but is precipitated by mercury chloride, iodine and all the mineral acids; like pepsin it is precipitated by neutral acetate of lead and does not give any precipitate with copper sulphate and iron chloride. The active principle so separated is named papain. It is most useful in deficiency of gastric juice, excess of unhealthy mucous in the stomach, in dyspepsia, intestinal irritation and the like, in doses of one to five grains; it is also used in solution to dissolve the fibrinous membrane in croup or diphtheria, a solution in glycerine being painted on the pharynx every five minutes; and also applied with good results to ulcers and fissures of the tongue and, in the form of a pigment prepared with borax and water, to remove warts and corns and other horny excrescences of the skin; in psoriasis and chronic eczema especially of the palms of the hands: Papain 12 grains, powdered borax 5 grains, and distilled water 2 drachms. Mix and make a solution. Apply it to the part affected.

The juice from the raw fruit is said to be more efficacious in dissolving albumen than pepsin. The raw fruit is scraped longitudinally and the milky juice is collected; this is put on a sand bath; after 24 hours or so a dull white powder is left; this is the best preparation for internal use; one or two grains with sugar or milk after meals should be given to adults. The tincture does not keep well and is disagreeable to taste; syrup of the powder may be made, if required, for children and women. It is most efficacious in dyspepsia. The fruit is useful in chronic diarrhœa; the green fruit is laxative and diuretic; its juice is emmenagogue and in large doses it acts as ecbolic; it dissolves coagulated albumen. The fresh milky juice is rubefacient and is an application for ringworm; it is a certain remedy in cases of scorpion stings; the seeds are also similarly useful; the seeds are powerfully emmenagogue; they and the milky juice form the best vermifuge especially for round worms in children. The ripe fruit is alterative and if eaten regularly corrects habitual constipation; it is useful in piles (bleeding piles) and dyspepsia.

Boiled and mixed with lime-juice and sugar it makes a good sauce. The dried and salted fruit reduces enlarged spleen and liver. The unripe fruit is made into a curry and eaten by women to stimulate secretion of milk. The leaves dipped in hot water or warmed over a fire and applied to the painful parts for nervous pains. Bruised leaves applied as a poultice are said to reduce elephantoid growths; inspissated juice of the fruit in pill form, in doses of 2 to 4 grains, is given internally for the same disease.

89. CARUM COPTICUM.

(*N. O.*—UMBELLIFERÆ.)

Sans.—Yamani. *Hind.*—Ajowan. *Ben.*—Jowan. *Ben.*—Ajwân.

Habitat.—This plant is largely cultivated in Eastern India.

Properties and Uses.—This is a source of the valuable antiseptic *Thymol*, a stearoptene which is contained in the oil yielded by its seeds sometimes to the extent of 20 or 30 per cent. It is identical with that obtained from *Thymus vulgaris*. This crystalline substance is well-known in the bazaars of India as *Ajwain-ke-phul* and a distilled water from the seeds, which is known as *Omum* water or *Ajwain-ka-arrack*, also contains it as an active principle.

The seeds have an aromatic smell and warm pungent taste. They are used as spices along with betelnuts and *pan* leaves as a carminative in flatulence, dyspepsia and spasmodic affections. *Ajwain-ke-phul* is used in small doses for the same purposes and in cholera to some extent. Applied externally in alcoholic solution, it is useful in allaying nervous pains. The oil distilled from the seeds is also used medicinally for the purposes indicated above. A tea-spoonful of *ajowan* with a little rock salt is a common domestic remedy for indigestion from irregular diet.

The following compound powder is given by Chakradatta as useful in cases of colic or pain in the bowels. Take of *ajowan*, rock salt, *sonchal* salt, *yavakshâra*, asafœtida and chebulic myrobalan equal parts; powder the ingredients and mix. Dose—grains 10 to 20 to be taken with wine. *Ajowan* taken daily with treacle is said to cure urticaria within a week.

90. CASSIA ALATA.

(*N. O.*—LEGUMINOSÆ)

Sans.—Dadrughna. *Eng.*—Ringworm Shrub. *Hind.* and *Ben.*—Dadmurdan. *Mah.*—Dadamurdana. *Tel.*—Sheema, Metta tamara. *Tam.*—Vendukolli. Sheemai agatti. *Can.*--Sheemigida, Agase-gida. *Mal.*—Seemagati. *Kon.*—Daddupâna.

Habitat.—It is cosmopolitan in the tropics, met with all over Bengal and many other parts of India.

Properties and Uses.—The leaves bruised into a paste with an equal weight of simple ointment or borax is a specific for ringworm and similar other skin affections; to be more effective it should be mixed with a little lime-juice or common salt; or the juice of the leaves mixed with a little lime juice, makes an equally efficacious application. The leaves in decoction is considered as a cure for herpes and other skin diseases, even venereal affections and all poisonous insect bites. The decoction is tonic, expectorant and astringent and is used as a mouth-wash in stomatitis. A tincture of the dried leaves or an extract from the leaves acts as a purgative like that of senna or colocynth.

---

91. CASSIA AURICULATA.

(*N. O.*—LEGUMINOSÆ.)

Eng.—Tanner's Cassia. *Hind.* and *Duk.*—Tarwar. *Guz.*—Awal. *Mah.*—Taravada. *Tel.*—Tangaedu. *Tam.*—Avarai. *Can.*—Avarike, Châkusina-gida. *Mal.*—Aveeram, Jimute.

Habitat—It grows wild in the Central Provinces, Western Peninsula, South India and Ceylon.

Properties and Uses.—The seeds are a valued local application to purulent ophthalmia or conjunctivitis known as "Country Sore Eye"; the seeds with their testa and their kernels are *finely* powdered and this powder is generally blown into the eyes or the powder mixed with cocoanut or gingelly oil is applied to the sore eyes. The bark is astringent in effect. The plant is used in diuresis and diabetes and the decoction, especially of the flower buds, is administered in diabetes with excellent results. The twigs are used as tooth-brushes.

---

92. CASSIA FISTULA.

(*N. O.*—LEGUMINOSÆ.)

Sans.—Râjavraksha, Suvarnaka. *Eng.*—Pudding-pipe tree, Purging Cassia. *Hind.* and *Duk.*—Amaltâs, girmalah. *Ben.*—Sundâli. *Guz.*—Garmâlâ. *Mah.*—Bâhâvâ. *Tel.*—Raelachettu, Aragvadhamu, Koelapenna. *Tam.*—Konai, Irajviruttam. *Can.*—Kakkae-mara. *Mal.*—Konna. *Kon.*—Kakkâyi.

Habitat.—A moderate sized deciduous tree indigenous to and common throughout India and Burma.

Properties and Uses.—The well-known brown pendulous pods of this tree, about 1 to 1½ feet in length, are used in medicine. The pulp of the fruit, the root-bark and the powdered seeds and leaves possess purgative properties. The pulp is an agreeable mild laxative, safe for children and pregnant women. It is best used combined with other purgatives as a confection or electuary as by itself it requires to be taken in doses of from one to two ounces to produce any effect. It is an ingredient in the confection of senna. Cassia pulp is also employed in the essence of coffee. For household use it is administered in combination with tamarinds. The confection made of the pulp is given in cases of diabetes. *Gulkhand* of which it forms an ingredient is a cooling laxative especially for delicate women; dose is half an ounce with warm milk taken at bed time. The pulp of the ripe pod mixed with tamarind pulp taken at bed time acts on the bowels mildly causing one or two soft motions the following morning. In the flatulent colic of children it is commonly applied round the navel to produce motions. The flowers in decoction are given in stomach affection. Externally the leaves ground into a paste are applied to ringworm; the bark and leaves mixed and rubbed with oil are applied to pustules, ringworm, chilblains, &c.

93. CASSIA LANCEOLATA.

(*N. O.*—LEGUMINOSÆ.)

Eng.—Tinnevelly Senna, Indian Senna. *Hind.*—Sunnâmakki, Sana. *Arab.*—Sana-e-Hindi. *Ben.*—Sonna-makki, senpât *Duk.*—Nat-ki-sonâ. *Guz.*—Senamakki. *Mah.*—Mulkacha Shonamakki. *Tel.*—Naelaponna. *Tam.*—Nilâvirai. *Can.*—Nelâvare. *Mal.*—Nilavâka.

Habitat.—This plant is largely cultivated in Southern India, at Tinnevelly and in the Bombay Presidency.

Properties and Uses.—The purgative properties of senna are well-known and it is the most commonly employed of all cathartics; it is sure in its operation but rather heating and apt to gripe and cause nausea; therefore an aromatic should generally be given with it. It should not be administered when there is irritation and fever, nor during pregnancy nor the existence of piles. It may be given to children and elderly persons quite safely when a tolerably active purge is required; and it is good to combine a saline aperient with it. The powdered leaves are sometimes administered; the dose varies from ½ to 2 drachms. The confection, a mild laxative, commonly called Lenative electuary is given from 1 to 4 drachms; the syrup, a good preparation for young children, from 1 to 2 drachms; tincture from 1 to 4 drachms; the compound infusion, an excellent family medicine, may be prepared as follows:—Senna leaves 4 drachms; raisins (stoned) 1 ounce; ginger (bruised) and cloves (powdered), each one drachm and boiling water a pint; macerate four hours in a covered vessel and strain: dose is 1 to 2 ounces; with the addition of milk and sugar it will taste like tea and will be readily taken by children. A tablespoonful of brandy will add to its stomachic properties and make it keep better, but, if for children, this should not be added. The infusion should be kept in a cool place. The pods of the senna tree also possess purgative property but in a less degree than the leaflets; 6 to 12 pods for adults and 3 to 6 for children and the aged. They are best infused in a glassful of cold water for 6 to 8 hours and the whole taken.

---

94. CASSIA OCCIDENTALIS. ✓

(*N. O.*—LEGUMINOSAE.)

Sans.—Kâsamarda. *Eng.*—Negro Coffee. *Hind* and *Duk.*—Kâsundâ. *Ben.*—Kâlakáshundâ. *Guz.* and *Mah.*—Hikâl. *Tel.*—Kasinda. *Tam.*—Paeyâvirai, Ponnavirai.—*Mal.*—Ponnâveeram. *Can.*—Doddatagache. *Kon.*—Hodu taikilo.

Habitat.—A common weed scattered from the Himalayas to the Western Peninsula, Bengal, South India, Burma and Ceylon.

Properties and Uses.—The seeds roasted and ground have been used as a substitute for coffee. The medicinal properties are destroyed in the roasting process. The leaves, roots and seeds, are purgative. They are useful in cough and whooping cough; the dose of the leaves is

90 grains. Externally they are applied smeared with grease to slight sores, itch, &c; the seeds are used in France and West Indies as a febrifuge in the form of vinous tincture. The infusion of the root is considered as an antidote to various poisons. The root is considered diuretic and is used in incipient dropsy.

Chemical composition of the seeds :—

Fatty matters.	4·9 per cent.	Calcium sulphate and phosphate, Chrysophanic acid,	0·9 per cent.
Tannic acid.	0·9 ,,		
Sugar ...	2·1 ,,		
Gum ...	28·8 ,,	Malic acid, Sodium chloride, Magnesium sulphate, Iron, Silica together,	5·4 per cent.
Starch ...	2·0 ,,		
Cellulose ...	34·0 ,,		
Water ...	7·0 ,,	Achrosine.	13·58 per cent.

95. CASSIA SOPHORA.

(*N. O.*—LEGUMINOSÆ.)

Sans. and *Can.*—Kásamarda, *Eng.*—Senna Sophera, Sinna Esculenta, Senna purpurea. *Hind.*—Bás-ki-Kasunda. *Duk.*—Jangli-takla. *Mah.*—Rán tankála. *Tel.*—Paidi-tangaeǒu. *Tam.*—Peria takarai. *Mal.*—Ponnántakara.

Habitat.—This plant is common throughout the tropics and well-known in India.

Properties and Uses.—The bark, leaves and seeds are cathartic in action; the juice of the leaves made into a plaster with sandlewood or a paste made from the root or powdered seeds is viewed as a specific for ringworm, also for dhobie itch; it is given internally as an expectorant for coughs; given with black pepper the root is a remedy for snake-bite. Bark in infusion or the powdered seeds with honey are given in diabetes. The ointment of the bruised seeds, leaves and sulphur or the root-bark ground into a paste with honey is an application for ringworm and patches of pityriasis and psoriasis. This virtue seems to be due to the chrysophanic acid which it and other species of Cassia contain. The infusion of the fresh leaves is a useful injection in gonorrhœa in the sub-acute stage; when it is administered internally it acts as an anthelmintic. Externally it is used for washing syphilitic sores. The infusion of the leaves is administered also in rheumatic and inflammatory fevers; mixed with sugar it is given in cases of jaundice.

---

96. CASSIA TORA.

(*N. O.*—LEGUMINOSÆ.)

Sans.—Tagā, Ayudham, Prabhoonata, Chakramarda.—*Hind.*—and *Ben.*—Chakundā, Panevār *Duk.*—Tarota. *Guz.*—Kovariya. *Mah.*—Takala. *Tel.*—Tagirisa. *Tam.*—Tagarai, Aendu. *Can.*—Tagache, Taragashee. *Mal.*—Takara. *Kon.*—Taikilo.

Habitat.—This plant is common everywhere in Bengal and widely spread and abundant throughout the tropical parts of India.

Properties and Uses.—Both leaves and seeds contain chrysophanic acid and therefore constitute a valuable remedy in skin diseases especially ringworm and itch; seeds steeped in the juice of *Euphorbia Nerifolia* and then made into a paste with cow's urine is an application to cheloid tumours; also useful in leprosy, psoriasis, &c.; ground with sour buttermilk and applied to ease the irritation of itch or eruptions. The root rubbed into paste with lime-juice is said to be a specific for ringworm. The mucilaginous and foetid smelling leaves are gently aperient and prescribed in decoction in 2 ounce doses for children suffering from feverish attacks while teething; boiled in castor oil they are applied to foul ulcers.

97. CEDRUS DEODARA.

(*N. O.*—CONIFERAE.)

Sans.—Devadâru. *Eng.*—Pinus Deodara, Himalayan cedar. *Hind.*—Deodâr, Toona. *Ben.*—Toon. *Tam.*—Toon-maram.

Habitat.—This tall and graceful tree is found all over the Northern Himalayas and is largely cultivated in India as an ornamental tree.

Properties and Uses.—The bark is powerfully astringent and a good remedy in remittent and intermittent fevers, diarrhœa and dysentery and though not bitter it is a fair substitute for Peruvian bark particularly when united with powdered *Bonduc* nut. Its powder is applied with much benefit in the treatment of ulcers. It is considered especially useful in bilious fevers and inveterate diarrhœa arising from atony of the muscular fibre.

The wood yields an oleo-resin known as *Kelu-ka-til* and a dark colored oil or tar resembling crude turpentine is obtained by destructive distillation. These are applied to ulcers and skin diseases. They are valuable in mange in horses and sorefeet of cattle. The leaves are also regarded as having mild terebinthinate properties. The wood is carminative.

98. CERA ALBA AND CERA FLAVA.

Sans.—Madujam. *Eng.*—Wax. *Hind.* and *Ben.*—Moni.

Wax is collected all over India as the product of wild and domesticated bees—*Apis Mellifica* and other species.

The honey combs are usually deposited on shrubs or trees. After extraction of the honey, the yellow wax is cut into fine shreds, bleached in the sun and remelted and this forms white wax.

Properties and Uses.—The principal use of bee-wax in medicine is in the preparation of many ointments and plasters of which it forms an important constituent. It forms the basis of all *cerates*.

---

99. CICER ARIETINUM.

(*N. O.*—LEGUMINOSÆ.)

Sans.—Chanaka. *Eng.*—Chicken-pea, Bengal gram. *Hind.*—and *Guz.*—Chanā. *Ben.*—Chota but, Butkalai. *Mah.*—Harbar. *Tel.*—Senagalu. Chanakamulu. *Tam.* and *Can.*—Kadalai. *Mal.*—Katala. *Kon.*—Chano.

Habitat.—Extensively cultivated throughout India especially in the Northern Provinces.

Properties and Uses.—The plant is employed as refrigerent in fevers; it is also employed in the treatment of dysmenorrhœa, the fresh plant is put into hot water and the patient sits over the steam. The free use of the vegetable owing to the abundance of oxalic acid is apt to do harm to persons liable to calculus as it leads to the formation of oxalate of lime in the bladder. It is said to increase biliary secretions. The seeds are considered antibilious; fried seeds are said to be diuretic in action and they relieve flatulence. The acid liquid obtained by collecting the dew drops from the leaves by means of spreading a cloth over-night on the tree or by any other means contains oxalic, acetic and malic acids and it is a useful astringent given in dyspepsia, vomiting, indigestion and costiveness; also in diarrhœa and dysentery. The boiled leaves are a nice application to sprains and dislocated limbs. When roasted like coffee the pulse is considered to be aphrodisiac, and it relieves flatulance and retention of urine as it stimulates diuresis. The liquid obtained from macerating the seeds is a tonic; it also allays vomiting and is antibilious. In bronchial catarrh the seeds in a parched condition given at night followed by a cup of warm milk give great relief.

Chemical Composition of common gram :—

	Percentage Composition :—		in 1 lb. of Husked Grain.		
	Husked Grain.	With Husk.	Ounces.	+	Grains.
Water	11·39 to 11·5	11·2	1	,,	367
Albuminoids	21·7 to 22·7	19·5	3	,,	207
Starch	59·0 to 63·18	53·8	9	,,	192
Oil	3·76 to 4·2	4·6			
Fibre	1·0	7·8	0	,,	294
Ash	1·5	2·3	0	,,	70
Phosphoric Acid	1·1	0·8	0	,,	182

100. CINCHONA CORTEX.

(*N. O.*—RUBIACEÆ.)

Eng.—Cinchona Bark, Peruvian Bark, Jesuits Bark.—*Vern.*—Cinchona.

Habitat.—The most important species of cinchona indigenous to tropical South America are now thoroughly acclimatised in India. Yellow cinchona bark (*Cinchona Calisaya*) : This species grows best at the Himalayan plantations where it is cultivated almost exclusively. Pale Cinchona bark (*Cinchona Officinalis, Cinchona Pallidae Cortex*) : This is chiefly cultivated on the Nilgiris; and Red Cinchona bark (*Cinchona Succirubra,*

Cinchona Rubrae cortex) : This tree which yields the red bark of commerce grows well both in Bengal (in Sikkim) and in the Madras Presidency.

Properties and Uses.—These are well-known. The barks and all preparations of cinchona are powerfully antiperiodic specially valuable in intermittent fevers. They are most extensively prescribed as tonics. The alkaloids quinine, quinidine, cinchonidine, cinchonine are similarly valuable as antipyretics. As a tonic and antiperiodic quinine stands unrivalled; in agues of all kinds it is indispensible; in neuralgic affections and those arising from debility its good effect is generally marked and decided. If has lately been recommended in cases of typhoid fever and in the sinking stage, combined with Port Wine is certainly beneficial. The common dose is 1 to 2 grains three times a day dissolved in 2 to 4 minims of *dilute* sulphuric acid often given in some bitter infusion such as gentian or calumba.

101. CINNAMOMUM MALABATHRUM.

(*N. O.*—LAURACEÆ.)

Sans.—Tilaka. *Eng.*—Country cinnamon. *Hind.*—Jangli-Dalchin. *Tam.* and *Mal.*—Ilavangam, *Can.*—Kadu dalchini. *Kon.*—Tikke.

Habitat.—This tree is found generally in the Peninsula, the Concans and Malabar Coast.

Properties and Uses.—The seeds bruised and mixed with honey or sugar are given to children in dysentery or coughs and combined with other ingredients in fevers. The bark is used as a condiment in curries. The inner bark when fresh has an aromatic odour and taste. The dried buds are employed with various combinations in diarrhœa, dysentery and coughs. They partake of the carminative properties of cinnamon and cassia.

102. CINNAMOMUM TAMALA.

(*N. O.*—LAURACEÆ.)

Sans.—Tejpatra, Tamalapatra. *Eng.*—Cassia Lignea. *Hind.*—Taj-kalam (bark), Tajpat (leaves). *Ben.*—Dálchini, Tejpat (leaves).

Habitat.—This tree is common on the Himalayas and in Eastern Bengal and Burma.

Properties and Uses.—The bark has an aromatic odour and possesses aromatic, carminative and stimulating properties; it is commonly used as a substitute for the more expensive cinnamon. The leaves have similar properties and are largely used as a condiment. The bark yields an essential oil resembling that of Ceylon Cinnamon. An oil is also distilled from the leaves which is a powerful stimulant much used in flavouring sweets and confectionary.

103. CINNAMOMUM ZEYLANICUM.

(*N. O.*—LAURACEÆ.)

Sans.—Gudetvak. *Eng.*—Cinnamom. *Hind.*, *Duk.*, *Punj.*, *Kash.*, *Guz.*, *Ben.*, *Mah.* and *Can.*—Dálchin. *Tel.*, *Tam.*, and *Mal.*—Lowangapatta. *Malay.*—Kulit-manis. *Cing.*—Kurundo. *Burm.*—Timbotik-yobo.

Habitat.—The true cinnamon is indigenous to Ceylon and Southern India, but it is cultivated mostly in Ceylon.

Properties and Uses.—It possesses cordial, carminative and astringent properties and is prescribed in dyspepsia, flatulency, diarrhœa and vomiting, although frequently employed as an adjunct to bitter tonics, purgatives and vegetable and mineral astringents. As a stimulant of the uterine muscular fibre it is employed in menorrhagia and in tedious labour due to defective uterine contractions. Powdered cinnamon in 20 grain doses is a reputed remedy given in dysentery. It is also very largely used as a spice. A combination of cinnamon, cardamoms and *tejapatra* leaves passes by the name of *trijataka*, these three aromatics being often used together. As a powerful stimulant cinnamon is given in cramps of the stomach, toothache and paralysis of the tongue. The essential oil is used in flavouring sweets and confectionary and as a powerful stimulant in amenorrhœa, &c., the bark chewed also gives much relief. The oil is locally applied with much benefit in neuralgia and headache.

The different oils prepared from cinnamon are :—(1) Oil from the bark (Ceylon) of golden yellow colour largely used in perfumery. (2) Oil from the leaves of clove-like odour called clove oil. (3) Oil from the root, of yellow colour and lighter than water.

The clove oil is used externally in rheumatic pains, headache and toothache. It is a frequent ingredient of pill-masses. It strengthens the gums and perfumes the breath. It contains about 70 to 80 per cent. of *eugenol* the remainder being cinnamic aldehyde.

104. CITRULLUS COLOCYNTHIS.

(*N. O.*—CUCURBITACEÆ.)

Sans. and *Can.*—Indràvaruni, Chitraphala. *Eng.*—Colocynth or Bitter Apple. *Hind.*, *Duk.*, and *Ben.*—Indràyan. *Tel.*—Paperabudama. *Tam.*—Paedicari, Attuttummatti. *Mal.*—Paikummata Katuvelleri. *Kon.*—Kàvandali.

Habitat.—The colocynth gourd is found wild in the arid tracts of the North West in the Punjaub and Sind and on the Coromandal Coast.

Properties and Uses.—This is a hydrogogue cathartic, useful in constipation, hepatic and visceral congestions, dropsy and the root in jaundice, ascites, rheumatism, &c. The drug constitutes the internal pulp of the dried peeled fruit, the seeds having been removed. It is bitter, acrid and cathartic, useful in biliousness, constipation, fever and worms; the juice of the fruit mixed with sugar is a household remedy in dropsy. The root is useful in cough and asthmatic attacks of children. A poultice of the root is said to be useful in inflammation of the breasts. The oil obtained from the seed is used for snake-bites, scorpion-stings, any bowel complaints, epilepsy, &c.; and also for the growth of hair; it is employed generally for blackening grey hairs.

The active principle is glucoside *colocynthin.* The colocynth pulp has an intensely bitter taste and is poisonous in excessive doses. In small doses it is expectorant, diuretic and alterative. The dose of the powder is from 2 to 8 grains; in this form it is seldom given; of the pill or extract the dose is from 5 to 10 grains. The powder is often used as an insecticide. The extract should never be given without some aromatic to correct its griping tendency.

Native Indian Preparations.—*Jvaraghni gutika*: Take of mercury one part, sulphur, colocynth pulp, cardamoms, long pepper, chebulic myrobalan and pellitory root each four parts. Rub these ingredients with the juice of *indrávaruni* root and make into pills weighing about 20 grains each. These pills are administered with the fresh juice of *gulancha* in recent fever. They move the bowels and reduce the fever.

---

105. CITRUS AURANTIUM.

(*N. O.*—AURANTIACEÆ.)

Sans.—Nàgranga. *Eng.*—Sweet orange. *Hind.*—Naringi. *Ben.*—Kamlà-neboo. *Tel.* —Nárangamu. *Tam.*—Nárangam, Kamalàranj. *Can.*—Kittale. *Mal.*—Madhuranàrakam. *Kon* — Sonnáringa.

Habitat.—The orange tree is originally a native of Northern India; the different varieties of the sweet orange are now grown all over India chiefly throughout the warmer moist regions.

Properties and Uses.—It is a blood purifier and appetiser. The juice of the sweet orange consists principally of mucilage, sugar and citric acid and is one of the most wholesome vegetable juices known; it is peculiarly grateful to invalids who, however, should not swallow the cellular pulp in which it is enclosed as this is indigestible and is likely to produce disorders of the bowels through which it passes unchanged. The dried orange peel or rind is an agreeable aromatic bitter possessing stomachic, tonic and astringent properties valuable in checking vomiting and preventing worms; it is generally used in the form of tincture or infusion which is a mild carminative tonic and is usually employed in combination with stronger bitters such as gentian and quinine. The infusion makes one of the best vehicles for the administration of Epsom and other neutral salts which it renders less offensive to the palate and stomach. Orange marmalade upon bread is a good breakfast diet for dyspeptic patients and the confection of orange peel in doses of 1 to 4 drachms may also be taken with advantage.

Water distilled from the orange flowers is a stimulant and refreshing drink. The finest quality is that distilled from the petals of the bitter orange. It is invaluable in scurvy. It and the syrup of orange flower are also very frequently used as pleasant flavouring agents. The rind pulverised and added to magnesia and rhubarb affords a grateful tonic to the stomach in gout and dyspepsia. The oil obtained from the rind and flowers may be taken as a stomachic on sugar in doses of from 1 to 3 drops; it is also used for flavouring chiefly. Externally it forms an excellent stimulating liniment, useful in gout, rheumatism, &c. The roasted pulp is an excellent application to foetid ulcers. Orange flowers and their distilled oil and waters are chiefly used as perfumes, but they are also regarded as antispasmodic and to some extent anodyne; the water is given in Europe for hysteria in doses of from 1 to 2 ounces.

---

106. CITRUS BERGAMIA OR CITRUS ACIDA.

(*N. O.*—AURANTIACEÆ.)

Sans.—Jambha, Jambeeram. *Eng.*—Acid Lime, Bergamotte. *Hind.*, and *Duk* —Limu, Neemboo. *Ben.*—Neboo. *Kash.*—Niumb. *Punj.* and *Guz.*—Limbu. *Mah.*—Limboo. *Tel.*—Nimmapandu. *Tam.*—Elumichhai. *Can.*—Limbe. *Mal.*—Cherunárakam. *Kon.*—Nimboovo. *Cing.*—Dehi. *Burm.*—Sámyasi.

Habitat.—Several varieties of the lime are indigenous to the Himalayas and largely cultivated in Upper India and Bengal.

Properties and Uses.—The fruit is refrigerent; the juice of the fruit is a valuable antiscorbutic; also useful in rheumatism. The antiscorbutic property is due to the presence of citric acid in the juice. It is a most agreeable acid with which pleasant effervescing draughts and beverages are made. The juice has not only a curative effect in scurvy, but it is also preventive; it is therefore most valuable for seamen, emigrants and others who undertake long sea-voyages. The oil expressed from the rind is called Bergamot oil. The essential oil of the leaves and flowers obtained by distillation is used for adulterating Bergamot oil. It is employed as a very useful refrigerent drink in small-pox, measles, scarletina, &c. where there is a hot, dry skin and much thirst. Lemons are an excellent remedy in pulmonary diseases; from six to nine a day are used in cases of lung troubles; in cases of hæmorrhage from the lungs, stomach, bowels, uterus, kidneys and other internal organs. Lime juice taken in ½ ounce dose allays hysterical palpitation of the heart. Lime juice is most useful in dysentery with sloughing of the mucous membranes. Twelve ounces a day have been given with success in a hopeless case. Lime juice diluted with its equal quantity of water forms an excellent gargle, useful in cases of scorbutic and other ulcerations of the mouth and sponginess of the gums. Lemon oil mixed with glycerine is applied on the eruption of acme. Lime pickle is very beneficial in cases of enlarged spleen. A squeeze of lime juice added to sauces, soups, gravies or stews after cooking improves the flavour and is a great help to digestion. The juice of the baked lemon is an excellent remedy for a cough, when mixed with an equal quantity of sugar or honey and taken in tea-spoonful doses. Lemonade may be made by pouring a pint of boiling water on five or six peeled limes cut in thin transverse slices. When cool, strain, sweeten to taste, and let the patient drink as plentifully as he likes. In diabetes, weak lemonade is preferable to plain water for allaying the great thirst; like other fluids, in this disease, it is better taken during the intervals between, than at meals.

In poisoning by croton oil seeds, castor oil seeds, the physic nut and the fresh root of the bitter cassava, mandioc or tapioca plant, a drink of lime juice 4 or 5 ounces at a time diluted with an equal quantity of *conjee* or plain water gives immediate relief to the purging, vomiting and other urgent symptoms. It is an antidote which should always be first tried; it seldom fails to afford more or less relief. A full dose of castor oil should be subsequently given.

For relieving the irritation, &c., of Mosquito bites, the local application of lime juice often proves more effectual than anything else. Applied to the surface at nights before going to bed it is believed also to afford protection, from the attacks of mosquitoes.

---

107. CITRUS MEDICA.

(N. O.—AURANTIACEÆ.)

Sans.—Mâtulang. *Eng.*—Citron. *Hind.*—Máphal. *Ben.*—Chholongo nebu, Karuna nebu. *Mah.* and *Can.*—Mádala. *Tel.*—Mádeephalamu. *Mal.*—Mádalanárakam. *Kon.*—Mávalinga.

Habitat.—It is a garden plant chiefly cultivated for its valuable fruit and met with chiefly in the South-west of India.

Properties and Uses.—The fruit is an expellent of poisons. The yellow pulp is an excellent aromatic and stomachic. Its juice makes a pleasant refrigerent drink in allaying febrile heat and thirst. It is useful in bilious and remittent fevers when combined with port wine and cinchona bark. The rind is made into an excellent marmalade and is an antiscorbutic; its preserve is used in dysentery. It is also made into a pickle which is useful as an appetiser in various kinds of fevers, dyspepsia and inflammatory affections. The distilled water of the fruit is a sedative. An oil is obtained from the rind of the fruit both by distillation and expression and is known as *cidrat.* The extract of cidrat is the oil of citron dissolved in spirits to which bergamot is sometimes added.

Native Indian Preparations.—In rheumatic affections such as pleurodynia, sciatica, lumbago, pain in the hip joints, &c., Sarangadhara recommends the administration of lemon juice with the addition of *Yavakshara* (impure carbonate of potash) and honey.

Rasayanamrita Lacha.—Take of long pepper, black pepper, ginger, the 3 myrobalans, bâberang seeds, cumin and nigella seeds, *ajowan,* and the seeds of *Cuedium diffusum* (*vanajamâni*), chiretta, *trivrit,* root of *Baliospermum Mantanam* (*danti*), *nim* bark and rock salt each two tolas, prepared iron sixteen tolas, sugar two seers, decoction of the myrobalans four seers and lemon juice two seers. Boil all these ingredients together till the watery portion is evaporated; lastly add clarified butter half a seer and prepare a confection. Dose:—one to two tolas in enlargement of the abdominal viscera, anaemia, jaundice, anasarca and chronic fever.

In fever complicated with pain in the head, throat and chest the following mixture is directed to be used as a snuff for promoting discharge of phlegm:—Take of lemon juice, ginger juice, rock salt, black salt and *sonchal* salt equal parts, and mix. The mixture should be warmed a little before use.

108. CLEOME VISCOSA.

(*N. O.*—CAPPARIDEÆ.)

Sans.—Adityabhakta. *Eng.*—Wild mustard. *Hind.*—Jangli-Hurhur. *Ben.*—Hurhuria. *Tel.*—Naelaváminta. *Tam.*—Náyvælai. *Can.*—Kádusásiva. *Mal.*—Aryavál. *Kon.*—Sirikála.

Habitat.—A common weed found all over India and plentifully in Bengal.

Properties and Uses.—These seeds have properties resembling those of mustard for which they are regarded as an efficient substitute. They are anthelmintic, carminative and stimulant in action. Externally they act as rubefacient and vesicant; they are useful in all cases in which mustard is indicated. As anthelmintic they are used in doses of 30 grains to 1 drachm in powder with sugar twice a day for two days and then followed by a dose of castor oil; they are specially useful in cases of round worms. The seeds yield on expression a fixed oil. The seeds are applied to the skin as poultice or paste or being bruised with vinegar, lime-juice or hot water for producing rubefacient action and the leaves applied to boils prevent the formation of pus; and their juice pressed out by bruising them with hot water is used as ear drops in earache; but in case of otorrhœa its instillation produces smarting pain; when mixed with oil it is a popular remedy for purulent discharges from the ear; it also forms an application for recent wounds and ulcers; for this purpose leaves boiled in ghee are also used.

109. CLITORIA TERNATIA.

(*N. O.*—LEGUMINOSÆ.)

Sans.—Aparàjita, Vishnu krànta. *Hind.* and *Ben.*—Apràjita. *Mah.*—Gokurna-mula (root), Gokurna-beeja (seeds). *Tel.*—Dintena. *Tam.*—Kàkkanam, Kavàchhi, Karuvilài. *Can.*—Shankapuspa. *Mal.*—Aral, Shankhapuspam. *Kon.*—Shankapuspi.

Habitat.—A very common plant found all over India and cultivated in flower gardens.

Properties and Uses.—The seeds have a powerful cathartic action like that of Jalap; they are recommended in the form of powder in 30 to 60 grain doses, as purgative and diuretic in cases of ascites and enlargements of the abdominal viscera; generally administered in combination with cream of tartar and ginger. They are also employed in weakness of sight, sore throat and mucous disorders, in tumours, affections of the skin and in dropsy. The alcoholic extract of the root is also a useful preparation in doses of 5 to 10 grains. The dose of the dry bark in powder is from 1 to 2 drachms.

Native Indian Preparations.—Take of the roots of *Aparajita, Pladera decussata* (*sankhini,*) *Baliospermum Montanum* (*Danti*) and *Indigofera tinctoria* (*nilini*) in equal parts, rub them together into an emulsion with water and administer with cow's urine. This preparation is given in ascites and enlargements of the abdominal viscera (Chakradatta).

110. COCCULUS CORDIFOLIUS.

(*N. O.*—MENISPERMACEÆ.)

Sans.—Guloochee, Amrita. *Eng.*—Heart-leaved moonseed, *Hind.* and *Ben.*—Gulancha. *Duk.* and *Guz.*—Gulbel. *Punj.*—Gilo, Gulanch. *Kash.*—Bekhgillo. *Tel.*—Tippateega. *Burm.*—Singo-mone. *Cing.*—Rasakinda. *Malay.*—Piturali. *Tam.* and *Can.*—Amradavalli. *Mal.*—Chittamratam, Paiyamratam.

Habitat.—A common climbing shrub growing in *nim* and other high trees in tropical India and Burma and Ceylon.

Properties and Uses.—The entire plant—stem, leaves and root are used in medicine, preferably in the fresh state; the root and stems should be collected in the hot season when the bitter principle is most abundant and concentrated. It is obtained in the dried state in bazaars. It is a very valuable tonic and is best given in infusion with or without milk; the tincture and extract have also been valued as alterative and tonic and, in a less degree, antiperiodic and diuretic, and are used in general debility, fever, jaundice, skin diseases, rheumatism, acidity of urine and urinary diseases, some forms of dyspepsia, chronic gonorrhœa, leucorrhœa, &c. It is used as a febrifuge and tonic in gout. In large doses the root is a powerful emetic; it is a popular remedy for snake-bite; and the watery extract is administered for leprosy; it is probably the most useful preparation and acts as tonic, antiperiodic and aphrodisiac. Combined with acetate of ammonia its infusion (1 ounce of the bruised stem macerated for 3 hours in half a pint of cold water and strained) is administered in intermittent and other mild forms of fevers. It is rendered more agreeable by the addition of cinnamon, cloves and other aromatics. The dose is 2 to 4 ounces three times a day. The juice mixed with powdered long-pepper and honey is a common household remedy for gonorrhœa. The juice forms one of the ingredients in *poushtiks* given in phthisis. The root and stem and especially the *extract* thereof is most useful in fevers, secondary syphilis and rheumatism, chronic inflammation of the bladder and splenic affections. It has been reckoned as a specific tonic, anti-periodic and diuretic. The dose is 5 grains. Several oils for external application are prepared with *gulancha* and are much used in skin diseases, rheumatic affections and other nervous complaints.

Native Indian Preparations:—*Guduchyadi taila*: Take of fresh *gulancha* 8 seers, water 64 seers, boil till reduced to one-fourth and strain. To the strained decoction add prepared sesamum oil 4 seers and *gulancha* beaten to a paste with water 1 seer, boil together till the water is evaporated. This oil is a favourite application in eruptive skin diseases from impure blood. The *Vrihat Guduchyâdi taila* is prepared by the addition of a number of other medicines in the form of paste, to the decoction of *gulancha* and the oil. Another compound oil called *Vata Gudachyadi taila* is thus prepared: Take of *gulancha* 12½ seers, water 64 seers; boil till reduced to one-fourth. Take of the fresh juice of *Adhatoda Vasica* (*Vâsaka*) and of datura leaves each 4 seers, prepared mustard oil 4 seers, aromatics in the form of paste 1 seer. Boil together the decoction of *gulancha* with the vegetable juices, oil and paste in the usual manner. This oil is recommended by Charaka in eruptive skin diseases with troublesome itching as also in diseases of nervous origin.

A decoction of *gulancha* or its fresh juice is given with the addition of long pepper and honey in chronic fever with cough. A compound decoction as described in *Bhavaprakash* is thus prepared:—Take of *gulancha*, *Hedyotis biflora* (*parparta*), *Cyperus rotundus* (*mustaka*), chiretta and ginger each one drachm, water half seer. Boil down to one-fourth. It is said to be useful in fevers caused by deranged air and bile. Practically it is found very useful in chronic fevers, which have resisted other antiperiodics and which are apt to recur after apparent recovery. In chronic fever with loss of appetite the following confection is recommended by many writers:— *Dhâtrimodaka*:—Take of chebulic and emblic myrobalans, ginger and long-pepper 1 part each, watery extract of *gulancha* 4 parts, water 16 parts. Boil till reduced to one-fourth and prepare a confection with 8 parts of sugar. When of proper consistence divide the mass into boluses of about a drachm each. One of these is taken every morning, in chronic fever with enlarged spleen, cough, loss of appetite etc.

---

111. COCCULUS SUBEROSUS.

(*N. O.*—MENISPERMACEÆ.)

Sans.—Kâkanâshikâ. *Eng.*—Cocculus Indicus. *Hind.*, *Duk.* *Ben.*, *Tel.*, and *Mah.*—Kâkmari. *Guz.*—Kâkphal. *Tam.*—Kâkakulli, Pen-kottai. *Can.*—Kâgemâri. *Mal.*—Meennanu, Pollakkaya. *Kon.*—Gardaphala. *Cing.*—Titt-taval.

Habitat.—Found in Southern and Eastern India and Burma.

Properties and Uses.—The poisonous berries constitute the *Cocculus Indicus* of commerce which is the source of picrotoxin; they also contain 50 per cent. of oil. The juice of the fresh fruit is a good application to scabies and foul ulcers. The dried fruit is a powerful narcotic; its active principle is *picrotoxin* which is a crystalline substance and a powerful poison irritating the respiratory and other centres in the medulla and producing violent spasmodic muscular contractions. It has been used in the smallest doses in epilepsy, especially in the nocturnal variety; in paralysis affecting the muscles of the pharynx and in sick headache. It is, however, to check the night-sweating of phthisis that this drug has been much used and good results are obtained in doses of $\frac{1}{200}$ to $\frac{1}{100}$ grain, three times a day; it may be given in pills and the dose gradually increased to $\frac{1}{32}$ grain; or it may be administered in solution with a little acetic acid and water or hypodermically $\frac{1}{50}$ grain. It is an antidote in morphine and chloral poisoning. Externally, in the form of ointment (1 grain of picrotoxin or 10 grains of the seeds to 1 drachm of simple ointment), it is an insecticide and destroys pediculi or lice which infest the body; it is useful in obstinate chronic skin diseases. In applying this ointment care should be taken to avoid all abraded or ulcerated surfaces on account of the danger of absorption of the poisonous principle of the seeds. In the form of an oil solution of the berries (1 drachm to 1 ounce of cocoanut oil) it is a useful external application.

112. COCCUS LACCA.

Sans.—Laksha. *Eng.*—Lac. *Hind.*—Lakh. *Ben.*—Gâlâ.

This important article of commerce is obtained from incrustations on the branches of various trees, chiefly the *Butea frondosa* which is called *Lâksha taru* (lac plant) in Sanskrit. It is produced by the lac insect *Coccus lacca* which punctures the bark. The resinous incrustation is formed only by the female insect and the portions of branches so covered are termed "stick-lac."

Properties and Uses.—The fluid lac-dye obtained by dissolving the crushed stick-lac in water is called *Alakta.* It is used in coloring silk. Cotton colored with this dye and pressed into flat, circular pieces is sold in the bazaars under the name of *Alta* and is used in painting the hands and feet of Hindu females. Shell lac is used in the preparation of sealing wax, varnish for carpenters and ornaments for women. Shell lac finely powdered, half-a-tola mixed with honey and prepared in the form of an electuary is given in Haematemesis.

Native Indian Preparations:—A decoction of shell lac is much used in the preparation of several medicinal oils, such as *Lâkshâdi taila, Chandanâdi taila, Angârka taila,* &c.

Lâkshâdi taila:—Take of shell-lac 2 seers, water 16 seers, boil till reduced to 4 seers and strain. To this decoction of shell lac, add 4 seers of prepared sesamum oil, 16 seers of whey, and two tolas each of the following substances, namely *Withania Somnifera* (*Asvagandha*), turmuric, *Devadâru* wood, root of *Sanseviera Zeylanica* (*murva*) *Pandanus Odoratissimus* (*Ketaki*), *Vanda Roxburghia* (*râsna*), dill seeds and liquorice root in the from of a paste and prepare an oil in the usual way; lastly add 4 tolas of camphor. This oil is much used for inunction in chronic fever and consumption. The other oils containing lac are prepared in a similar way with the addition of various medicinal substances in the form of paste.

---

113. COCOS NUCIFERA.

(*N. O.*—PALMACEAE.)

Sans.—Tranarâj. Deerghavraksha, Sadâphala, Rasâyanataru, Narikela. *Eng.*—Cocoanut Palm. *Hind.*—Nârival. *Ben.*—Narikel. *Tel.*—Tenkâyichettu. *Tam.*—Tengu. *Can.*—Tenginamara. *Mal.*—Ten. *Kon.*—Mâddo.

Habitat—This graceful palm is extensively cultivated in Southern India and Ceylon. It is not found in the Upper Provinces of Hindustan, but is plentiful in Eastern Bengal, Burma towards the sea coast, in Malabar and Coromandel Coasts and the islands of the Indian Archipelago.

Properties and Uses.—The whole tree is of great economical value to the people of the sea-board districts of India almost every part being utilised. The juice extracted from the flowering spikes is made into a palm wine or toddy. It is very refreshing and possesses laxative properties. It is said that its continued use twice or thrice weekly during pregnancy has a marked effect on the colour of the infant which is born of a fair complexion, *i.e.*, if of dark parents, comparatively fair; if of lighter colored parents, the offspring generally assumes European complexion. From the unfermented juice of the tree a coarse sugar is prepared somewhat different from cane-sugar. The fresh juice is considered refrigerent and diuretic. The fermented juice constitutes the spirituous liquor called toddy. The milk of the fresh kernel is useful in debility, incipient phthisis and cachexia; in large doses it is aperient. The water of the unripe fruit is a cooling, refrigerent drink useful in thirst, fever and urinary disorders. The tender milk of the fruit is nourishing, cooling and diuretic. The pulp of the ripe fruit is hard and indigestible. The fresh oil prepared by boiling the milk of cocoanut is a useful application in baldness and also for burns. The cocoanut oil prepared from fresh pulp is a good substitute for Cod-liver oil; it is largely used in American hospitals in wasting diseases of children; the dose is from 20 to 30 minims rising to a drachm thrice daily; the only drawback is its indigestibility. As hair-oil it is much used, and is said to promote the growth of hair. The milk of the green fruit is cooling and allays vomiting in bilious fevers. The terminal bud of the tree is esteemed as a nourishing, strengthening and agreeable vegetable. The root of the cocoanut is used as a diuretic in uterine diseases. The ashes of the leaves are used in medicine. They contain a good deal of potash. The cleared shell of the nut or portions of it are burnt in a fire and, while red-hot, covered by a stone cup. The fluid deposited in the interior of the cup is rubefacient and is an effectual domestic remedy for ring-worm.

Native Indian Preparations.—A delicious and nutritious confection is prepared from the pulp of cocoanut with the addition of some aromatic and carminative substances; it is called *Nárikelkhandu* and is prepared thus:—Take of the pounded pulp of cocoanut half-a-seer, fry it in 8 tolas of clarified butter and afterwards boil in 4 seers of cocoanut water till reduced to a syrup consistence. Now add coriander, long pepper, bamboo manna, cumin seeds, nigella seeds, cardamoms, cinnamon, *tejapatra*, the tubers of *Cyperus rotundus* (*mustaka*) and the flowers of *Mesua ferrea* (*nagakesara*) one tola each in fine powder and prepare a confection. Dose 2 to 4 tolas in dyspepsia and consumption.

114.—COFFEA ARABICA.

(*N. O.*—RUBIACEAE.)

Eng.—Coffee. *Hind.*—Kâfi, Bun. *Ben.*—Coffee. *Arab.*—Kahwa. *Guz.* and *Mah.*—Caffi. *Tel.*—Kâpivittulu. *Tam.*—Kapikottai. *Can.*—Kafi, Bunnu. *Mal.*—Bunnu.

Habitat.—*Coffea Arabica* and several other species of the plant are cultivated in Southern India, Mysore and Coorg.

Properties and Uses.—The dried seeds "Coffee beans" yield the crystalline principle *Caffeine* which is identical with the *Theine* contained in tea. The Coffee seed is a stimulant to the nervous and vascular systems. It produces a feeling of buoyancy and exhilaration, increases the heart's action, stimulates the system so as to sustain prolonged and severe muscular exertion; caffeine has the power of checking the waste of the tissues. It has the power of preserving wakefulness, it gives rise to increased vigour of imagination and intellect without any subsequent stupor; in nervous affections manifesting deficient energy of the brain it is very useful; it is a palliative in spasmodic asthma, in whooping cough, hysterical affections and in palpitation of the heart; it is highly recommended in cholera infantum; successful in chronic diarrhœa. It is said that, in early stages of typhoid fever, coffee is almost a specific. In the French Colonies where coffee is more used than in the English, as well as in Turkey, where it is the principal beverage, not only gravel but gout is scarcely known. Roasted coffee has the disinfectant and deodorant properties. A strong infusion of black coffee is useful as an antisoporific in cases of poisoning by opium, alcohol and other stupefying or narcotic poisons. It is a good vehicle for the administration of quinine and sulphate of magnesia as it conceals the bitter and nauseous taste of those medicines. A strong cup of coffee is considered a good protection from the effects of Malaria. In their raw state coffee berries possess febrifuge properties and are prescribed medicinally most frequently for Hemicrania and intermittent fevers.

Chemical Composition of Coffee (Payen):—

In 100 parts:

Cellular tissue	... 34·0	Mineral constituents	...6·69
Hygroscopic Moisture.	12·0	Chlorogenate of Potash and Caffeine	... 3·5 to 5
Fat ...	... 13·0	Nitrogenous matter	... 3
Starch, Sugar, dextrin.	15·0	Free Caffeine	... 0·80
Legumen ...	... 10·0		

115.—CORDIA MYXA.

(*N. O.*—BORAGINEÆ.)

Sans.—Slesmàtakam, Selu. *Eng.*—Sebesten fruit. *Hind.*—Losorá. *Pers.*—Sapistàn. *Ben.*—Bahubàr. Bal-phal. *Tel.*—Peddanakkaeru. *Tam.*—Periyanaruvili. *Can.*—Mannadike. *Mal.*—Naruvari. *Kon.*—Sharpala.

Habitat.—A small deciduous tree growing nearly all over India and cultivated in Bengal.

Properties and Uses.—The fruit is very mucilaginous and the mucilage is demulcent and is highly esteemed in coughs, in diseases of the chest, the uterus, the urethra, &c. The bark is a useful astringent and used in infusion in the form of a gargle. The kernels are a good remedy for ringworm; they are powdered, mixed with oil and applied. The juice obtained from the bark and administered in cocoanut milk is said to relieve severe colicky pains.

---

116. CORIANDRUM SATIVUM.

(*N. O.*—UMBELLIFERÆ.)

Sans.—Kustumbari, Dhânyaka. *Eng.*—Coriander. *Hind.*—Dhania. *Arab.*—Kusbara. *Ben.*—Dhane. *Pers.*—Kishniz. *Tel.*—Kotimiri. *Tam.*—Kottumalli. *Can.* and *Kon.*—Kottumbari. *Mal.*—Kottampàlari.

Habitat.—A herbaceous plant extensively cultivated in all parts of India for its seeds.

Properties and Uses.—Coriander fruit is aromatic, stimulant, carminative and antispasmodic; it contains ½ per cent. of volatile oil to which it owes its aromatic odour. The oil has also a stimulant carminative property, very useful in flatulent colic, &c., the dose is from 1 to 4 minims on sugar or in emulsion; the dried fruit has also similar effect; it is generally used in infusion or decoction. An eye-wash is prepared by Mahommedans for preserving the sight in small-pox; it is also useful in chronic conjunctivitis. The seeds are generally chewed to correct foul breath; roasted seeds are useful in dyspepsia. They are made into a paste and applied to relieve pain in cephalalgia; as a gargle they are useful in thrush and as a poultice for chronic ulcers and carbuncles. The juice of the fresh plant is an application to erythema. A strong decoction with milk and sugar to taste is given in cases of bleeding piles. Cold infusion of seeds or powder of fried seeds is very useful in colics of children. Coriander is considered to lessen the intoxicating effects of spirituous liquors.

---

117. CORYPHA UMBRACULIFERA.

(*N. O.*—PALMACEÆ.)

Sans.—Alpàyushi, Katkàli, Tali. *Eng.*—Tali-pot or Fan-Palm. *Hind.*—Bhajarbettu. *Ben.*—Talee. *Tel.*—Shreetàlamu. *Tam.*—Sheedàlam. *Can.*—Shreetâli. *Mal.*—Kutapana, Talipana. *Kon.*—Talat màddo.

Properties and Uses.—A kind of sago is obtained from the pith of this tree. People beat it in mortars to flour and bake cakes of it which taste much like white bread; it serves them instead of corn before their harvest is ripe; it is generally used by poor classes; it is also prepared in the form of *conjee* which is like that of sago, arrowroot, barley or oatmeal and almost equally nutritious.

---

118. COSTUS SPECIOSUS.

(*N. O.*—ZINGIBERACEÆ.)

Sans.—Pushkara, Káshmeera, Kemuka. *Hind.*—Kená, Kust. *Ben.*—Ken. *Tel.*—Kashmeeramu. *Tam.*—Koeshtam. *Can.*—Pushkaramoola. *Mal.*—Channakkoova, Narunchana.

Habitat.—An elegant climbing plant found plentifully all over Bengal and some other parts of Eastern India.

Properties and Uses.—The root is bitter, astringent and digestive, useful in catarrhal fevers, coughs and skin diseases; it is also anthelmintic, depurative and aphrodisiac. The tuber is cooked and made into a syrup or preserve which is considered to be very wholesome.

---

119. CRATAEVA NURVALA, C. RELIGIOSA.

(*N. O.*—CAPPARIDACEÆ.)

Sans.—Pashugandhá, Ajápa Varuna, Asmarighna. *Hind.*—Tapia, Birmi. *Ben.*—Barun. *Mah.*—Vàyavarna. *Tam.*—Mávilingu. *Can.*—Nàrumbele, Mavalanga. *Mal.*—Nirvála.

Habitat.—This tree is usually cultivated in the vicinity of temples in Central India, Bengal and Assam.

Properties and Uses.—The leaves are aromatic, bitter and stomachic; the root possesses alterative properties. The leaf-juice in doses of ½ to 3 tolas is given in rheumatism mixed with cocoanut milk and ghee; and externally the bark and leaves pounded and tied in a cloth are applied as a fomentation; the root and the bark are also used in the form of embrocation which is prepared by boiling them in oil. They form the principal medicine for calculus affections; they have the property of promoting appetite, increasing the secretion of bile, acting as laxative and removing disorders of the urinary organs. The bark is specially useful in urinary complaints and fevers and also to relieve vomiting and symptoms of gastric irritation; it is generally administered in the form of decoction; the decoction is prepared by bruising and boiling 4 ounces of it in 1½ pints of water till reduced to 1 pint and then strained and cooled; the dose is from 2 to 4 ounces. The fresh leaves bruised well with a little vinegar, lime-juice or hot water, and applied to the skin as poultice or paste act as rubefacient and vesicant as efficiently as mustard flour; it takes 5 to 15 minutes to obtain rubefacient effect; if kept longer it acts as vesicant.

120. CRINUM DEFLEXUM.

(*N. O.*—AMARYLLIDEÆ.)

Hind.—Chindar. *Ben.*—Sookhdursun. *Guz.* and *Mah.*—Nag-down. *Tel.*—Kesarichettu. *Tam.*—Tudaiváchi, Vishamoongil. *Can.*—Vishamoonguli. *Mal.*—Valutta polatàli. *Kon.*—Kirtmári.

Habitat.—A large plant with handsome white inflorescence and graceful foliage much cultivated in Indian gardens.

Properties and Uses.—The leaves and root possess emetic virtues and are a good substitute for ipecacuanha. The succulent leaves bruised and mixed with castor oil form a useful application for repelling whitlows and other inflammations at the end of toes and fingers. The juice of the leaves is used for the earache after being slightly roasted. The bruised leaves are generally kept in cattle sheds as they are supposed to have the property of driving away noxious insects and parasites; the smoke of the burnt leaves is regarded as poisonous to mosquitoes.

121. CROCUS SATIVUS.

(*N. O.*—IRIDEÆ.)

Sans.—Bhavarakta, Agnishikha, Kumkuma. *Arab.*, *Hind.* and *Ben.*—Jafrán. *Mah.* and *Guz.*—Keshar. *Tel.*—Kunkumamu. *Tam.* and *Mal.*—Kunkumam. *Can.* and *Kon.*—Kunkuma-kesara.

Habitat.—The safron crocus, a native of Asia Minor is cultivated on a small scale in Kashmir.

Properties and Uses.—As medicine it is used for its stimulant, antispasmodic and stomachic properties: in over-doses it is a narcotic poison. It is used in small doses, in fevers, melancholia, enlargement of the liver and in catarrhal affections of children. It has also emmenagogue virtues. In European medicine it is used chiefly as a coloring and flavouring agent. The dose of the drug is from 1 to 3 grains and of the tincture it is ½ to 2 drachms. It is given to cage birds when they are moulting or otherwise sickly a few threads being infused in the water which they drink.

---

122. CROTON TIGLIUM.

(*N. O.*—EUPHORBIACEÆ.)

Sans.—Naepâla, Jayapala. *Eng.*—Purgative croton, Croton-oil seed. *Hind.*, *Guz.* and *Duk.*—Jamâlgoet. *Ben.* and *Punj.*—Jaipâl. *Mah.*—Jeyaphal. *Tel.*—Naepalvaema. *Tam.* and *Mal.*—Naervâlam, Chiduram. *Can.*—Japala beeja. *Kon.*—Japhal.

Habitat.—The croton plants are found wild and widely distributed throughout India and plentiful in Eastern Bengal extending to Assam and Burma.

Properties and Uses.—The croton seed is a powerful drastic purgative; in overdoses it is an acro-narcotic poison. It should be given only when a strong purgative is required as in apoplexy, convulsions, insanity, ardent fevers, &c. Externally it is of great value, especially the officinal liniment, as a stimulant rubefacient and counter-irritant. A useful liniment is made by mixing half an ounce of croton oil with three and half ounces of sesamum, cocoanut or other bland oil. The oil is a powerful vesicant producing pustular eruptions. It proves very useful in chronic rheumatism, paralysis, diseases of the joints, phthisis and chronic bronchitis. Internally it is useful in dropsy, obstinate constipation and apoplexy, the dose being one drop on sugar or in emulsion or made into a pill with bread crumb; should it cause griping, vomiting or too violent purging, a good large draught of lime-juice is the best antidote and it may be safely repeated in half-an hour if the vomiting, &c., continue. In lock-jaw and mania it is of great advantage, a few drops placed at the base of the tongue will produce catharsis. It is particularly valuable in cases where a minute and effectual dose is required; but it must not be resorted to generally except in cases where it is desirable that a speedy irritant action on the intestines should be produced. The seeds are also used as a drastic purgative. They are boiled 2 or 3 times in milk and their outer skin and embryo (the little leaf-like body found between the two halves of the kernal) are removed before being used internally. The seeds are employed in very minute doses in the form of pills prepared with great care, the dose being $\frac{1}{4}$ to $\frac{1}{2}$ grain mixed with extract catechu and honey or gum acacia. The seeds half roasted over a lamp or candle flame and the smoke inhaled through the nostrils relieves a fit of asthma. The oil diluted with 9 or 10 parts of mustard oil or olive oil is a useful liniment in infantile bronchitis, asthma, paralysis, chronic rheumatism and arthritis. The oil is also diuretic, purgative and rubefacient. The seed is frequently applied over the temples for headache and eye affections.

Its principle constituents are:—a fatty fixed oil, tiglinic acid, crotonic or quartenylic acid and croton oil.

Native Indian Preparations:—*Ichhâbhedi vatika:*—Take of mercury, sulphur, borax and black pepper one part each, ginger three parts, croton seeds nine parts; rub them together with water and make into two-grain pills. These are given in fever with constipation as also in ascites and anasarca.

Rukkeshee Rasa:—Take of chebulic myrobalan five parts, croton seeds one part, soak them in the milky juice of *Euphorbia nerifolia* (*snuhi*) and make into four-grain pills. These are given with a decoction of the root of *Ipomæa Turpethum* (*trivrit*) or *Baliospermum Montanum* (*danti*) as a drastic purgative in obstinate constipation. (Rasendrasarsangraha).

Mahánárácha Rasa:—Take chebulic myrobalan, pulp of *Cassia Fistula*, emblic myrobalan, root of *Baliospermum montanum* (*danti*), Picrorrhiza Kurroa (tiktâ), milky juice of *Euphorbia nerifolia* (*snuhi*), root of *Ipomœa Turpethum* (*trivrit*) and the tubers of *Cyperus rotundus* (*mustaka*) each one tola; pound them to a coarse powder and boil in 4 seers of water till the latter is reduced to one-eighth. Then take a tolâ of husked croton seeds, tie them in a piece of thin cloth and boil them in the above-mentioned decoction till the latter is reduced to the consistence of a fluid extract. To this extract add a powder composed of 8 parts of purified croton seeds, three parts of ginger and two of black pepper, mercury and sulphur, in quantity sufficient to make a pill-mass; rub them together for twelve hours and make into two-grain pills. These are given with cold water in tympanitis, colic, ascites, &c., as a drastic purgative. After the operation of this medicine rice should be given with curdle milk and sugar.

123. CUBEBA OFFICINALIS.

(*N. O.*—PIPERACEÆ.)

Sans.—Suganda-muricha. *Eng.*—Cubebs. *Hind.* and *Ben.*—Kabàb-chini. *Guz.*—Tadamiri. *Mah.*—Kankola, Himsimiri. *Pers*—Kibabeh. *Arab.*—Kababah. *Tel.*—Toka-miriyàlu, Chalava-miri-yàlu. *Tam.* and *Mal.*—Vàl-milaku. *Can.*—Gandha-menasu, Bàl-menasu.

Habitat.—This climbing woody bush indigenous to Java and Sumatra is cultivated to a small extent in India; but the cubebs, the dried unripe full-grown fruits of the shrub, are easily obtainable in the Indian bazaars, being imported from Singapore.

Properties and Uses.—It has stimulant, carminative and diuretic properties; it is used as a carminative spice, as stimulant to the mucous membrane in diseases of the genito-urinary organs such as gonorrhœa, gleet, leucorrhœa and other vaginal discharges of women; as expectorant in the coughs of old age. It produces tension of the vocal cords and clears the throat of the tenacious mucous and, therefore, it is much used by singers. Cubeb powder is best taken in milk and the oil in mucilage.

---

124. CUCUMIS MELO.

(*N. O.*—CUCURBITACEÆ.)

Sans.—Kharvuja. *Eng.*—Sweet Melon. *Hind.* and *Mah.*—Khurbuz. *Ben.*—Khermuj. *Guz.*—Turbuch. *Tel.*—Velàpandu. *Tam.*—Velàpalam. *Can.*—Kalangida. *Kon.*—Bachang.

Habitat.—This plant is extensively cultivated in gardens as well as in the sandy basins of rivers on account of its fruit; found particularly in Northern Bengal and also Kashmir and Afghanistan.

Properties and Uses.—The flattened and elliptic seeds yield a sweet edible oil which is nutritive and diuretic and given in painful discharge and suppression of urine. The same may be said of the seeds of all the species of cucumis. Bruised seeds are applied as poultice in cases of tympanitis in children. The pulp of the fruit is also a powerful diuretic very beneficial in chronic, as well as acute eczema. The whole fruit is eaten daily in chronic eczema with much benefit.

125.—CUCUMIS SATIVUS.

(*N. O.*—CUCURBITACEÆ.)

Sans.—Trapusha. *Eng.*—Common cucumber. *Hind.* and *Duk.*—Khira. *Ben.*—Sasà. *Guz.*—Kàkri. *Mah.*—Kàkdi. *Tel.*—Dosekâya. *Tam.*—Mulluvellari. *Can.*—Mullusavte. *Mal.*—Mullanvellari, Kakkari. *Kon.*—Towshe.

Habitat.—Its original home is Northern India, found wild in the Himalayas from Kumaon to Sikkim; now it is cultivated throughout.

Properties and Uses.—The seeds yield an oil like that of the seeds of other species of cucumis. The leaves, boiled and mixed with cummin seeds, roasted and powdered, are administered in throat affections in doses of 30 grains or more. Powdered and mixed with sugar they are powerfully diuretic. In sun-stroke pieces of cucumber are put in the head so that the patient may breathe moistened air in order to neutralise the heat of his body.

126.—CUCURBITA MAXIMA.

(*N. O.*—CUCURBITACEÆ.)

Sans.—Punyalatha, Dadhiphala. *Eng.*—Squash gourd. *Hind.*—Mithakaddu. *Guz.* and *Mah.*—Làl-Bhopla. *Tel.*—Gummadi Kàyi. *Tam.*—Pooshani. *Mal.*—Chakkerakumpalan. *Can.*—Cheenikâyi. *Kon.*—Duddini.

Habitat.—This creeper is extensively found very frequently on the roofs of houses all over India.

Properties and Uses.—The fruit is largely used by Indians in their curries. The seeds yield an oil which acts as a nervine tonic. The pulp of the fruit is often used as a poultice to boils, carbuncles, unhealthy ulcers, &c. The dried pulp is a remedy in hæmoptysis and hæmorrhages from the pulmonary organs given in the form of a confection. The part of the fruit stalk which is in *immediate* contact with the ripe gourd is removed and dried, and when it is made into a paste by rubbing in water it is considered a specific for bites of venomous insects of all kinds, chiefly for that of the centipede.

127.—CUMINUM CYMINUM.

(*N.O.*—UMBELLIFERÆ.)

Sans.—Jeeraka, Hrásvanga. *Eng.*—Cummin seed. *Hind.* and *Ben.*—Jeerà. *Pers.*—Zira. *Guz.*—Jirautmi. *Mah.*—Jiregire. *Tel.*—Jeelakara. *Tam.* and *Mal.*—Cheerakam. *Can.*—Jeerige. *Kon.*—Jeera.

Habitat.—This is extensively cultivated in most provinces of India except perhaps Bengal and Assam.

Properties and Uses.—The cummin seeds are largely used by the people of India as a spice in curries; they are aromatic, carminative and stimulant; also stomachic and astringent, useful in dyspepsia and diarrhœa; the dose is from 10 to 30 grains. They yield an essential oil to which they owe their bitter taste and aromatic odour. The seeds are also cooling and therefore form an ingredient of most prescriptions for gonorrhœa; externally they are applied in the form of poultice to allay pain and irritation, the seeds reduced to powder mixed with honey, salt and clarified butter are applied externally for scorpion bites. The seeds mixed with lime juice are administered in cases of bilious nausea in pregnant females. White cummin seeds taken internally shortly after child-birth increases the secretion of milk. A quantity of the seeds lightly smeared with ghee put into a pipe and smoked relieves hiccup. The essential oil contained in the seeds is a mixture of Cymol and Cuminol and other hydro-carbons.

---

128. CUPRUM.

Sans.—Tàmra. *Eng.*—Copper. *Hind.*—Tàmbà. *Ben.*—Tama. *Mah.* and *Kon.*—Tàmbe. *Tel.*—Râgi. *Tam* and *Mal.*—Sembu, Seppu. *Can.*—Tàmra.

Copper ore is found in the districts of Singbhum and Hazaribagh in Western Bengal, and smelting is carried on on a small scale. The salts of copper, although poisonous, are employed medicinally, being astringent, tonic and emetic in their operations; externally they are caustic and detergent. The principal salt used in medicine is the sulphate of copper commonly known as blue stone or *nilatutá* in Hindustanee and Punjabi, *mayiltutta* in Dravidian languages and *tuttha* in Sanskrit. It is prepared in a fairly pure state by roasting the copper pyrites and crystallizing from solution in water. It may be obtained in all the bazârs. It is a powerful astringent and tonic given in doses of from $\frac{1}{8}$ to 1 grain or more; in larger doses, *i.e.*, 5 to 10 grains it is an emetic; it acts very promptly and is, therefore, used in cases of poisoning by narcotics. Applied locally it acts as stimulant, styptic and escharotic; it is useful in the ophthalmia of children attended with copious discharge, leucorrhœa, gonorrhœa and ulcerations of the mouth, &c., 3 to 5 grains of the finely powdered sulphate incorporated with half an ounce of honey is a very useful application, or a lotion of 1 to 2 grains of the sulphate dissolved in one ounce of water. Obstinate indolent ulcers will often yield, when other measures have failed, to the persevering application of the solutions of the sulphate and of graduated strength from 2 to 10 grains to the ounce of water. In chronic diarrhœa and dysentery the following pills are of great benefit:—Take finely powdered sulphate of copper and opium, of each 6 grains; thoroughly mix them with a little of honey and divide into 12 pills, of which one should be taken thrice daily. These pills have been found very useful in controlling diarrhœa in the advanced stages of consumption. In the chronic diarrhœa and dysentery of children, a better form is 2 grains of the sulphate dissolved in 12 drachms of omum water; of this the dose is 1 tea-spoonful thrice daily. In diphtheria and croup of young children a solution of the sulphate of copper (5 grains in one ounce of water) is given in tea-spoonful doses every half hour till vomiting is produced. In ringworm and scald head the following ointment has been found useful:—sulphate of copper in powder, 20 grains; powdered galls, 1 drachm; ceromel, 1 ounce. Mix them thoroughly and rub well into the diseased part. In prickly heat a lotion of the sulphate of copper (10 grains to one ounce of water or rose water) often gives more relief than any other application. In bleeding from the nose a weaker solution, *i.e.*, 4 grains to an ounce of water, is sometimes introduced into the nostril with success when alum fails. Excessive bleeding from leech bites may often be speedily arrested by the application of a little powdered sulphate of copper. In cases of poisoning when it is of the greatest importance to empty the stomach as rapidly as possible, such as in poisoning by opium, datura, nux vomica, cocculus indicus, aconite, arsenic, &c., where the poison has been swallowed, sulphate of copper, 5 grains in a pint of tepid water, taken at a draught is a good emetic. If this does not operate in half an hour it may be repeated; and a third dose even may be given, if necessary, but this quantity should not be exceeded. Its operation should be promoted by copious draughts of warm water. The white of egg is the best remedy if the sulphate causes any unpleasant effects.

129. CURCULIGO ORCHIOIDES.

(N. O.—HYPOXIDACEÆ.)

***Sans.*—Bhoomitàla, Tàlamulika, Mushali. *Hind.*, and *Guz.*—Musalikand, Kalimusali. *Ben.*—Tàlamul. *Tel.*—Nelaladi-chettu or gadda. *Tam.* and *Mal.*—Nilappanai. *Can.*—Neladàli. *Mah.* and *Kon.*—Bhuyimaddi.**

Habitat.—It is a native of the greater part of hotter regions of India and Ceylon.

Properties and Uses.—The tuberous roots constitute the *kali* (black) *musli* and the white variety *safed musli* of the bazârs. They are considered demulcent, diuretic, tonic and restorative useful in gonorrhœa, piles, debility and impotence. They are prescribed usually combined with bitters and aromatics in the form of electuary the dose being one tea-spoonful twice a day; sometimes the drug is given with milk and sugar in doses of two drachms in 24 hours. The tubers are usefully administered in cases of asthma, jaundice, diarrhoea and colic as follows:— The tubers are washed and freed from rootlets, cut in slices by a wooden knife and dried in the shade, and then given in doses of 180 grains beaten up with an equal quantity of sugar in a glass of milk until it forms a thick mucilage.

Native Indian Preparations.—The tubers enter into the composition of several medicines intended to act as aphrodisiacs. The following is an example:—Take of the root of *Asparagus racemosus (satávari). Sphaeranthus mollis (munditikà)*, *gulancha*, seeds of *Butea frondosa* (*hastikarna*), and the tuberous roots of *mushali* equal parts; powder and mix. Dose is about a drachm with honey or clarified butter useful in the debility of old age.

130. CURCUMA AMADA.

(N. O.—ZINGIBERACEÆ.)

Sans.—Karpura haridrâ. *Eng.*—Mango ginger. *Hind.*—Ama-haldi. *Ben.*—Amàdà. *Mah. Can.* and *Kon.*—Ambe-halad. *Tel.*—Kasturi pasupu. *Tam.*—Kasturi-manjal.

Habitat.—This ornamental and beautiful plant, when in flower, is found in Bengal and on the hills on the West Coast.

Properties and Uses.—The root is used as a perfume, also medicinally when fresh and dried. The tubers have an agreeable fragrant smell and aromatic taste. They are regarded as cooling and carminative and are useful in prurigo. The fresh root possesses the smell of green mango and is used as a condiment and vegetable. The infusion of the root is employed to produce the flavour of the mango artificially in confectionary. The rhizomes are also used externally in the form of paste as an application for bruises and skin diseases generally combined with other medicines useful in improving the quality of blood.

---

131. CURCUMA ANGUSTIFOLIA.

(N. O.—ZINGIBERACEÆ.)

Sans.—Tavakshri. *Eng.*—East Indian Arrow-root. *Hind* and *Ben.*—Tikkur. *Mah.*—Tavakeera. *Tam.*—Artimâvu, Kookai. *Mal.*—Koova. *Can.*—Koove hittu.

Habitat.—This plant is found plentifully in Bengal, in the Central Provinces extending to Bombay; grows wild in jungles.

Properties and Uses.—The tubers of this and other species are the chief source of East Indian Arrow-root which is so highly valued as an article of diet. It is largely manufactured and exported in Malabar and Travancore. The tubers are dried and powdered and a flour is prepared which forms a very cooling, demulcent and nutritious food; it is an excellent diet in the form of *conjee* in cases of dysentery, dysuria, gonorrhoea, &c., also useful in typhoid fevers, ulcerations of the bowels and bladder. For its demulcent and cooling effect in cases of difficult and painful micturition it is best administered in the form of thin *conjee* prepared like barley water with milk and sugar added. Made into a confection with the addition of a small quantity of cardamoms it forms a cooling, stomachic food useful especially in cases where a demulcent is needed; it may be safely administered as a substitute for barley and used in all cases where barley is indicated.

132.—CURCUMA AROMATICA.

(N. O.—ZINGIBERACEÆ.)

Sans.—Vanaharidra. *Eng.*—Wild Turmuric, Yellow Zedoary, Cochin Turmuric. *Hind.*—Jangli-haldi. *Ben.*—Ban-halad. *Tel.*—Adavi-pasupu. *Tam.* and *Mal.*—Kâttu-manjal. *Can.*—Kâdarasina.

Habitat.—Found wild all over in Bengal and largely cultivated in gardens.

Properties and Uses.—The rhizomes are of a pale yellow colour, have an agreeable fragrant smell and yield a yellow colouring matter like turmuric, and the fresh root has a camphoraceous odour. The dried rhizome is used as a carminative and aromatic adjunct to other medicines. It is also used externally, bruised in oil as an application to sprains and bruises.

133. CURCUMA LONGA.

(*N. O.*—ZINGIBERACEÆ.)

Sans.—Karidrá, Nishá. *Eng.*—Turmuric. *Hind. Duk.* and *Punj.*—Haldi. *Kash.*—Lidar. *Ben. Mah. Guz.* and *Kon.*—Halad. *Pers.*—Zerd-chubu. *Tel.*—Pasupu, Haridra. *Tam.* and *Mal.*—Manjal. *Can.*—Haldi, Arasina. *Cing.*—Kahá. *Burm.*—Tanun. *Malay.*—Kooneit.

Habitat.—The turmuric plant is indigenous and extensively cultivated all over India on account of its rhizomes.

Properties and Uses.—The rhizomes are employed largely as a coloring agent and condiment entering largely into the composition of Indian curry powders. The root contains a yellow essential oil and starch, and acts as a stimulant aromatic tonic and carminative, usefully administered in intermittent fevers and dropsy; it is sometimes given in doses of 15 to 20 grains twice a day for flatulence and week state of the stomach; it is used both externally and internally in skin diseases due to impurity of the blood. Turmuric paste mixed with a little lime juice and saltpetre and applied hot is a popular application to sprains and bruises. In small-pox and chicken-pox a coating of turmuric is applied to facilitate the process of scabbing. A decoction of turmuric (1 ounce of the bruised root to 20 ounces of water) is applied to relieve the burning in catarrhal and purulent ophthalmia popularly known as "country sore eye." A piece of rag soaked in it should be kept constantly over the affected eye; it relieves the burning and moderates the urgency of the symptoms. Its powder is sprinkled on ulcers to stimulate them to healthy action. A paste made of the flowers is used in ringworm and other parasitic skin diseases. In piles an ointment made of turmuric, hemp leaves, onions, and warm linseed oil gives great relief when the piles are painful and protruding. In catarrh and coryza the inhalation of the fumes of the burning turmuric from the nostrils causes a copious mucous discharge and gives instant relief; the fumes are also used to relieve hysterical fits. The inhalation is taken at night and no fluid is allowed for some hours afterwards. The smoke produced by sprinkling powdered turmuric over burnt charcoal will relieve scorpion sting when the part affected is exposed to the smoke for a few minutes. Turmuric and alum powder in the proportion of 1 to 20 is blown into the ear in chronic otorrhoea.

Native Indian Preparations:—A paste of turmuric and the leaves of *Justicia Adhatoda* (*vâsaka*) with cow's urine is rubbed on the skin in prurigo (Chakradatta). Several other combinations of the sort are in vogue, such as turmuric and *nim* leaves, turmuric and the ashes of the plantain tree, &c. Turmuric is also given internally with cow's urine in prurigo and eczema (Chakradatta).

Haridrakhanda:—Take of turmuric 64 tolas, clarified butter 48 tolas, milk 16 seers, sugar 12 tolas and boil them together over a gentle fire in an earthen pot. Then add black pepper, long pepper, ginger, cinnamon, cardamom, *tejapatra*, *bâberang* seeds, root of *Ipomœa Turpethum* (*trivrit*) the three myrobalans, flowers of *Mesua ferrea* (*Nâgakesara*), tubers of *Cyperus rotundus* (*mustaka*) and prepared iron, each 8 tolas in fine powder and prepare a confection. Dose—one tola every morning in prurigo, boils, urticaria, etc. A cure is said to be effected in 7 days.

---

134. CURCUMA ZEDOARIA OR ZERUMBET.

(N. O.—ZINGIBERACEÆ.)

Sans.—Kachura, Shati. *Eng.*—The Round Zedoary. *Hind.*—Kakhur. *Ben.*—Sati. *Pers*—Kazhur. *Duk*—Katchoor. *Mah. Can.* and *Kon.*—Kachora. *Tel.*—Kachœramu. *Tam.*—Kastorimanjal, Nirvisham. *Mal.*—Adavi-kachhola.

Habitat.—This plant is cultivated in gardens in many parts of India for its root.

Properties and Uses.—The root possesses an agreeable, aromatic, camphoraceous smell, has stimulant and carminative properties, useful in flatulence and dyspepsia and as a corrector of purgatives. It is generally chewed by Indians to correct a sticky taste in the mouth, especially by singers for clearing the throat; it is also used in cases of irritation of the fauces and upper part of the wind-pipe. In cases of cold and fever it is given in decoction together with long pepper, cinnamon, liquorice and honey or sugar-candy to relieve cough and bronchitis; the pounded root combined with alum is applied to bruises. As demulcent, expectorant and aromatic its dose is about one drachm. It is an odoriferous ingredient of the cosmetics used for the cure of chronic skin diseases caused by impure or deranged blood. It is generally used in combination with other medicines as also in the preparation of medicated oils. The dry root powdered and mixed with the powdered wood of the *Caesalpinia sappan* makes the red powder called *abir* which is mixed with water and thrown over the person during the *Holi* festival of the Hindus.

---

135. CYNODON DACTYLON.

(*N. O.*—GRAMINEÆ.)

Sans., and *Mah.*—Doorvá. *Eng.*—Huriallee grass, Couch grass, Creeping panic grass. *Hind.*, and *Ben.*—Durbá. *Tel.*—Garike. *Tam.*—Arugu, Mooyarpul. *Can.*—Garikæ, Ambate-hullu. *Mal.*—Karukapullu. *Kon.*—Jirbankura.

Habitat.—This elegant perennial grass grows everywhere throughout India.

Properties and Uses.—The creeping root-stock is used medicinally. The fresh expressed juice of the grass is astringent and is useful in hæmaturesis and as an application in catarrhal ophthalmia, also to cuts and wounds; for this purpose bruised grass may also be applied; the juice when sniffed up in case of epistaxis proves a valuable styptic and stops bleeding. The fresh juice also acts as diuretic and is used in cases of dropsy and anasarca and as astringent in chronic diarrhœa and dysentery. The decoction of the roots is also diuretic and valuable in cases of vesical calculus and in secondary syphilis. A cold infusion of the grass stops bleeding from piles ; it is generally given with milk ; useful in irritation of the urinary organs. The roots crushed and mixed with curds are given in cases of chronic gleet ; the dose is two drachms of the root.

136. CYPERUS ROTUNDUS.

(*N. O.*—CYPERACEÆ.)

Sans.—Musta, Dhanakoota, Bhadramusti. *Hind.* and *Ben.*—Moothoo. *Guz.* and *Mah.*—Motha. *Tel.*—Tungamusti. *Tam.*—Korai kilangu. *Can.*—Koranarigadde, Abdahullu. *Mal.*—Kari-muttan.

Habitat.—It is a plentiful species occurring throughout the plains of India.

Properties and Uses.—The tubers have tonic and stimulant effect ; also demulcent, diuretic, diaphoretic, astringent, emmenagogue and vermifuge properties useful in fever, diarrhœa, dysentery, dyspepsia, vomiting, cholera, &c. The bulbous roots are scraped and pounded with green ginger, mixed with honey and given in cases of dysentery in doses of about a scruple. The fresh tubers are applied to the breast in the form of paste or plaster as a galactagogue. It is applied to scorpion stings and when dried to spreading ulcers.

Native Indian Preparations.—*Shadanga Paniya:*—Take of the tubers of *Cyperus Rotundus*, red sandle-wood, root of *Andropogon Muricatus* (*usira*), *Oldenlandia herbaceæ* (*perpáta*), *Pavonia Odorata* (*bála*) and dry ginger each one drachm, water two seers; boil down to one seer. This decoction is given as a drink for appeasing thirst and relieving heat of body in fever. It may be taken *ad libitum.*

---

137. DATURA ALBA AND D. FASTUOSA.

(*N. O.*—SOLANACEÆ.)

Sans.—Dhustoora, Unmatta. *Eng.*—Thorn-apple, Datura. *Hind.*, *Duk.*, *Ben.*, *Punj.*, and *Guz.*—Dhatoora. *Pers.*—Kouzmasab. *Tel.*—Umetta, Dhaturamu. *Tam.*—Umattai. *Can.* and *Mal.*—Ummattam. *Kon.*—Duturo. *Kash.*—Dáthir. *Burm.*—Padáyin. *Cing.*—Attana. *Malay.*—Kachubang.

Habitat.—This datura plant, of which the generic names have been given above, exists in different species which are distinguished by prefixes denoting the colour of the flowers—white, purple, &c. These species are found growing commonly on waste places throughout India.

Properties and Uses.—The different species of this plant possess the same medicinal properties although the purple variety is generally regarded as the more valuable. Although it is a powerful medicine much caution is necessary in its employment as, in overdoses, it acts as a violent narcotic poison. This plant has long been known to Indians for its intoxicating and narcotic properties as it produces a temporary insensibility in ordinary doses. The seeds are in popular use in India by the dissipated and the depraved in combination with *sabja*, toddy, *majum*, *ganja* and the like to increase their stupifying effect. The plant, as a whole, has narcotic, anodyne and antispasmodic properties. It has properties analogous to those of belladonna; it also causes the dilatation of the pupil of the eye when locally applied in watery solution which is, at a rough estimate, about equal in effect to a four grain (to the ounce) solution of atropine. The smoking of the dried leaves and stem (10 to 20 grains to begin with, subsequently increased to 30 grains) in a pipe or in cigarettes is found successful in relieving spasmodic asthma and kindred affections. When the leaves fail, the dried seeds which are thought to be more powerful, may be tried. The earlier in the attack it is employed he greater are the chances of success; it has little effect when the attack has lasted for some hours. For a person subject to asthma a good plan is to adopt the habit of smoking the drug the last thing at night whether an attack is threatening or not; at any rate he should keep a cigarette or a pipe of it already filled and ready by his bed-side for lighting to use it immediately on the commencement of the attack. But in all cases it should be immediately discontinued if it produces giddiness, a feeling of sickness or any other unpleasant symptom. The smoking has also proved beneficial in chronic coughs, hard and dry, with violent paroxysms and scanty expectoration.

For Rheumatic swellings of the joints, lumbago, painful tumours, nodes, glandular inflammations such as mumps, &c., the local application of datura leaves proves most serviceable in relieving pain, when applied in the form of poultice (made by bruising the fresh leaves into a pulp and mixing them with the aid of a little water, with an equal weight of rice flour to the consistence of a poultice) or epithem which consists of steeping a few entire leaves in arrack or other spirit and placing them whilst wet over the seat of pain and securing them in that position by a bandage or as fomentation made by infusing the leaves in boiling water in the proportion of one ounce to each pint of liquid, and applied as hot as can be borne by means of two or more thickly folded clothes or preferably flannels alternating with one another. The liniment (prepared by macerating for seven days one ounce of the bruised seeds in a pint of sesamum or other bland oil and straining) is also similarly useful. These preparations are useful in relieving the pain attendant on painful or difficult menstruation, and in some painful affections of the uterus they are more advantageously placed on the lower part of the abdomen. They also prove beneficial in relieving neuralgic pains, especially of the face; for this the liniment is best adapted, well rubbed in over the seat of pain and along the space immediately in front of the year or rather in the narrow space between the ear and the jaw.

The tincture, extract, liniment, plaster and poultice are the chief preparations of datura. The tincture is a useful and cheap substitute for opium, twenty drops being equal to one grain of opium. The extract is a convenient substitute for the extract of belladonna in $\frac{1}{4}$ to $\frac{1}{2}$ grain doses employed successfully in mania and epilepsy. In tetanus or lock-jaw consequent on a wound, local application of the poultices of the leaves to the wound previously cleansed by the irrigation of tepid water and renewed three or four times a day, together with the internal administration of the tincture of datura, in doses of 20 to 30 drops in water, three or four times daily, and continued, unless the spasms previously yield, till the full dilatation of the pupil is produced with some degree of giddiness, drowsiness or confusion of ideas, is found worthy of trial in the absence of more effective agents. If the spasms abate *i.e.*, if they recur at more distant intervals and are less severe and prolonged when they do occur, the medicine in smaller doses at longer intervals may be continued till the spasms cease altogether; but if, under the use of the remedy, after it has produced its specific effects on the system the spasms shew no sign of abatement, no good but perhaps harm will result from continuing it. In addition to the above means datura liniment should be well rubbed in along the spine several times daily. The further details of treatment are the same as those advocated in the use of belladonna to which datura bears a very close resemblance in its effects on the system. Employed as above directed, datura may be used with safety, provided that the case is carefully watched and the medicine diminished or discontinued on the full development of its physiological effects. In cases of guineaworm a datura poultice is said to be the most useful in relieving the pain and hastening the expulsion of the worm.

The fresh juice of the leaves is a popular household application to subdue pain and inflammation in glandular swellings such as mumps, in ophthalmia, ear-ache, to relieve pains of gout and rheumatism and to inflamed breasts. The fresh juice may be used alone or mixed with opium. The leaves are also applied as anodyne poultice to inflamed breasts to check the inflammation and excessive secretion of milk in cases where an abscess is threatened. The leaves boiled in oil or the oil itself are rubbed on in rheumatic and other pains of the limbs, &c. Internally the juice of the leaves is administered with curdled milk in gonorrhœa. It is also a popular internal remedy for the prevention of hydrophobia. The treatment consists in giving the medicine previous to the time of the development of hydrophobia. Usually hydrophobia comes 40 days after the patient has been bitten by the mad dog. The treatment is to give the following medicine two weeks after the patient has been bitten, *i.e.*, between the 15th and 25th days. In the morning after the 15th day a dessertspoonful of wood charcoal powder is given; half-an-hour after an ounce of the juice of the *black* datura leaves is given which is soon after followed with palmyra jaggery or something else to check vomiting. Then the patient is bound lest he does mischief to others and is kept in the sun for 4 or 5 hours until noon. Then, the patient gradually becomes mad and does many things like the mad dog (evidence of the patient having been bitten and of his total recovery). In the afternoon many pots of cold water are poured over his head; this causes great annoyance to the patient and he resents it to the utmost protesting loudly. Food is now given such as pork, salt-fish, brinjal, horse-gram, Bengal-gram, &c., &c. The patient is then considered out of danger and is given a simple light diet. In case of treating a person already suffering from hydrophobia the front part of his head is scratched with a lancet so as to make it bleed a little and the ground leaves of the black datura rubbed and the juice given internally.

The above method of treatment is one of the several modes employed by Hindu Vaidyans and it is the one adopted and recommended by a well-known popular physician of South India.

The seeds have a more powerful narcotic property and they are considered to have a strong aphrodisiac effect. They are employed by Hakims in the preparation of a medicated ghee which is believed to contain strong aphrodisiac properties, and is rubbed on the genitals twice a day to stimulate them, and about 4 grains of the ghee is also taken internally once a day. The seeds ground and made into pills and laid upon the decayed tooth are said to relieve tooth-ache, but greatest caution should be taken in applying the medicine, since it is a powerful narcotic drug. The seed contains an alkaloid called *daturine* which is a powerful narcotic anodyne and antispasmodic especially useful in asthma and bronchitis, also in insanity and ophthalmia.

---

138. DAUCUS CAROTA.

(*N. O.*—UMBELLIFERÆ.)

Sans.—Garjara. *Eng.*—The Carrot. *Hind.* and *Ben.*—Gâjar, *Pers.*—Zardak. *Tel.*—Gajjara-gedda. *Tam.*—Gajjara-kilangu.

Habitat.—The carrot is indigenous to Cashmere and Western Himalaya, and is now largely cultivated in India for culinary purposes.

Properties and Uses.—The seeds are used as a nervine tonic. Externally the fresh root when scraped forms a good stimulating poultice for foul ulcers. The seeds yield a yellowish colored volatile oil which is regarded as a nervine tonic.

---

139. DIOSPYROS EMBRYOPTERIS.

(*N. O.*—EBENACEÆ.)

Sans.—Tinduka. *Eng.*—Wild mangosteen. *Hind.*—Tendu. *Ben.*—Gab. *Tel.*—Tumikichettu, Tumil. *Tam.*—Tumbika. *Can.* —Bandada or Tumaki-mara. *Mal.*—Panichhimaram. *Kon.*—Bandâ-rooku.

Habitat.—This tree grows commonly all over India.

Properties and Uses.—The rind of the fruit and the bark have astringent properties. As infusion or decoction it is an efficient remedy for chronic dysentery and diarrhœa, for hæmorrhages from the internal organs. It is also used as a gargle in aphthæ and sore throat. The juice of the fruit is a good application to fresh wounds as it is astringent and styptic in effect. It is rich in tannin. The oil extracted from the seeds is used in dysentery and diarrhœa with success.

---

140. DIPTEROCARPUS TURBINATUS.

(*N. O.*—DIPTEROCARPEÆ.)

Eng.—Gurjun oil tree, Wood oil tree. *Hind.* and *Ben.*—Garjan, Tihya-garjan, Teli-garjan. *Cing.*—Horatel. *Burm.*—Kanyensi.

Habitat.—This magnificent ever-green tree grows plentifully in Eastern Bengal, Burma, Chittagong and Pegu to Singapore.

Properties and Uses.—This tree is famous over East India and Malaya Islands on account of a thick honey-like oleo-resin or liquid which it yields, and which is known as garjan balsam. It is usually found in the bazaars in three principle varieties—the pale, the red or reddish brown and the black or dark brown. It has a simple aromatic copaiba-like odour and taste without the persistent acridity of copaiba. It is soluble in water and more freely in alcohol. It has all the advantages of copaiba as an expectorant without the disadvantage of exciting an eruption. Half to two drachms of the balsam in an ounce of the malt extract three times a day given in cases of chronic bronchitis acts admirably. Its essential oil has been successfully administered in the treatment of gleet, gonorrhœa in the advanced stages, leucorrhœa and other vaginal discharges, leprosy and certain other skin diseases. The dose is about a teaspoonful twice or thrice daily, given floating on omum or other aromatic water or, made into an emulsion with lime water; the oleo-resin is applied to indolent ulcers, leprosy, psoriasis, &c., in the form of an emulsion made with three parts of lime water to one of the oil, with which the affected parts are rubbed diligently twice a day, and each time for about two hours. Also internally it is given in leprosy in two-drachm doses with lime water twice daily. Mixed with *dámer* it is applied to timber to prevent the attack of white-ants.

141. DOLICHOS UNIFLORUS.

(*N. O.*—LEGUMINOSÆ.)

Sans.—Khalakula, Kulastha. *Eng.*—Horse-gram plant. *Hind.* and *Ben.*—Kulti. *Tel.*—Ulavalu. *Tam.*—Kollu. *Can.*—Huruli. *Mal.*—Kollu, Mutira. *Kon.*—Kulithu.

Habitat.—A common twining plant growing all over India.

Properties and Uses.—The decoction of this grain is used by females in leucorrhoea and menstrual derangements. It is also given to females during parturition to promote discharge of the lochia. The pulse is a demulcent in calculus affections, coughs, &c. Its employment is said to reduce corpulence.

---

142. ECLIPTA ERECTA.

(*N. O.*—COMPOSITÆ.)

Sans.—Bhringarâj, Kesharâj, Superna. *Hind.*—Bungrâh, Mochrand. *Ben.*—Kesooria, Kesuti. *Tel.*—Guntagalijæru. *Tam.*—Karishâlankanni. *Can.*—Ajâgara, Garunga. *Mal.*—Kanni. *Kon.*—Kâjalamâvu.

Habitat.—This weed is found abundantly throughout India and plentiful on the Himalaya.

Properties and Uses.—The root is tonic and deobstruent in hepatic and splenic enlargements and in various chronic skin diseases; in these cases it is powdered and applied externally. The root is given to relieve scalding of the urine in doses of 180 grains mixed with salt. It is anodyne and absorbant and relieves headache, when applied with a little oil. The root has also emetic and purgative properties. The expressed juice of the leaves in combination with aromatics such as *Ajavan* seeds is used as a tonic and deobstruent, and 2 drops of it given with 8 drops of honey is a popular remedy for new born children suffering from catarrh. The fresh plant mixed with sesamam oil is applied externally in elephantiasis. The juice is administered in teaspoonful doses in jaundice and fevers. The leaves form an excellent remedy for scorpion stings; they are bruised and rubbed on the painful and inflamed part around the bite and then tightly applied to the wound itself; by so doing they are said to draw forth all the poison from the wound. The juice of the leaves mixed with gingelly or cocoanut oil and boiled together makes an excellent preparation for annointing the head and is said to render the hair black and luxuriant.

143. ELLETARIA CARDAMOMUM.

(*N. O.*—SCITAMINEÆ.)

Sans.—Ela. *Eng.*—Cardamom. *Hind.*—Chhoti Elâchi. *Ben.*—Elachi. *Guz.*—Elachi. *Tel.*—Elákaya. *Tam.*—Elakay. *Mah.*—Elachi. *Can.*—Elakki.

Habitat.—This plant is cultivated for its fruit in many parts of Southern India and Ceylon.

Properties and Uses.—The Cardamom seeds are valuable as a warm cardial and aromatic, carminative stimulant due to an essential oil which is their characteristic constituent.

144. ELEUSINE CORACANA.

(*N. O.*—GRAMINACEÆ).

Sans.—Râjika, Krishnâ. *Eng.*, *Hind.*, *Tel.*, *Can.* and *Mal.*—Râgi. *Ben.*—Muroora. *Tam.*—Irâgi. *Kon.*—Nânchano.

Habitat.—This grain is grown almost in all parts of India.

Properties and Uses.—This grain is rather difficult of digestion but highly nourishing; it is most suitable to hard-working classes. It forms a principle diet given to prisoners in some of the Indian jails.

Chemical Composition (Professor Church):—

	In 100 parts.		In 1 pound.	
	Husked.	Whole.	Ounces.	Grains.
Water ...	13·2	12·5	2	0
Albuminoids ...	7·3	5·9	0	413
Starch ...	73·2	74·6	11	409
Oil ...	1·5	0·8	0	56
Fibre ...	2·5	3·6	0	252
Ash ...	2·3	2·6	0	182

The percentage of phosphoric acid in the whole grain is about 0·4

145. EMBELIA RIBES AND E. ROBUSTA.

(*N. O.*—MYRSINEAE.)

Sans.—Vidanga. *Hind.*—Bâberang. *Ben.*—Biranga. *Tel.* and *Tam.*—Vayu, Vilamgan. *Bom.*—Vaivarang.

Habitat.—The former is a large climber abundant in the hilly parts of India from the Central Himalaya to Ceylon and Singapore; the latter is found chiefly in Bengal and Burma extending to the Lower Himalaya.

Properties and Uses.—The dried berries of both varieties are carminative, stomachic and stimulant useful in dyspepsia and skin diseases. They also act as a certain anthelmintic specially useful in expelling tape-worms. They contain the active principle called *Embelic acid.* For expelling intestinal worms the powder of the seeds is given in drachm doses with honey or with an infusion of the seeds.

Native Indian Preparations.—*Bâberang* enters into the composition of several applications for ring-worm and other skin diseases. The following is an example :—Take of *baberang*, rock salt, chebulic myrobalan, *bakuchi*, mustard, turmuric and the seeds of *Pongamia glabra* (*karanja*), equal parts and make them into a thin paste with cow's urine (Chakradatta).

146. EMBLICA OFFICINALIS.

(*N. O.*—EUPHORBIACEAE.)

Sans.—Dhâtri, Amraphalam. *Eng.*—Emblic Myrobalan. *Hind.*—Amlikâ, Anvurah. *Ben.*—Amlâ. *Mah.*—Avalâ. *Tel.*—Nelli, Amalakamu. *Tam.*, *Mal.* and *Can.*—Nellikay. *Cing.*—Nelli, Nellika. *Burm.*—Ziphiyu-si.

Habitat.—This tree is chiefly met with in the Deccan and in the sea-coast districts of India.

Properties and Uses.—The fresh fruit or its juice is considered cooling, refrigerent, diuretic and laxative; as diuretic, the juice is generally given with honey; the dose is from 1 to 3 drachms. The dried fruit is astringent, containing a large proportion of gallic acid and is, therefore, very useful in hæmorrhage, in diarrhœa and dysentery; with iron it is a valuable remedy in anæmia, jaundice and dyspepsia. A paste of the fruit is a useful external application over the pubic region in irritability of the bladder. An infusion of the seeds is applied with benefit to recent inflammations of the conjunctiva and other eye complaints. The dried fruit immersed in water in a new earthen vessel a whole night yields a decoction which is used as a collyrium in ophthalmia. It may be applied cold or warm. A fermented liquor prepared from the root is used in jaundice, dyspepsia, cough, &c. The fresh fruit is a gentle purgative and a sherbat prepared from it is a favourite, cooling drink which is said to have a diuretic effect. The bark has an astringent property and its juice combined with honey and turmuric is a remedy for gonorrhœa. The leaves are used as infusion with fenugreek seeds in chronic dysentery and as a bitter tonic. The decoction of the leaves is useful as a mouth-wash in aphthæ. The milky juice is a good application to offensive sores. A fixed oil obtained from the berries has the effect of strengthening and promoting the growth of hair. The essential oil distilled from the leaves is largely employed in perfumery. The tender shoots given in butter-milk cure indigestion and diarrhœa; green fresh leaves combined with curds have also similar effect. The fruit is preserved or made into confection when it is a pleasant purgative, useful in habitual constipation; it is employed with much benefit in various complaints connected with digestive organs.

Native Indian Preparations.—*Dhâtri Leha*—Take of powdered emblic myrobalan 64 tolas, prepared iron 32 tolas, liquorice powder 16 tolas, mix them together and soak in the juice of *gulancha* for seven times successively. This preparation is given in doses of 20 to 40 grains in anæmia, jaundice and dyspepsia. *Dhatri Arishta* or fermented liquor of emblic myrobalan :—Take the fresh juice of two thousand emblic myrobalans, honey in quantity equal to one-eighth of the juice, powdered long pepper 16 tolas, sugar six seers and a quarter; mix them together, boil for a while and leave the mixture to ferment in an earthen jar. This liquor is used in jaundice, dyspepsia, indigestion, cough, &c.

---

147. ERIODENDRON ANFRACTUOSUM.

(*N. O.*—BOMBACEÆ.)

Hind.—Huttian. *Ben.*—Spimool. *Can.*—Apoorani. *Mal.*—Poola.

Habitat.—This tree is met with generally in forests in almost all parts of India.

Properties and Uses.—The gum or dried juice which the tree yields has tonic, alterative and aphrodisiac properties; it contains tannic and gallic acids, and therefore it is astringent. It is useful as a styptic; given with benefit in diarrhœa, dysentery and menorrhagia; ground to powder and taken in milk it acts like a good tonic, given to children as a cooling laxative. The dried flowers are used as demulcent. They are boiled with poppy seeds, goat's milk and sugar and then inspissated and of this conserve two drachms are given three times a day in hæmorrhoids. The roots have stimulant and tonic properties and, in large doses, act as emetic. The young roots dried in the shade and powdered form a chief ingredient in a medicine highly reputed as aphrodisiac; the gum is also given in impotence. In 20 to 30 grain doses with equal quantity of sugar it is useful in diarrhœa of children. The tap-root of the young plant is useful in gonorrhœa and dysentery.

148. ERYTHRINA INDICA.

(*N. O.*—LEGUMINOSÆ.)

Sans.—Parijata. *Eng.*—Indian Coral tree. *Hind.*—Ferrud, Pangra. *Ben.*—Palita-madar. *Tel.*—Barijamu, Machhikara. *Tam.*—Kaliyana marukkà. *Can.*—Hongara, Pongara. *Kon.*—Pangiro.

Habitat.—This tree is common in Bengal and many parts of India often grown in gardens as a support for black-pepper vines.

Properties and Uses.—The bark is antibilious and febrifuge, useful as a collyrium in ophthalmia. The inner side of the bark is smeared with ghee and held over the flame; the soot thus deposited is used in watery eye, tinea-tarse, and purulent conjunctivitis, being applied to the inner side and edges of the lower lid. The fresh juice of the leaves taken in two ounce doses is a good vermifuge and cathartic; it is also used as an injection into the ear for the relief of ear-ache and as an anodyne for toothache. The leaves are externally applied to disperse venereal buboes and to relieve pain in the joints.

---

149. ERYTHROXYLON COCA.—(*The Coca plant.*)

(*N. O.*—ERYTHROXYLACEÆ.)

Habitat.— This South American shrub is now being cultivated in India and Ceylon in the tea districts with some success.

Properties and Uses.—The leaves contain cocaine and have remarkable sustaining power. The alkaloid cocaine and its salts are stimulant and restorative; it is injected hypodermically and painted externally to produce local anæsthesia. Cocaine produces mydriasis and is therefore much used in minor operations and in ophthalmic surgery. The action commences in about three minutes and lasts for about half-an-hour.

---

150. EUCALYPTUS GLOBULUS.

(*N. O.*—MYRTACEÆ.)

Eng.—The Australian or Blue Gum tree.

Habitat.—This tree which is a native of Australia and Tasmania has now been cultivated in India on the highlands, chiefly on the Nilgiris.

Properties and Uses.—The red gum or Eucalyptus kino is an astringent, less astringent and more demulcent than catechu or kino; found effectual in the treatment of chronic bowel-complaints and especially in the chronic dysentery of Europeans. The dose is from 5 to 10 grains as powder or in the form of syrup. The essential oil distilled from the leaves is called *Eucalyptol*. It has an agreeable, fragrant, aromatic odour and is greatly valued for its antiseptic, rubefacient, stimulating and antispasmodic properties much used as an inhalant. Large doses cause headache and fever with accelerated respiration and thirst. Upon anaemic persons it acts as narcotic. In Australia it is a popular remedy for fevers and in Europe it has been used successfully in the treatment of diseases prevalent in marshy districts. It produces marvellous results in cases of intermittent fevers, especially obstinate ones where quinine has failed. The tincture, infusion, and decoction of the Eucalyptus leaves are used for disinfecting the dressings of wounds. Dilute essence or distilled water of the leaves are also used as astringent and hæmostatic. They are also employed with success in purulent catarrhal affections of the urethra and vagina. Fresh young leaves are applied as a local stimulant to small wounds slow to cicatrise. The leaves when masticated perfume the breath and harden spongy and bleeding gums.

---

151. EUGENIA JAMBOLANA.

(*N. O.*—MYRTACEÆ.)

Sans.—Jambula. *Eng.*—Jambul, the Black plum. *Hind.*—Jaman. *Ben.*—Kâla-jam. *Guz.*, *Mah.* and *Kon.*—Jambul. *Tel.*—Nærædu. *Tam.* and *Mal.*—Nâval. *Can.*—Næralu.

Habitat.—This tree is found all over India extending from the Himalaya to Southern India.

Properties and Uses.—The bark is astringent and is used as such in decoction in cases of chronic diarrhœa and dysentery and as a gargle in sore throat, spongy gums, &c. The juice of the tender leaves either alone or combined with carminatives such as cardamoms and cinnamon is given in goat's milk in the diarrhœa of children. The expressed juice of the leaves together with that of the leaves of mango and emblic myrobalan about a drachm each is administered in goat's milk and honey in cases of dysentery with bloody discharge. The seed or stone of the fruit is used as a remedy in diabetes and is believed to check the diastasic conversion of starch into sugar in that form of the disease depending on increased production of glucose. For this the liquid extract is the most suitable preparation. The dried seeds in combination with those of *Mangifera Indica* are administered with very good effect in the form of powder in cases of diarrhœa and dysentery. An unstable glucoside named *Jambulin* has been said to exist in the seeds which also contain gallic acid. The dose of the extract is half to two drachms and that of the powder 5 to 30 grains. The syrup or vinegar prepared from the ripe fruit is an agreeable stomachic and carminative, useful in spleen enlargement and an efficient astringent in chronic diarrhœa.

---

152. EUPHORBIA ANTIQUORUM.

(*N. O.*—EUPHORBIACEÆ.)

Sans.—Snuhi, Vajri, Sehunda. *Eng.*- Triangular Spurge. *Hind.*—Tidhára, Sehund. *Ben.*—Narsij, Tikáta sij. *Mah.*—Narasija. *Tel.*—Bommajemudu. *Tam.* and *Mal.*—Chaturkalli. *Can.*—Bonthekalli. *Kon.*—Nivali, Chaturkalli.

Habitat.—A small tree common in India chiefly in Bengal.

Properties and Uses.—The fresh milky juice or gum which flows from the branches is an acrid irritant applied externally to relieve pain of gout, rheumatism, toothache, &c. When mixed with cantharides it forms what is called gout plaster; but it must be used with great caution as it is a dangerous irritant application. Internally it is a powerful emetic and a violent purgative. A plaster made from the roots and mixed with asafœtida is applied externally to the stomachs of children suffering from worms. The bark of the root is purgative and the stem in decoction is given in gout but with much care. When taken internally it acts as a drastic purgative; it is employed in nervous diseases, dropsy, palsy, deafness and amaurosis. The stem fried, powdered or sprinkled over old ulcers promotes healing; the stem warmed and applied as a covering to whitlows or felons at the ends of fingers has the effect of fomentations and warm poultices rendering the nail and skin supple and favouring the formation and discharge of the matter. The gum resin boiled in oil forms an effective application to scrofulous and other inveterate ulcers. But all the preparations of this plant should be employed with much care.

---

153. EUPHORBIA NERIFOLIA.

(*N. O.*—EUPHORBIACEÆ.)

Sans.—Patrasnuk, Svarasaná. *Hind.*—Thohar. *Ben.*—Mansásij. *Mah.*—Thora. *Tel.*—Akujimudu. *Tam.*, *Can.* and *Mal.*—Ilaikkalli. *Kon.*—Pânnànivali.

Habitat.—A small tree found in Central India and cultivated in Bengal.

Properties and Uses.—The white, acrid, milky juice is internally a purgative and externally it has rubefacient properties. As drastic purgative it is given in combination with other medicines such as chebulic myrobalan, long-pepper, *trivrit* root, &c., and which are kept steeped in it in cases of ascites, anasarca and tympanitis. The juice is also applied to remove warts and similar excrescences and to afford relief in ear-ache; mixed with soot it is used as an *anjan* in ophthalmia. The juice is largely used with clarified or fresh butter as an application to unhealthy ulcers and scabies. Applied to glandular swellings it prevents suppuration.

Turmuric powder mixed with the juice of *Euphorbia nerifolia* is recommended to be applied to piles. Thread steeped in the above-mentioned mixture is used in ligaturing external hæmorrhoids (Chakradatta). The root-bark boiled in rice water and arrack is given in dropsy. The root mixed with black-pepper is employed in snake-bites both internally and externally.

---

154. EUPHORBIA TIRUCALLI.

(*N. O.*—EUPHORBIACEÆ.)

Sans.—Trikantaka, Vajradruma. *Eng.*—Milk-hedge, Indian Tree-spurge. *Ben.*—Lankasij. *Tel.* and *Tam.*—Kalli. *Can.*—Mondukalli. *Mal.*—Tirukalli. *Kon.*—Baddinivali.

Habitat.—This plant is a native of America but has become acclimatised and grows freely in all parts of India.

Properties and Uses.—The milky juice obtained by pricking the succulent stems and fleshy leaves is applied to itch and scorpion bites. It is also a warm, rubefacient remedy in rheumatism, toothache, &c. The milky juice being an acrid irritant is employed to raise blisters; given with butter it is said to cure affections of the spleen and to act as a purgative in colic and bowel complaints. It has also emetic and antisyphilitic properties. The decoction of the tender branches as also that of the root is administered in colic.

---

155. FERONA ELEPHANTUM.

(*N. O.*—RUTACEÆ.)

Sans.—Kapitha. *Eng.*—Elephant or Wood-apple. *Hind.* and *Duk.*—Khaet. *Ben.*—Kathbel. *Burm.*—Mahan. *Mah.*—Kavitpâna. *Tel.*—Velāga. *Tam.*—Vilakpittam, Vellil. *Can.*—Baelada-phala. *Mal.*—Vilâv. *Kon.*—Belpatri-phal.

Habitat.—The wood-apple tree is met with throughout India, cultivated for its fruit.

Properties and Uses.—The pulp of the ripe fruits is edible and it is aromatic, antiscorbutic and in the form of sherbat or chutney made with the addition of salt, tamarind and spices is an excellent stomachic. A jelly much resembling black-currant jelly but with a more astringent taste is made from it. The pulp is also useful in some affections of the gums and throat. The unripe fruit is a useful astringent employed alone or in combination with *bela* and other medicines in diarrhœa and dysentery. The transparent gummy substance exuding from the stem when cut or broken resembles and may be used in the place of the true gum arabic; reduced to powder and mixed with honey it is given in dysentery and diarrhœa. The leaves when bruised have a fragrant smell like anise. They are aromatic, carminative and astringent, used as such in the bowel complaints of children.

Native Indian Preparations.—*Kapithashtaka Churna.*—Take of the pulp of unripe wood-apples eight parts, sugar six parts, pomegranate juice, tamarind pulp, *bela* fruit, flowers of *Woodfordia floribunda* (*dhâtaki*), *âjmad* and long-pepper each three parts, black-pepper, cumin seeds, coriander, long-pepper root, root of Pavonia adorata (*bàlà*), *sonchal* salt, *ajowan*, cardamoms, cinnamon, *tejapatra*, flowers of *Mesua ferrea* (*nàgakesara*), ginger and plumbago root, each one part, powder the ingredients finely and mix. Dose, about one drachm. This preparation is used in chronic diarrhœa and dysentery with loss of appetite and in affections of the throat.

---

156. FERULA ASAFŒTIDA.

(*N. O.*—UMBELLIFERÆ.)

Sans. and *Can.*—Hingu. *Eng.*—Asafœtida. *Hind.*, *Duk.*, *Ben.*, *Punj.*, *Guz.*, *Mah.* and *Kon.*—Hing. *Kash.*—Yang. *Tel.*—Inguva. *Tam.* and *Mal.*—Perungáyam. *Cing.*—Perunkayam. *Burm.*—Shinka or Shingu. *Malay.*—Hingu.

Habitat.—This small plant grows wild and plentifully in Persia and Afghanistan. The gum-resin (asafœtida) is found in all the Indian bazaars.

Properties and Uses.—Asafœtida, the concrete juice obtained from the plant is a carminative, antispasmodic, expectorant, stimulant and slightly laxative drug. It is in popular use in India for many centuries, especially as an ingredient in condiments. It is a valuable remedy for hysteria, flatulence, flatulent colic and spasmodic affections of the bowels especially when connected with hysteria, in fainting, nervous palpitations, hypochondriasis and other affections due to hysteria, in the spasmodic, and in the obstinate coughs of childhood remaining after attacks of inflammation and also, in the advanced stages of whooping cough and, in the chronic bronchitis and asthma of adults. It is fried before being used. Raw and unfried asafœtida is said to cause vomiting. It may be given in the form of pill or in that of mixture prepared by rubbing down in a mortar five drachms of asafœtida in a pint of hot water and straining and setting aside to cool. Of this solution, which is thick and milky, the dose is from one to two tablespoonfuls. In typhoid fever, cholera, convulsions and flatulent diseases of children it is used as an enema, two drachms of the gum being added to a pint of water or thin gruel. A tea-spoonful of the mixture with a little omum water is often very effectual in relieving the flatulent colic of children. It may also be tried in the convulsions of pale, weakly children. The plaster of asafœtida is a good stimulant application to the chest of children suffering from whooping cough. Asafœtida is useful as an anthelmintic for round worms in children; asafœtida enema is an effectual means of removing thread-worms from the rectum and lower bowel. As anæsthetic asafœtida is employed in hemicrania and dental caries. An emulsion (5 grains of the gum to one drachm of water) is dropped into the nostrils to relieve the pain of hemicrania; in dental caries a mixture of opium and asafœtida is placed in the hollow tooth to relieve the ache. In the early stages of cholera asafœtida combined with camphor, black-pepper and opium is said to be of great value. Asafœtida is given to increase the lochial discharge after child-birth; it is prepared and administered thus: it is first fried; a small quantity is then mixed with garlic and palmyra jaggery and a bolus is made and given to the patient every morning.

Native Indian Preparations.—*Hingvashtaka Churna.*—Take of fried asafœtida, ginger, long-pepper, black-pepper, *ojowan*, cumin seeds, nigella seeds and rock salt, equal parts; reduce them to powder and mix. Dose, ten to twenty grains, to be taken with the first morsel of rice and clarified butter taken at breakfast. Thus administered it is said to increase the appetite and digestive powers and to cure flatulence (Bhaishajya Ratnavali). Some writers recommend the above powder to be made into pills with lemon juice. In the flatulence of infants a powder composed of asafœtida, rock salt, cardamoms, ginger and the root of *Clerodendron siphonanthus* (*Bhârgi*) in equal parts is prescribed by several writers. In flatulent colic with costiveness, a suppository made of asafœtida, rock salt and honey and smeared over with clarified butter is introduced into the rectum (Chakradatta).

In hemiplegia, stiff-neck, facial palsy, sciatica and other diseases of the nervous system, fried asafœtida is given along with a compound decoction called *Mâshabalâdi.* A bit of warm asafœtida, placed in the cavity of a carious tooth, is said to relieve pain (Chakradatta).

---

157. FICUS BENGHALENSIS.

(*N. O.*—URTICACEÆ.)

Sans.—Vata. *Eng.*—Banyan tree. *Hind.* and *Ben.*—Bar. *Burm.*—Pyi-nyoung. *Mah.*—Vata-vraksha. *Tel.*—Marichettu, *Tam.* and *Can.*—Alamaram. *Mal.*—Paerâl, Vatam. *Kon.*—Goeli-ruku.

Habitat.—This well-known tree is wild in the Lower Himalaya and is now found all over India.

Properties and Uses.—The milky juice is useful as external application to pains and bruises, in rheumatism and lumbago to the soles of the feet when cracked or inflamed, to the teeth and gums for toothache. Internally it is astringent, useful in dysentery and diarrhœa. An infusion of the bark is a powerful tonic and has specific properties in the treatment of diabetes. A decoction of the bark, which contains about 10 per cent. of tannin, is used as an astringent lotion in leucorrhœa, with advantage. The seeds are cooling and tonic. The leaves are heated and applied as a poultice to abscesses to promote suppuration and discharge of pus. The root-fibres in the form of decoction are supposed to resemble sarsaparilla in action; they are useful in gonorrhœa. The infusion of the small branches is useful in hæmoptysis. The tender ends of the hanging roots are given for obstinate vomiting. The young buds like the milky juice are astringent and useful in cases of dysentery and diarrhœa. The concentrated juice in combination with fruit is an aphrodisiac and also believed to be of much value in spermatorrhœa and gonorrhœa.

---

158. FICUS CARICA.

(*N. O.*—URTICACEÆ.)

Sans.—Anjira. *Eng.*—The Fig tree. *Hind.*, *Ben.*, *Pers.* and *Mah.*—Anjir.

Habitat.—This tree is cultivated throughout India for its fruits. Fresh figs are to be found in all the Indian bazaars.

Properties and Uses.—The figs when ripe contain 60 to 70 per cent. of grape sugar. They are employed medicinally, but are demulcent, emollient, nutritive and laxative. The pulp is occasionally used in the form of a poultice to promote suppuration.

159. FICUS GLOMERATA AND F. RACEMOSA.

(*N. O.*—URTICACEÆ.)

Sans. and *Mah.*—Audumbara. *Eng.*—The Gular Fig or Country Fig tree. *Hind.*—Gular. *Ben.*—Jajnà-dumar. *Tel.*—Attimánu, Moydi. *Tam.*, *Mal.* and *Can.*—Atti. *Kon.*—Rumdi-ruku.

Habitat.—This tree is found in the sub-Himalayan ranges extending to all parts of India.

Properties and Uses.—The bark, leaves and unripe fruit are astringent and used as such externally and internally in dysentery. The fruit is given in aphthous complaints and when boiled in milk it is a good remedy for visceral obstructions. The fruit is said to be efficacious in diabetes. A bath made of the fruit and bark is regarded as a cure for leprosy. The bark is slightly astringent used in the form of fine powder, and, in combination with gingelly oil, it is applied to cancerous affections. The infusion of the bark is given in diabetes, and the young leaves reduced to powder and mixed with honey are administered in bilious affections. The fluid which yields on incision in the root is given as a tonic by Hindu Vaidyans.

160. FICUS RELIGIOSA.

(*N. O.*—URTICACEÆ.)

Sans.—Pippala, Shreevraksha. *Eng.*—The Peepul tree. *Hind.*—Pipal. *Ben.*—Ashwath. *Guz.*—Jàri. *Duk.*—Anipeepul. *Mah.*—Pimpala. *Tel.*—Ravichettu. *Tam.*—Arashamaram. *Can.*—Ashvathamara. *Mal.*—Arayál.

Habitat.—This sacred peepul is a large tree found wild and cultivated in Bengal, Central India and the Lower Himalaya.

Properties and Uses.—The seeds have cooling and laxative properties and are prescribed in the form of electuary and powder. The bark is astringent and is useful in gonorrhœa. The fruit is laxative and helps digestion. It forms a very nutritious food for cattle. The fruit dried and powdered and taken in water for 14 days is said to remove asthma. The leaves of young shoots are used as purgative and are useful in skin diseases. The tender shoots boiled in milk and administered together with a sufficient quantity of sugar added to taste makes a very nutritious and cooling morning drink. The juice is useful in cracked feet. The powder of the dried bark is used in cases of anal fistulæ. The leaves are said to be a food for silkworms. The decoction of the leaves and bark is used for tanning leather.

---

161. FLACOURTIA CATAPHRACTA.

(*N. O.*—FLACOURTIACEÆ.)

Sans., *Tel.*, *Tam.*, *Can.* and *Mal.*—Tâlispatram. *Hind.*—Tâlis patri, Paniâmlak. *Ben.*—Paniyala. *Mah.*—Tâleespatra.

Habitat.—This plant is found in Bengal and on the sea-coasts of India.

Properties and Uses.—The dried leaves are carminative, expectorant, stomachic, tonic and astringent, useful in asthma, bronchitis, phthisis and catarrh of the bladder. The powdered leaves, half to one drachm, are often given along with the juice of the leaves of *Adhatoda vesica* (Malabar Nut tree) and honey and a confection called *Talisadya churna* is prepared from the *Talis-patri* along with pepper, ginger, bamboo-manna, cardamoms, cinnamon and sugar. The juice of the fresh leaves and of their tender stalks is useful in fevers as antiperiodic for infants, the dose being 5 to 10 drops in water or mother's milk; it is also used in affections of the chest, phthisical cough, dysentery, diarrhœa and indigestion caused during dentition. In Bengal it is given as a tonic in parturition.

---

162. GARCINIA MANGOSTANA.

(*N. O.*—GUTTIFERÆ.)

Eng.—The Mangosteen. *Hind.* and *Ben.*—Mangustin. *Bom.*—Mangostin, Mengut. *Mal.*—Manggusta. *Bur.*—Mengkop, Mengut. *Malay.*—Mangusta.

Habitat.—This tree is a native of the Straits Settlement and Singapore, extensively cultivated in British Burma and the Malayan Peninsula and to a certain extent in the Madras Presidency.

Properties and Uses.—The mangosteen fruits, which are largely imported into India, are of the size and shape of a small apple with thick, woody, astringent rind; it is much esteemed as a table fruit in India. The rind contains tannin, resin and a principle named *Mangostin*. The bark of the tree and young leaves are also very astringent. The rind or entire dried fruit are employed as remedies in chronic diarrhœa and dysentery, usually in the form of a syrup, the drug being boiled in water and sugar added to the strained decoction previouly evaporated to a suitable volume. It may also be employed in powder given in doses of 10 to 15 grains in port wine, or made into a paste with a little sugar and, in either form, may be improved by the addition of aromatics. In the Straits Settlement the fruit is regarded as a remedy in gonorrhœa and gleet and is stated to lessen both the irritation and the discharge of matter.

163. GARCINIA PICTORIA.

(*N. O.*—CLUSIACEÆ.)

Eng.—Mysore Gamboge tree. *Tam.*—Mukki. *Can.*—Jorige-huli mara. *Mal.*—Kurukapuli. *Kon.*--Vatamba.

Habitat.—Malabar Coast and Mysore.

Properties and Uses.—The well-known gum resin of this tree which is known as gamboge is a powerful hydragogue cathartic and anthelmintic. It forms an ingredient of most remedies employed for the expulsion of the tapeworm. It is not given *alone* as a purgative on account of its tendency to produce vomiting and griping; in combination with other cathartics it operates more favourably; combined with bitartrate of potash it is useful in dropsical affections; in solution with alkalies it acts as a diuretic. The dose of the powdered gum as a full purgative is from 2 to 6 grains; as an alterative from half a grain up to six grains, of the compound gamboge pill and that of gamboge and scammony the dose is from 5 to 10 grains. For the expulsion of worms, the following is a good formula:—of gamboge 10 grains, sulphate of iron 6 grains, lump sugar 20 grains and oil of peppermint 3 drops and water 3 ounces:—one ounce to be taken every 4 hours until the desired effect is produced.

164. GARCINIA PURPUREA.

(*N. O.*—GUTTIFERÆ.)

Eng.—Mate Mangosteen. *Hind.*—Kokam. *Guz.* and *Mah.*—Kokambel. *Tam.*—Murgal mara. *Can.*—Murginahuli-mara. *Mal.*—Punampuli. *Kon.*—Beerunda.

Habitat.—This tree grows plentifully in the Konkan and Canara districts of Western India.

Properties and Uses.—The seeds yield a concrete oil known as kokum oil or kokum butter. This oil or butter consists chiefly of *tristearin* and is of much use as nutritive, demulcent and emollient; it is useful as an ointment. The fruit has an agreeable acid flavour and is eaten by poorer classes as a substitute for ghee. It has been recommended as a substitute for cod-liver oil. This oil has a healing property and might be usefully employed in such wounds and sores as are accompanied with inflammation.

165. GARDENIA GUMMIFERA & G. LUCIDA.

(*N. O.*—RUBIACEÆ.)

Hind., *Ben.*, *Guz.*, *Mah.* and *Can.*—Dikamali. *Eng.*—Dikamali or Cambi resin. *Tel.*—Tella manga. *Tam.*—Kumbai.

Habitat.—Both these trees are common in many parts of India, particularly in the Central and Southern Provinces.

Properties and Uses.—The resin obtained from these trees is carminative and antispasmodic; externally it is antiseptic and stimulating. It is mostly employed internally in hysteria, flatulent dyspepsia and nervous disorders due to dentition; externally it is applied to foul and callous ulcers and to keep off flies from sores. It is a successful anthelmintic in cases of round worms.

166. GAULTHERIA FRAGRANTISSIMA.

(*N. O.*—ERICACEÆ.)

Eng.—Indian Wintergreen.

Habitat.—This plant is found in the Nilgiris, also in Burma and Ceylon.

Properties and Uses.—The leaves yield a fragrant volatile oil which is practically identical with that of the true wintergreen. It is aromatic, stimulant and carminative, given with success in acute rheumatism and sciatica in doses of 10 minims, gradually increased, in capsules. The oil is also applied externally in liniments or ointments. It has powerful antiseptic properties and may be used in small quantity for preserving vegetable preparations. It is also used as a pleasant flavouring agent, especially for dentifrices.

167. GENDARUSSA VULGARIS.

(*N. O.*—ACANTHACEÆ.)

Sans.—Krishna nirgunda. *Hind.* --Kálà-báshimb. *Tel.*—Nallanochili. *Tam.* and *Mal.*—Karunochbhi. *Can.*—Karinekkigida. *Kon.*—Kalo-negundu.

Habitat.—This plant is to be found chiefly in Canara and Travancore.

Properties and Uses.—The bark is considered a good emetic. The leaves are scattered among clothes to preserve them from insects. The infusion of the leaves is given in fevers; also a bath in which the leaves are saturated is very efficacious in fever cases. The juice of the leaves is administered in coughs of children and the same mixed with oil is a useful embrocation in glandular swellings of the neck and throat; mixed with mustard seed it makes an effective emetic. The leaves and tender stalks put in a bag together with some salt, warmed and applied externally, are useful in diseases of joints, in chronic rheumatism and similar complaints.

168. GENTIANA KURROO.

(*N. O.*—GENTIANACEÆ.)

Eng.—Indian Gentian. *Hind.* and *Ben.*—Karu, Kutki. *Bom.*—Pâshânveda.

Habitat.—This species abounds round Simla, extending to Kashmir at altitudes of 5 to 10 thousand feet.

Properties and Uses.—The root is an efficient substitute for the imported gentian, as it contains the same principles, gentian bitter, gentianic acid, pectin and an uncrystallizable sugar as the European root. It is a valuable bitter tonic, the tincture and infusion corresponding closely to that of the European gentian.

---

169. GLORIOSA SUPERBA.

(*N. O.*—LILIACEÆ.)

Sans.—Lánglikà, Agnisikkâ, Kalikari. *Hind.*—Carihari. *Ben.*—Bishalánguti. *Guz.*—Khadyanag. *Mah.*—Karianag. *Tel.*—Agnishikha, Langali. *Tam.*—Kartikka-kilangu. *Can.*—Nângulika. *Mal.*—Macttoenni, Kandal *Kon.*—Vàgàuànkta.

Habitat.—This elegant climbing plant is common in Bengal and in low jungles throughout India.

Properties and Uses.—The tuberous root is regarded as tonic and stomachic in doses of 5 to 10 grains. . It has been employed as an anthelmintic for cattle. A salt is produced from the root by repeated washing and grinding, throwing away the liquor and washing the residue carefully. The white powder so found is bitter and is given in gonorrhœa up to 12 grains. It is not poisonous. It is alterative, tonic and antiperiodic; in large quantities it might be poisonous. The root powdered and reduced to a paste is applied to the navel, supra-pubic region and vagina with the object of promoting labour pains.

In cases of retained placenta a paste of the root is applied to the palm and soles while powdered nigella seeds and longpepper are given internally with wine.

170. GLYCERRHIZA GLABRA.

(*N. O.*—LEGUMINOSÆ.)

Sans. and *Ben.*—Yashti-madhu. *Eng.*—Liquorice. *Hind.*—Mulhatti. *Guz.* and *Mah.*—Jeshtimadh. *Tel.*—Yashti-madhukam. *Tam.*—Ati-madhuram. *Can.*—Jestamaddu.

Habitat.—This is not indigenous to India but the root is cultivated to some extent around Peshawár, from where it is imported to Bombay. The liquorice root is found in all the bazaars of India.

Properties and Uses.—The root is sweet, demulcent, cooling and useful in inflammatory affections, cough, hoarseness, sorethroat, &c.; it is much used in pharmaceutical preparations as an adjunct; also used for flavouring decoctions, oils and *ghritas*. The liquid extract is specially useful in disguising the taste of nauseous medicines.

171. GMELINA ARBOREA.

(*N. O.*—VERBENACEÆ.)

Sans.—Gandhari, Shripani, Káshmiri. *Hind.*—Kambhar. *Ben.*—Gamari. *Guz.*—Shewan. *Mah.*—Shivanasâl. *Tel.*—Gumar tek. *Tam.*—Gummudu teku. *Can.*—Kâshmiri-mara.

Habitat.—This tree is common on the Lower Himalaya and in the Nilgiris and on the East and West Coasts of India.

Properties and Uses.—The root is an ingredient of the *dasamula*, a compound decoction of ten plants which is in great repute among Hindu physicians. It is a bitter tonic, stomachic and laxative, useful in fever, indigestion, anâsarca, &c. It is used in the form of infusion or weak decoction. The tender leaves are demulcent, used in infusion, in gonorrhœa and catarrh of the bladder. The root, taken with liquorice, honey and sugar increases the secretion of milk. The fruits are sweetish bitter and cooling. They enter into the composition of several cooling and refrigerent decoctions for fever and burning of the body. The following is an example:—Take of the fruits of *Gmelina Arborea, Grewia Asiatica (parushaka)*, liquorice root, red sandal wood and the root of *Andropogon muricatum (ushira)*, equal parts, in all two tolas, water 32 tolas, and boil till reduced to one-half. This decoction is used as a drink in bilious fever.—(*Chakradatta.*)

172. GOSSYPIUM INDICUM.

(*N. O.*—MALVACEÆ.)

Sans.—Anagniká, Karpas. *Eng.*—Indian Cotton plant. *Hind.*—and *Guz.*—Rui. *Ben.*—Kapâs, Tula. *Burm.*—Wah. *Duk.*, *Mah.* and *Kon.*—Kàpus. *Tel.*—Patti. *Tam.*—Partti. *Can.*—Hatti. *Mal.*—Karuparutti.

Habitat.—This is extensively cultivated in India in various species.

Properties and Uses.—In the United States the cotton seed is a popular remedy successfully employed in cases of intermittent fevers. A pound of the seeds is boiled in a quart of water to a pint and a teacupful of the decoction is given to the patient in bed an hour or two before the expected return of the chill. The seeds in the form of emulsion are given in dysentery. They are laxative, demulcent, expectorant and aphrodisiac; as a nervine tonic they are given internally in headache and brain affections; deprived of their outer coat they are powdered and given in milk in doses of two drachms of the powder. Pounded and mixed with ginger and water they are applied to orchitis. The seeds in the form of poultice make a good application to burns and scalds. The oil expressed from the seeds and known as the cotton seed oil is an important vegetable, largely consumed in England and in America; it makes a good liniment in rheumatic affections; it is useful in clearing the skin of spots and freckles. The juice of the leaves is useful in dysentery. A tea or infusion of young leaves is recommended in lax habits and for preparing a vapour bath for the anus in cases of tenesmus. The leaves externally in the form of poultice hasten the maturation of boils, and with oil they are applied as a plaster to gouty joints. The root has emmenagogue properties, useful in dysmenorrhœa and suppression of the menses produced by cold. It may be given in large doses with impunity, especially during the first stage of labour. In Gynæcological practice, gossypium is far better and safer than ergot, since rapidity of action is not so necessary, and, it is said, that it can be given without any unpleasant secondary or after-effects, frequently complained of during a prolonged course of ergot subcutaneously or per os. In cases of dysmenorrhœa and suppression of the menses due to cold, a decoction of 4 ounces of the bark in two pints of water boiled down to one pint, may be used in doses of two ounces every twenty to thirty minutes or the fluid extract in doses of half to one drachm. A syrup of the flowers is useful in hypochondriasis on account of its stimulating and exhilarating effect. A poultice made of them is applied to burns and scalds. The young fruit is given to check dysentery. The cotton wool is a filterer of atmospheric germs, preventing their access to wounds, cavities of the nose, ear &c. It is used in the preparation of gun-cotton or pyroxyllin which, in turn, is the source of collodion.

173. GREWIA ASIATICA.

(*N. O.*—TILIACEÆ.)

Sans.—Parush. *Hind.* and *Ben.*—Phalsá. *Guz.*—Phalsa. *Mah.*—Phalasi. *Tel.*—Pitiki.

Habitat.—This tree is found throughout India, chiefly cultivated for its fruit.

Properties and Uses.—The small acid fruit is much esteemed by the people. A *sherbat* is prepared from it and a spirit is also distilled after fermentation. The fruit is one of the *phala-traya* or fruit-triad of Sanskrit writers and possesses astringent and cooling properties. The bark contains a mucilaginous juice and the infusion is used as a demulcent.

174. GUIZOTIA ABYSSYNICA.

(*N. O.*—COMPOSITÆ.)

Eng.—Niger seed, Kersani seed. *Hind.*—Kala-til. *Ben.*—Râm-til, Surguja. *Mah.* and *Guz.*—Kesani, Kersani. *Tel.*—Valesulu. *Tam.*—Kàttellu. *Can.*—Kâdellu.

Habitat.—This annual herbaceous plant is cultivated in many parts of India, chiefly in Bengal, Bombay and the Deccan.

Properties and Uses.—The oil expressed from the seeds is employed in cooking and for anointing the body and it may be used in place of sessamum or olive oils. It is frequently employed in India as an adulterant of more valuable oils.

175. GYMNEMA SYLVESTRE.

(*N. O.*—ASCLEPIADEÆ.)

Sans,—Meshasringi. *Hind.* and *Ben.*—Mera-singi. *Guz.* and *Mah.*—Kavali. *Tel.*—Boda-patra. *Tam.*—Shiru kurunja.

Habitat.—A shrubby climbing plant common in Central and Southern India and on the Western side, plentiful about Bombay.

Properties and Uses.—The root has long been held in great repute by the Hindus as a remedy for snake-bite, the powder being dusted upon the wound and a decoction given internally. The leaves, when chewed, deaden the sense of taste. They contain a glucoside named *Gymnemic acid*, of which it forms about six per cent., combined with an inorganic base. It is related in some particulars to glycerrhizic acid, but has some distinctly peculiar reactions and has the anti-saccharine property ascribed to it. Tartaric acid and a neutral principle were also found to be present.

---

176. GYNANDROPSIS PENTAPHYLLA.

(*N. O.*—CAPPARIDEÆ.)

Sans.—Arkapushpika, Surjavarta.. *Eng.*—Caravella seeds. *Hind.*—Hurhur. *Ben.*—Hurhuria, Sàdâ-hurhuria. *Mah.*—Hulhul. *Tel.*—Velakura. *Tam*'—Velai. *Can.*—Shrikâla. *Mal.*—Kârvela.

Habitat.—This annual plant, common on cultivated ground, is met with in the warmer parts of India.

Properties and Uses.—The small kidney-shaped black seeds resemble those of *Cleome Viscosa.* The whole plant has an odour somewhat resembling black currant leaf, and when crushed in the fresh state yields an acrid essential oil resembling that of garlic or mustard. The powdered seeds, in doses of 30 grains to one drachm, are anthelmintic and administered internally, for the expulsion of round worms, combined with sugar, twice daily for two days and followed on the third morning by a dose of castor oil. They have also great antispasmodic virtues and are useful in cases of sprains, &c; bruised with vinegar, lime-juice or hot water, they can be made into a plaster or poultice, which forms a useful application externally. Bruised leaves are rubefacient and also vesicant, producing much serous exudation. The juice of the leaves is used occasionally as an anodyne instillation for the relief of otalgia and catarrhal inflammations of the middle ear; but it produces a burning sensation. The leaves are applied externally to boils to prevent the formation of pus.

---

177. GYNOCARDIA ODORATA.

(N. O.—BIXINEÆ.)

Eng., Hind., Ben. and *Bom.*—Chaulmugra. *Pers.*—Birinjmogra.

Habitat.—This evergreen tree grows on the Lower Himalaya, abounds in Sikkim, extending to Rangoon and Chittagong.

Properties and Uses.—The seeds of the fruit yield on expression a fixed oil to the extent of about 30 to 35 per cent., which is of a light brown colour when fresh, and of a peculiar odour. Chaulmugra oil, as obtained in the bazaars, is of a more or less dark colour, thick, obtained by hot expression and usually adulterated. The oil is in great repute in India as a remedy for leprosy; it has also been advantageously administered in scrofula, skin diseases and chronic rheumatism. The dose of the seeds coarsely powdered is about six grains thrice daily, in the form of pill, gradually increased to three or four times that amount or until it causes nausea, when the dose should be diminished or the use of the remedy suspended for a time. This is the best form of administration. The dose of the oil is from five to six drops *gradually* increased to thirty minims, given in emulsion or in milk or cod-liver oil, preferably in capsules. During its use it is advisable to avoid all salt meats, acids, spices and sweetmeats; on the other hand its operation is aided by butter, ghee and oily articles of diet. It has been successfully given in phthisis, and also applied externally to the chest. The *gynocardic acid*, which is its active constituent, is given in doses of ¼ to ½ grain. Magnesium gynocardate has been tried with some success in leprosy and is said to agree better than the oil. The action of the oil in leprosy, though believed to be, at the best, palliative, is nevertheless more marked than that of gurjun oil, as the prolonged and regular use of the oil might surely arrest the progress of the disease. The seeds of the allied *Hydrocarpus Inebrians* (*Gardapal*) yield an oil on expression, which is known as *Kavatel* (*Tel.*—Niradivittulu. *Tam.*—Neradimuttu) and used as a substitute for chaulmugra oil in leprosy in Malabar, the dose being half a tea-spoonful twice daily.

178. HELIANTHUS ANNUSES.

(*N. O.*—COMPOSITÆ.)

Sans., *Hind.*, and *Ben.*—Suriya-mukhi. *Eng.*—Sunflower. *Pers.*—Guli-aftab. *Tel.*, *Tam.* and *Can.*—Surya-kânti.

Habitat.—This annual plant with its large, coarse yellow flowers is common in Indian gardens.

Properties and Uses.—This plant is purposely grown and cultivated in gardens in swampy and malarious districts, as its presence is said to be efficient in purifying the air and removing malaria. The seeds yield on expression an oil which is equal to olive or almond oil for culinary and table purposes. It is also employed in industrial purposes such as for woollen dressing, for candle and soap-making, for which it is said to be superior to most other oils. In the form of oil-cake it is a valuable food for cattle and poultry.

179. HELICTERES ISORA.

(*N. O.*—STERCULIACEÆ.)

Sans.—Avatarni. *Eng.*—The Indian screw tree. *Hind.*—Morarphali. *Ben.*—Antmorà. *Pers.*—Kist-bar-kisht. *Guz.*—Mrigashinga. *Tel.*, *Tam.* and *Mal.*—Valumbari. *Can.*—Bhoothakaralu.

Habitat.—This shrub is common in Central and Western India.

Properties and Uses.—The fruits consist of spirally twisted carpels which form a very popular medicine. They are employed chiefly in intestinal disturbances such as colic, &c. The juice of the root-bark is a good remedy in disorders of the stomach. The seeds powdered and mixed with pure castor oil forms an excellent application in otorrhœa, ulcers in the ear, &c.

180. HELIOTROPIUM INDICUM.

(*N. O.*—BORAGINEÆ.)

Sans.—Hastisbundà, Nakràri. *Eng.*—Heliotrope. *Hind.*—Hatta-juri. *Ben.*—Hattisura. *Tel.*—Gurugu. *Tam.*—Nakkipoo. *Can.*—Chalukondee. *Mal.*—Telkata, Væenapacha.

Habitat.—A small fragrant plant, common in many parts of India.

Properties and Uses.—The juice of the leaves is used as an application to wounds and sores, to boils and to the bites of scorpions and stings of insects.

181. HELLEBORUS NIGER.

(*N. O.*—RANUNCULACEÆ.)

Sans.—Katuki, Katurohini. *Eng.*—Hellebore. *Hind.*—Kalikatuki. *Mah.*—Bálakadu. *Tel.*, *Can.* and *Mal.*—Katukarohini. *Tam.*—Katurohini.

Habitat.—This plant is to be found plentifully on the Ghauts and in the hilly districts of India.

Properties and Uses.—The root of this plant is a hydragogue cathartic, producing watery motions; it is also emmenagogue and anthelmintic. Formerly it was in high esteem and employed in apoplexy, amenorrhœa, epilepsy, dropsy, hypochondriosis, mania, melancholia and chronic skin affections and worms. It is now seldom prescribed, except under great care, as it is in large doses an acro-narcotic poison. The dose of the powdered root or of the extract is from 5 to 10 grains; and of the tincture, one drachm.

Kálikatuki is used chiefly as a bitter and antiperiodic for children, as its name *Bálkadu* indicates. It is not believed to have any drastic purgative properties by Hindu Vaidyans; if at all, very mild properties of this nature

182. HEMIDESMUS INDICUS.

(*N. O.*—ASCLEPIADEÆ.)

Sans., *Ben.* and *Punj.*—Anantamul. *Eng.*—Indian Sarsaparilla. *Hind.*—Magrabu, Hindi sâlsâ. *Mah.*—Anantâmul, Upasâra. *Pers.*—Aushbahe-hindi. *Tel.*—Sugandhipál. *Tam.* and *Mal.*—Nannâri-ver. *Can.*—Nâmada-beru. *Kon.*—Dudváli. *Cing.*—Irimusu.

Habitat.—This climbing plant is found plentifully throughout Northern India, common in Bengal and extending to Travancore and Ceylon.

Properties and Uses.—The fragrant root-barks of this plant possess demulcent, alterative tonic properties and are, therefore, prescribed in dyspepsia, loss of appetite. fever, skin diseases and ulcerations, especially those of syphilitic origin, constitutional syphilis, chronic rheumatism and leucorrhœa. The hemidesmus root powdered and mixed with cow's milk is given with much benefit in cases of gravel and strangury ; it is also given in infusion or decoction with or without cummin seeds, in two to three ounce doses thrice daily. It is said to purify the blood and correct the acrimony of the bile. It is also said to possess the sudorific and alterative properties of sarsaparilla and therefore useful in affections of the mucous membrane generally. In the form of syrup it has demulcent and diuretic properties. The root, roasted in plantain leaves, then beaten into a mass with cummin and sugar and mixed with ghee is a household remedy in genito-urinary diseases. The hot infusion of the root-bark with milk and sugar is a good alterative tonic especially for children in cases of chronic cough and diarrhœa. The root is generally used in combination with a number of other medicines.

Native Indian Preparations.—Take of *Anantamul*, root of *Pavonia odorata* (Bâlâ), tubers of *Cyperus rotundus* (*Mustaka*), ginger and the root of *Picrorrhiza kurroa* (*Katuki*), equal parts, in all two tolas, and reduce them to a paste with water. This dose, administered with warm water in the morning, is said to clear the bowels and relieve fever (Bhaishajyaratnavali).

A decoction of the roots of colocynth, *anantamul*, *sârivâ* and *Hedyotis biflora* (*Parpârta*) prepared in the usual way is administered, with the addition of powdered long-pepper and bdellium (*guggula*), in chronic skin diseases, syphilis, elephantiasis, loss of sensation and hemiplegia (Sharangadhara).

183. HERPESTIS MONNIERA.

(N. O.—SCROPHULARINEÆ.)

Sans.—Brahmi, Manduki. *Eng.*—Thyme-leaved Gratiola. *Hind.*—Barambhi, Safed-Kammi. *Ben.*, *Can.* and *Kon.*—Brahmi. *Mah.*—Báma. *Tel.*—Sâmbràni chettu. *Tam.*—Neerpirami. *Mal.* and *Can.*—Neerbrahmi.

Habitat.—This small annual creeping plant is found in the tropical regions all over the world.

Properties and Uses.—The whole plant including the root is employed medicinally. It is considered a nervine tonic, useful in insanity and epilepsy. Half a tola of the fresh juice of the leaves with two scruples of *pachak* root and honey is given in insanity. The leaves fried in clarified butter are taken to relieve hoarseness. The leaves and stalks are diuretic and aperient, particularly useful in that stoppage of urine which is accompanied by obstinate costiveness. A poultice made of the boiled plant is placed on the chest in coughs of children.

Native Indian Preparations.—A powder composed of equal parts of *brahmi*, Acorus calamus (*vachá*), chebulic myrobalan, root of Justicia adhatoda (*vásaka*) and long pepper is given with honey in the hoarseness of phthisis (Bhavaprakasa).

Brahmi ghrita: Take of old clarified butter four seers, fresh juice of *brahmi* four seers, Acorus calamus (*vacha*), *páchak* root and the root of *Canscora decussata* (*sankhapushpi*), equal parts, in all thirty-two tolas, in the form of a paste and boil them together till the watery portion is evaporated. This is used in insanity, epilepsy and hoarseness.

---

184. HIBISCUS ABELMOSCHUS.

(*N. O.*—MALVACEÆ.)

Sans.—Latàkasturikâ. *Eng.*—The Musk-mallow. *Hind.* and *Ben.*—Mushk-dána, Kasturi-dana. *Pers.*—Makstàn. *Tel.*—Kastoori-benda. *Bom.*—Mishkadána. *Mal.*—Kàtta-kasturi. *Tam.*—Vattilai-kasturi. *Can.*—Kadu-kasturi.

Habitat.—A herbaceous annual grown in many parts of India for its fibre, common in Bengal and found in most tropical regions.

Properties and Uses.—The seeds are medicinally stimulant, aromatic, tonic, carminative and antispasmodic, useful in nervous debility, hysteria and other nervous disorders, atonic dyspepsia and a few other conditions in which musk is indicated. The best efficacious method of using the drug is as a tincture which is given in 1 to 2 drachm doses. The scented seeds are used to some extent in perfuming medicinal oils. They enter into the composition of some compound prescriptions being regarded as cooling, emollient and demulcent. They are used as a drink in fevers, gonorrhœa &c., and as an inhalation in hoarseness, and dryness of the throat.

---

185. HIBISCUS ESCULENTUS.

(*N. O.*—MALVACEÆ.)

Sans.—Tindisha, Pàtali, Gandhamuia. *Eng.*—The Edible Hibiscus, Okra. *Hind.*—Bhendi, Rämturai. *Duk.* and *Punj.*—Bhandi. *Ben.*—Dheras. *Mah.*—Bhenda. *Guz.*—Bhinda. *Pers.*—Babniyáh. *Tel.*—Bendakäya. *Tam.*—Vendaikkäy. *Mal.*—Venda. *Can.*—Bendekäyi. *Cing.*—Bandakâ. *Burm.*—Youn-padi-si. *Malay.*—Kachang-lindir.

Habitat.—This tall herbaceous annual is naturalised in all tropical countries. It is much esteemed in India for its fruit, which is known as "ladies' fingers" and largely used both by Europeans and Indians.

Properties and Uses.—This well-known plant abounds in a copious bland viscid mucilage which consists chiefly of pectin and starch and possesses valuable emollient, demulcent and diuretic properties. The decoction prepared by boiling three ounces of the fresh capsules cut transversely in a pint and a half of water for twenty minutes, straining and sweetening to taste, is an agreeable drink, most serviceable in fevers, catarrhal attacks, irritable states of the genito-urinary organs, such as dysuria, gonorrhœa, leucorrhœa and in all cases attended with scalding pain and difficulty in passing urine. In dysentery, especially in the chronic form, the bland mucilage is often most beneficial. It is generally given in the form of soup. The mucilage, in which the whole plant abounds, is considered to have aphrodisiac effect. The tender pods are eaten in cases of spermatorrhœa. The mucilage from the fruit and seeds or the fresh capsules bruised form an efficient emollient poultice.

186. HIBISCUS ROSA SINENSIS.

(*N. O.*—MALVACEÆ.)

Sans.—Japa, Rudrapushpa. *Eng.*—China Rose or Shoe-flower plant. *Hind.*—Jasut. *Ben.*—Jaba. *Mah.*—Jasavanda. *Tel.*—Dâsanachettu. *Tam.*—Shamberattai. *Mal.*—Champarutti. *Can.*—Dâsanige.

Habitat.—This is very common in flower-gardens of India.

Properties and Uses.—The flowers of this plant are emollient and demulcent; fried in ghee, they are given in menorrhagia; the dark-red petals are demulcent, administered in the form of infusion in ardor-urinæ, strangury and irritable conditions of the genito-urinary tract; it is also a refrigerent drink in fevers. The seeds pounded into a pulp and mixed with water are given with much benefit in gonorrhœa. An oil made by mixing the juice of the fresh petals and olive oil in equal proportions and boiling till the water has evaporated is useful as a stimulating application for the hair.

---

187. HIBISCUS SABDARIFFA.

(*N. O.*—MALVACEÆ.)

Eng.—Roselle, Red Sorrel. *Hind.*, *Guz.* and *Mah.*—Làl-ambâri. *Ben.*—Mesta, Patwa. *Tel.*—Seemagogu, Erragonkáya. *Tam.*—Shivappukâychurai. *Mal.*—Pulicheera. *Can.*—Pundisoppu.

Habitat.—This plant is largely cultivated for its fibre in many parts of India.

Properties and Uses.—The emollient and demulcent qualities common to the *Malvaceæ* are present in this plant also, but are combined with a certain amount of acidity which stimulates and, at the same time, neutralises the bilious secretion and thus prevents oppression of the stomach during the administration of the mucilaginous decoction; a decoction of the seeds, in doses of 1 to 2 drachms three or four times a day, is useful in cases of dysuria and strangury and in some mild forms of dyspepsia and debility. The fruit has valuable antiscorbutic properties. From it or rather succulent calyx, a drink useful in biliousness may be prepared by boiling it with water and adding a little salt, pepper, asafœtida and molasses. For convalescence and in mild cases of fever it forms an acid refreshing drink.

---

188. HOLARRHENA ANTIDYSENTERICA.

(*N. O.*—APOCYNACEÆ.)

Sans.—Kutaja, Kalinga. *Eng.*—The Kurchi, Conessi or Tellicherry Bark. *Hind.*—Karchi, Kureyâ, Dudhi. *Ben.*—Kurchi. *Pers.*—Indar-javitalkh. *Bom.*—Pandhra-kura. *Tel.*—Kâkakodise, Kolamukki, Iudravrakshamu. *Tam.*—Veppalai. *Can.*—Korasi-gina-gida.

(The seeds): *Sans.*—Indrayava. *Hind.* and *Ben.*—Indrajab, Tita-indrajao. *Bom.*—Kurvà-indrajoa. *Tam.*—Kuluppalai-virai.

Habitat.—This small tree is common in the forests of India, indigenous to the tropical Himalaya.

Properties and Uses.—The bark of the stem and root, preferably of the young plants and the seeds, are well known as remedies in acute and chronic diarrhœa and dysentery. The bark contains an alkaloidal principle which has been named *Conesseine* and *Kurchiene* and which has been employed medicinally. The bark has astringent, anti-dysenteric, febrifuge and anthelmintic properties. It is used in the form of powder; other preparations are the solid and liquid extracts and the decoction.

---

189. HONEY—(Mel).

Sans. and *Ben.*—Madhu. *Hind.*, *Guz.* and *Mah.*—Madh. *Duk.*—Shapad. *Punj.*—Shad. *Pers.*—Angabin. *Arab.*—Aasl. *Kash.*—Mhách. *Tel.*—Téne. *Tam.* and *Mal.*—Tén. *Can.*—Jénu. *Cing.*—Piyáye. *Malay.*—Ayer-madu.

Properties and Uses.—Honey is a saccharine vegetable juice collected by the honey bee (*Apis mellifica*) and other species belonging to the insect order *Hymenoptera.* It occurs chiefly in the nectaries of many species of flowers which the bee collects and deposits in the honey-comb prepared from waxy substances elaborated within the body of the insect and collected from the surface of leaves. There are various sorts of honey as collected by different species of bees and from different kinds of flowers. But the one that is collected by the common bee called *Madhumakshiká* is the honey that is used in medicine. It is nutritious and demulcent. It is also a very useful laxative, especially for children, who take it readily. It has been a favourite vehicle for the administration of medicines such as powders, pills, &c., intended for children. It is used as a flavouring and sweetening agent in mixtures and as a basis for confections. When mixed with vinegar it forms oxymel, very useful in some forms of catarrh and cough; it may be used either alone or combined with other medicines. A mixture of equal parts of honey and distilled vinegar or lime-juice melted together by gentle heat is an excellent adjunct to cough mixtures, and in the coughs of childhood this combination, diluted with an equal quantity of water and with or without a few drops of Paregoric, forms a useful and pleasant mixture, which children will readily take. An ounce of yellow wax melted together with four ounces of clarified honey and strained forms what is termed '*Ceromel,*' which is an excellent stimulant application for indolent and other ulcerations. It is admirably adapted for use in hot climates, where animal fats, which form the basis of so many ointments, soon become rancid and unfit for medicinal use.

---

190. HORDEUM VULGARE.

(*N. O.*—GRAMINEÆ.)

Sans.—Yava. *Eng.*—Barley. *Hind.*—Jav, Jaoa. *Ben.*—Jab. *Pers.*—Jao. *Tel.*--Pachcha yavalu. *Tam.*—Barlhi arisi. *Mah.*, *Kon.* and *Guz.*—Bâjri. *Can.*—Javegodi.

Habitat.—This cereal is largely cultivated in several varieties in each of the provinces of India.

Properties and Uses.—Barley contains starch and nutritive constituents resembling those of wheat and in addition 3 per cent. of fixed oil. It contains a large amount of nitrogenous matter which makes it specially suitable as invalid's food in the form of powder. Barley is very nutriticus and demulcent. The partially germinated and dried grain is the source of malt extract which is more nutritious and demulcent than the unmalted barley. Malt extract consists chiefly of dextrin and malt sugar (maltose) and contains the ferment diastase which is developed during the malting process and which possesses the power of converting starch into dextrin and sugar, thus assisting in the digestion of starchy or farinaceous foods. It is a valuable vehicle for other medicines, especially cod-liver oil, with which it forms a palatable combination.

The decoction of barley (made by boiling 2½ ounces of pearl barley in 4 pints of water down to two pints and strained) is an agreeable demulcent in affections of the mucous membrane and an excellent diluent drink in fevers. It may be rendered more pleasant and useful as a fever drink by the addition of sugar and a few slices of lemon. If a laxative is required the compound decoction, prepared as follows, may be given : Sliced figs and stoned raisins, of each 2½ ounces; bruised liquorice root 4 drachms; water 1 pint; barley, as above, 2 pints; boil down to a quart and strain. The demulcent properties of either of the above formulas may be increased by the addition of an ounce of gum arabic to each pint of the liquor. As a food for infants brought up by hand, simple barley water and milk, equal proportions, sweetened with a little refined sugar, has been recommended; care should be taken to stop it if the bowels should become relaxed with this diet. A barley pudding good for invalids may be made as follows: Add to four table-spoonfuls of Robinson's Prepared Barley, sufficient cold milk to form a thin paste, pour on it a quart of boiling milk, then add a little of butter, a table-spoonful of powdered lump sugar, sufficient lemon peel to flavour it, and two eggs previously well beaten up; mix well and let the whole bake for an hour and a half in a slow oven. This is very nutritious and easy of digestion; it may be rendered more palatable to some by the addition of a slice or two of lemon.

191. HYDRARGYRUM.

Sans.—Rasa, Pârada. *Eng.*—Mercury. *Hind.*, *Ben.* and ***Mah.***—Pârâ. *Can.*—Pâdrasa. *Tel.*—Pâdarasam. *Tam.*—Rasa.

Properties and Uses.—Compounds of mercury have been in use among Hindus for many centuries, chiefly for the same diseases as those for which they are employed in modern medicine. The preparations now in use among *Vaidyans* and *Hakims* are:—Calomel (*Rasa-karpura*) Cinnaber (*Hingula*) and the Black Sulphide (*Kajjali*). Four preparations of mercury are described in Sanskrit books, namely black, white, yellow and red, called respectively *Krishna*, *Sveta*, *Pita* and *Rakta* bhasmas. The black preparation is the Black Sulphide. The white preparation is the *Rasa-karpura* or Perchloride of Mercury. The yellow preparation called *Pita bhasma* is prepared as follows:—Take of mercury and sulphur equal parts, rub them together for seven days with the juice of *Bhumyámálaki* (*Phyllanthus neruri*) and *Hastisundi* (*Heliotropium Indicum*). Place the mixture in a covered crucible and heat it in a sand-bath for twelve hours. The result will be a yellow compound. The red preparation, called *Rakta bhasma* or *Rasa sindura*, is prepared in a variety of ways. The following is one of them:—Take of mercury and sulphur equal parts, rub together with the juice of the red buds of *Ficus Bengalensis* (*Vata*) for three days successively, introduce the mixture within a bottle and heat it in a sand-bath for twelve hours. A red deposit will adhere below the neck of the bottle. It is taken out in the shape of dark-red shining scales.

Of these four preparations, three are sulphides, the black, the yellow and the red; of these the yellow preparation is not in use. The red and black preparations are largely used. The four preparations, namely, Cinnaber, the Black Sulphide called *Kajjali*, the red preparation called *Rasa sindura*, and the *Rasa-karpura* of the bazaar are the four principal forms in which mercury is used in Hindu medicine; that is, they constitute the basis of all the formulæ containing mercury. The medicinal uses of the mercurials are generally alterative tonic. Combined with other appropriate medicines, mercurial preparations cure a host of diseases, act as powerful tonics and improve the vision and complexion.

Native Indian Preparations:—In fevers of all descriptions, mercury is extensively used in combination with aconite, croton seed, *datura* and other medicines. The following are a few examples :—

Hingulesvara pills made up of cinnabar, aconite and long-pepper in equal parts rubbed together and made into pills of 4 grains each. They are given beaten up with a little honey in ordinary remittent fever (Bhaishajya-ratnavali). *Taruna Jvrari* are pills of 4 grains each, composed of mercury, sulphur, aconite and croton seeds, equal parts rubbed together with the juice of *Aloe Indica*. They act on the bowels and relieve fever. They are administered with sugar and water (Bhaishajyaratnavali).

In diarrhœa and dysentery mercury is used in a great variety of forms : – *Vajrakapáta-rasa* are pills of six grains, containing mercury, sulphur, opium, *mocharasa* (gum of *Bombax Malabaricum*), the three myrobalans, ginger, black-pepper and long-pepper, all in powder and equal parts, mixed together after soaking the powder seven times in the juices of the leaves of *Cannabis sativa* (*Vijaya*) and *Verbesina calendulacea* (*Bhringaraja*). Dose is from four to twenty-four grains, administered with honey in obstinate chronic diarrhœa (Bhaishajyaratnavali).

Rasa-parpati is the black sulphide of mercury obtained in the shape of round disks, prepared by melting together a mixture of equal parts of sulphur and mercury in an iron ladle, smeared with *ghee* (clarified butter). It is used alone or with the addition of other medicines in chronic diarrhœa. Other varieties of *parpati* or mercurial preparations in shape of disks are prepared with the addition of iron, gold, copper, etc.; and used in this complaint, as, for example, *Svarna parpati*, *Panchamrita parpati*, etc.

Panchámrita parpati is made up of sulphur 8 tolas, mercury 4 tolas, prepared iron 2 tolas, prepared talc 1 tola, prepared copper half a tola, all rubbed together in an iron mortar, melted in an iron ladle and prepared in disks like those of *Rasa-parpati*. Dose is 4 grains with honey and ghee, gradually increased to 16 or 18 grains. *Parpatis* of different sorts when given in cases of diarrhœa with anasarca are conjoined with a milk diet, *water and salt being prohibited* (Bhaishajyaratnavali).

Mahagandha-rasa is also a sulphide of mercury made into a *parpati*, with the addition of mace, cloves, nutmegs and *nim* leaves. It is administered in doses of about 4 grains in the acute diarrhœa of children (Rasendrasarsangraha). *Pándusudana-rasa* is a mixture of mercury, sulphur, prepared copper, croton seeds and bdellium in equal parts, rubbed together with ghee and made into two grain pills. They are given with the juice of *nim* leaves and honey in jaundice. Acids and cold water for drinking should be avoided.

In affections of the lungs mercury is used in a variety of combinations, of which the following are a few examples:—*Rasendra gutika*, which is prepared thus:—Take of purified mercury 2 tolas. Add to it 1 tola of the juice of *Jayanti* leaves (*Sesbania Aegyptica*) and of fresh ginger, rub together till the mixture thickens, then soak it in the juice of *Jussiœa repens* (*Kanchata*) and *Solanum Indicum* (*Vrihati*) respectively for 24 hours. Take of purified sulphur 8 tolas and soak in the juice of *Verbesina calendulacea* (*Bhringarája*). When dry, mix the sulphur with the mercury and rub together with sixteen tolas of goat-milk till the mass is fit for being made into pills. Dose is about four grains, to be taken with goat-milk and juice of ginger. This pill is useful in bronchitis and cough generally (Chakra). *Rájamrigánka rasa* is a mixture of *Rasa sindura* (red sulphide of mercury), prepared gold and copper, realgar, orpiment and sulphur in various proportions. Dose is about 4 grains with 2 grains each of long and black pepper, honey and clarified butter. It is said to be useful in phthisis and chronic bronchitis with fever (Bhaishajya-ratnavali).

In diseases of the nervous system, several combinations of mercury with gold, iron, talc, &c., are used, such as, the *Chaturmukha rasa*, *Chintámani chaturmukha*, *Yogendra rasa*, &c. They are all similar in composition with but slight variation in the proportions of the active ingredients and their adjuncts. *Chintámani chaturmukha* is a preparation containing the red sulphide of mercury, prepared talc, prepared iron, and prepared gold in proportion of two, two, one and half tola respectively, all rubbed together with the juice *of Aloe Indica* and made into two grain pills. This medicine is said to be useful in nervous diseases, insanity, cephalalgia, deafness, noise in the ears, paralysis of the tongue, diseases of the female and urinary organs, phthisis, fever, etc. It improves nutrition, increases the appetite and strength and brightens the complexion.

Two other preparations containing *Rasa sindura* are *Shadguna Balijárita Rasa sindura* and *Svarna sindura*. *Shadguna Balijárita Rasa sindura* is thus prepared: Take of mercury and sulphur in equal parts and prepare *Rasa sindura*, as already described, by sublimation in a glass bottle. On the second day mix this *Rasa sindura* with an equal quantity of sulphur and again sublime the compound. Repeat the process in this way six times. This preparation is considered superior to the ordinary *Rasa sindura*.

Svarna sindura is thus prepared:—Take of fine leaf gold one tola, purified mercury 8 tolas, mix together by rubbing in a mortar, add 12 tolas of sulphur and again rub together, till the mass is of a dark colour. Sublime in a glass bottle on the sand bath.

The three forms of *Rasa sindura* above mentioned are said to cure all sorts of diseases, but are particularly used in chronic fever, catarrh and cough of children, mental and bodily debility, anæmia, &c.

Mercury is used in syphilis both externally and internally. The following is one of the preparations used in this disease:—

Saptasâli vati:—Take of mercury and catechu each half a tola, pellitory root one tola, honey one and a half tola. Rub together till the globules of mercury disappear, and divide into seven pills or boluses. One pill is administered every morning with water in primary syphilis. Acids and salt should not be taken after the use of this medicine.

13

For external application about a drachm of mercury is recommended to be rubbed between the palms with the juice of the leaves of *Sida cordifolia* (*Bátyálaka*) till the globules of mercury are no longer visible. The palms are then to be warmed over the fire till perspiration breaks out from them (Bhavaprakash).

For fumigation in primary syphilis, about half a drachm of the black sulphide mixed with one-fourth part of wheat flour is employed daily for seven days in succession (Bhavaprakash).

In secondary syphilitic eruptions the following composition is used for fumigation: Take of cinnabar one tola, realgar half a tola, powder and mix. About 15 grains of this is used at a time. Powders for fumigation are heated over a fire of jujube tree wood and the vapour is applied to the skin under cover in a closed room.

Mercury enters into the composition of several applications for skin diseases, as in the following:—Take of cinnabar, sulphur, red oxide of lead, rock salt, seeds of *Cassia tora* (*Chakramarda*), *Baberung*, *Cleome felina* (*Svarnakshiri*) and the root of *Aplotaxis auriculata* (*Kushta*) in equal parts. Powder them and reduce to a thin paste with the juice of *datura*, *nim* or betel leaves. This application is said to cure ringworm, eczema, prurigo, psoriasis, &c. (Sarangadhara).

For lice in the hair, mercury rubbed with *datura* or betel leaf is recommended to be applied to the scalp (Chakra).

---

192. HYDROCOTYLE ASIATICA.

(N. O.—UMBELLIFERÆ.)

Sans.—Mandukaparni. *Eng.*—Indian penny wort. *Hind.* and *Duk.*—Vallári, Brahmamanduki. *Ben.*—Tholkuri. *Guz.*—Karinga. *Mah.* and *Kon.*—Brahmi, Ekpânni. *Tel.*—Manduka or Brahmichettu. *Tam.*—Vellärai. *Mal.*—Kutakam, Kodogam. *Can.*—Vondelaga. *Cing.*—Hingotu-kola. *Burm.*—Minkhua-bin. *Malay.*—Dawoon-pŭnga-gah.

Habitat.—This small weed is common all over India, growing plentifully in moist localities.

Properties and Uses.—The whole plant is used medicinally. It is a valuable alterative tonic and reliable local stimulant. As an internal and external remedy in ulcerations, chronic and obstinate eczema, leprosy and other cutaneous affections, such as chronic and callous ulcers, scrofulous ulceration, syphilis accompanied by gummatous infiltration and ulceration, enlargement of glands, in abscess and in chronic rheumatism, its efficacy has been highly valued, and as a stimulant to healthy mucous secretion in infantile diarrhœa and ozœna and as emmenagouge in amenorrhœa it has been successfully employed. For internal administration, the powder of the leaves, the fluid extract of the fresh plant and the syrup are suitable, and for external application are employed the powder, the plaster, the ointment and the bath. In elephantiasis, enlarged scrotum and affections of the cellular tissues the ointment prepared with lanoline or vaseline containing one drachm of the liquid extract or the powder in each ounce, is an external application, while internally the liquid extract, 1 to 5 drops thrice daily, will be found to check the periodic fever associated with these affections and known as 'moon-fever' in India. For leprous, scrofulous and syphilitic affections and ulcerations, the powder, in 3 to 5 grain doses, may be given thrice daily; at the same time some of the powder may be sprinkled on the ulcers or, which is better, poultices made of the fresh leaves bruised into a paste may be applied. As a remedy for leprosy it has considerable repute. Under its use the patient, in the course of a few weeks, improves in all respects. After continuing its use for some time this remedy causes great itching of the skin over the whole body; it should then be discontinued for a week, aperients administered and the medicine recommenced. Though it may not effect a cure it often does a great deal of good.

Of the whole plant, the root is believed to be the most active part. The constituents are oily and resinous together with mucilaginous principles and tannin. They have been collectively named *Vellarin*, which is the active principle of the plant.

The preparations in use of the plant are:—(1) The powder of the leaves, which is prepared as follows: The leaves are carefully separated as soon as possible after the plant is gathered, spread on a mat in the shade and then freely exposed to the air, but not to the sun nor heat, as it takes away all its virtues. They lose about nine-tenths of weight by drying. When thoroughly dried they should be finely powdered and kept in well-corked or stoppered bottles. Of this powder the dose is from 3 to 5 grains thrice daily. (2) The plaster or poultice prepared from the fresh leaves by trituration with *cold* water in a mortar to make it a thick paste; it is a stimulating application. (3) Syrup prepared from 90 grammes of powder, boiled in a quart of water till reduced to a pint, to which add 2 lbs.

of sugar and thoroughly mix at 31° C. till a syrup is formed : dose is 1 drachm, gradually increased. (4) Fluid extract of the fresh plant—one ounce of the extract representing one ounce of the powder: dose is 1 to 5 minims, gradually increased to 15 minims. (5) Ointment—4 grammes of the powder mixed with 30 grammes of vaseline or lanoline. (6) Decoction prepared from 30 grammes of the dried plant to one pint of water. (7) Bath (in skin diseases)—1,500 grammes of the fresh plant added to a tubful of hot water.

193. HYGROPHILA SPINOSA.

SYN.—ASTERACANTHA (Barleria) LONGIFOLIA.

(N. O.—ACANTHACEÆ.)

Sans.—Kokilâksha, Ikshugandhâ. *Hind.*, *Punj.*, *Kash.*, *Guz.* and *Mah.*—Tâlmakhân. *Ben.*—Kântakolika, Kuliâkhara. *Duk.*—Kolsi. *Tel.*—Neerugobbi. *Tam.*—Neermulli. *Can.*—Kolavalike. *Mal.*—Vayalchulli. *Cing.*—Ikkiri. *Burm.*—Soopadàn.

Habitat.—This little annual plant is common in moist places throughout India and Ceylon. The seeds and the root in the dried state are easily obtainable in the bazaars.

Properties and Uses.—The root is a cooling bitter tonic and a reputed diuretic and demulcent, employed in the form of decoction (1 ounce in one pint of water boiled for ten minutes) in rheumatism, in diseases of the genito-urinary tract and in dropsical affections. The leaves and seeds are also regarded as demulcent and diuretic, useful in jaundice and anasarca. The leaves are used as a pot-herb. The ashes of the plant are also used as a diuretic in dropsy. The roots are said to contain a principle which has been found to be a *cholesterol.* The following preparation is highly recommended by Dr. Kanny Lal Dey :—

Take of freshly dried Asteracantha leaves, 2 ounces; distilled water, 16 ounces; macerate for three days; press and strain. Of this the dose is from one to three tablespoonfuls in water thrice daily.

---

194. HYOSCYAMUS NIGER.

(N. O.—SOLANACEÆ.)

Sans.—Pàrasikaya. *Eng.*—Henbane. *Hind.*, *Ben.* and *Guz.*—Khoràsani-ajowan. *Tel.*—Kurashani-vàmum. *Tam.*—Kurasani-omum. (The seeds)—*Hind.* and *Ben.*—Buzrool.

Habitat.—This valuable medicinal plant grows wild throughout the Himalayan range at altitudes varying from 8,000 to 11,000 feet.

Properties and Uses.—The plant as found in the temperate Himalayan region may be regarded as practically identical in its chemical constituents with that cultivated for the drug markets of the world. Of cultivated henbanes the second year's growth of the *biennial* plant has usually been preferred. The active principle residing in the seeds, also in the leaves and green flowering tops, is *Hyoscyamine*. one of the three mydriatic alkaloids, atropine, hyoscyamine or daturine and hyoscine. It is isomeric with atropine, into which it can be converted. It may be split up into *hyoscine* and *Hyoscinic Acid*. Hyoscine is a volatile oily liquid about 5 times more powerful therapeutically than hyoscyamine. The seeds contain in addition about 25 per cent of a thick yellow fixed oil. In the *British Pharmacopœia* the fresh leaves and flowers and flowering tops and the dried leaves and flowering tops are official. From the fresh plant an extract and juice are prepared and the tincture is made from the dried herb. Hyoscyamine is sedative, anodyne, antispasmodic, stimulant and mydriatic (dilating the pupil of the eye) in effect. Its effects are milder than those of belladonna. Hyoscyamus is largely prescribed in mental excitement, insomnia, palpitation connected with debility and hysteria. It has a peculiarly sedative effect, particularly beneficial in irritable affections of the lungs, bowels and genito-urinary organs, such as cystitis, etc. The dose of the powdered leaves is from ½ to 2 drachms; of the fresh juice expressed and preserved, from ½ to 1 drachm; of the tincture ¼ to 1 drachm; of the extract (the most common form of administration), from 1 to 5 grains. There are also cataplasms, plasters and oil of hyoscyamus intended for external applications. In over-doses hyoscyamus is a narcotic poison, producing delirium, coma and death, and its operation is generally very rapid.

195. ICHNOCARPUS FRUTESCENS.

(*N. O.*—APOCYNACEÆ.)

Sans.—Sârivâ. *Hind.*--Dudhilatä. *Ben.*—Syâmalatâ. *Burm.*—Tansapai.

Habitat.—This climbing plant is widely distributed from the Western Himalaya to Bengal, Burma, the southern part of the Bombay Presidency, South India and Ceylon.

Properties and Uses.—The root is regarded as analogous in its properties to that of *Hemidesmus Indicus* and is often used as country sarsaparilla in the treatment of skin eruptions. The stalk and leaves are in common use, in the form of decoction, in simple fever.

Native Indian Preparations.—Take of *Anantamula*, root of *Pavonia odorata* (*bálá*), tubers of *Cyperus rotundus* (*mustaka*), ginger and the root of *Picrorrhiza* *kurroa* (*katuki*), equal parts, in all two tolas, and reduce them to a paste with water. This dose administered with warm water in the morning is said to clear the bowels and relieve fever (Bhaishajyaratnavali).

A decoction of the roots of colocynth, *Anantamul*, *sâriva* and *Hedyotis biflora* (*parparta*) prepared in the usual way is administered with the addition of powdered long pepper and bdellium in chronic skin-diseases, syphilis, elephantiasis, loss of sensation and hemiplegia (Sharangadhara).

196. INDIGOFERA ASPALATHOIDES.

(*N. O.*—LEGUMINOSÆ.)

Tam.—Shivanàrvembu. *Can.*—Shivamalli-gida, Neelamalli-gida. *Mal.*—Manali.

Habitat.—This plant is commonly met with in South India, mostly growing on waste and barren grounds.

Properties and Uses.—The leaves, flowers and tender shoots are cooling and demulcent and employed in leprosy and cancers. The root is chewed as a remedy for toothache and aphthæ. The whole plant rubbed with butter is applied to reduce œdematous tumours. A preparation is made from the ashes of the burnt plant to clean dandruff from the hair. The leaves are applied to abscesses and an oil is got from the root and is used to anoint the head in erysipelas.

197. INDIGOFERA TINCTORIA.

(*N. O.*—LEGUMINOSÆ.)

Sans.—Neela, Neelinee. *Eng.*—True Indigo. *Hind.* and *Ben.*—Nil. *Guz.*—Gali. *Mah.*—Nila. *Sind.*—Nil. *Tel.*—Neeli. *Tam.*—Nilam. *Pers.*—Nilah. *Can.* Neeli. *Mal.*—Amari, Avari.

Habitat.—This plant, which is usually not more than two or three feet high, is found wild and cultivated extensively in India, especially in Bengal, in the delta of the Ganges, in Madras, Sind and Bombay.

Properties and Uses.—The plant yields a valuable dye-stuff called indigo, of which it yields as much as 50 per cent. The leaves of the plant and indigo have been used in hepatitis, epilepsy and other nervous affections. They are used in the form of powder mixed with honey. The leaves rubbed upon water and applied to the abdomen are efficacious in promoting urine. Indigo itself is frequently applied to reduce swellings in the body. Powdered indigo sprinkled on foul ulcers is said to cleanse them. The juice of the young branches mixed with honey is recommended as application for aphthæ of the mouth in children. The decoction of the root is given in calculus; the root when boiled in milk is used as a purgative, and a decoction of the stem used as a gargle is considered efficacious in mercurial salivation. The plant is popularly regarded in some parts as a preventive of hydrophobia, administered internally in infusion and the juice applied externally to the part bitten.

198. IPOMÆA DIGITATA.

(*N. O.*—CONVOLVULACEÆ.)

Sans.—Virari, Ksheerakandâ, Vrushavalli. *Hind.*—Bilai-khand. *Ben.*—Bhuin-kumrá. *Mah.*—Bhui kohala. *Tel.*—Matta pal-tiga. Nelagummudu. *Tam.*—Phalmodika. *Mal.*—Mothalkanta. *Can.*—Nela kumbala.

Habitat.—This plant is indigenous to the hotter parts of India and largely cultivated as an ornamental plant.

Properties and Uses.—The root is regarded as tonic, alterative, aphrodisiac, demulcent and lactagogue. The powdered root-stalk is given with wine for the purpose of increasing the secretion of milk, to children in case of emaciation, debility and want of digestive power; also in spleen complaints. Powdered sun-dried root boiled in sugar and butter and administered, has the effect of promoting obesity, moderating menstrual discharge. The powdered root acts as purgative, also as cholagogue, useful in liver complaints.

---

199. IPOMÆA HEDERACEÆ.

(*N. O.*—Convolvulaceæ.)

Eng., *Hind.*, *Punj.*, *Ben.*, *Guz.*, and *Mah.*—Kalà-danà. *Arab.*—Hab-ün-nil. *Pers.*—Tukhm-i-nil. *Tel.*—Kolli-vittulu. *Tam.*—Kodi-kakkatan virai.

Habitat.—This plant, yielding the *kaladana* seeds, is found wild in some parts of India and cultivated in several places.

Properties and Uses.—The seeds are an efficient cathartic, closely allied to jalap; and an extract, tincture, compound powder and resin were made official in the *Pharmacopœia of India*. The active principle is a pale yellowish resin, *Pharbitisin*, existing to the extent of about 8 per cent., somewhat resembling resin of Jalap (*Convolvulin*) and corresponding to that body in its chemical characters. The dose of the seeds dried and powdered is from half to one drachm administered either alone or combined with cream of tartar and ginger; and that of the resin is from 2 to 8 grains. The following compound powder is preferable to the powdered seeds by themselves:—Powdered *Kaladana* seeds 7 drachms, rock-salt or cream of tartar 7 drachms powdered ginger 1 drachm, all in fine powder mixed together; pass through a fine sieve. Of this the dose, as a purgative, for an adult, is from 60 to 90 grains.

200. IPOMÆA TURPETHUM.

(*N. O.*—CONVOLVULACEÆ.)

Sans.—Trivrit, Triputá, Nandi. *Eng.*—Turpeth root, Indian Jalap. *Hind.*—Pithori. *Ben.*—Teori, Dhud. *Guz.* and *Mah.*—Nishotar, Phutkari. *Arab.*—Turband. *Tel.*—Tégada. *Mal.*, *Can.* and *Kon.*—Tigade. *Tam.*—Chivadai, Gunakandi.

Habitat.—This perennial plant grows wild nearly all over India.

Properties and Uses.—The root and root-bark of "white turpeth," which are obtainable in the bazaars, are in common use among Indians as cathartic and laxative; the darker variety, known as "black turpeth," is not used, as it is too drastic in its action. The dried and powdered root-bark of the white variety is best administered in doses ½ to 1½ drachms in combination with ginger and cream of tartar as in compound jalap powder; or about two scruples of the root are rubbed into pulp with water and taken with the addition of rock-salt and ginger or sugar and black-pepper. The bark of the fresh root is rubbed up with milk and administered as purgative. The root-bark contains about 4 per cent. of a brownish yellow glucosidal resin, 95 per cent. of which is *Turpethin*. The root contains, besides the resin, fatty substance, volatile oil, albumen, starch, a yellow colouring matter, lignin, salts and oxide of iron.

201. IRIS FLORENTINA or GERMANICA.

(*N. O.*—IRIDACEÆ.)

Eng.—Orris root. *Hind.* -Irsa. *Pers.*—Beg-i-banfsa (violet root).

Habitat.—This plant is cultivated in Kashmere and Kabul. Orris root is to be found in the bazaars of Calcutta and Bombay.

Properties and Uses.—Orris root contains an essential oil, otto of orris, highly valued in perfumery. Orris root is occasionally used in medicine as deobstruent and diuretic. The powdered root enters largely as a fragrant ingredient into the composition of dentifrices. The roasted seeds have been said to approach very nearly coffee in quality.

---

202. IRON, SULPHATE OF.

Hind. Guz. and *Duk.*—Hirà-kasis, Kashish. *Ben.*—Hiràkos. *Punj.* and *Kash.*—Sang-i-sabz. *Tam.*, *Tel.*, *Mal.* and *Can.*—Anna-bedi, Anna-bhedi. *Malay.*—Madukalpa.

Properties and Uses.—Pure sulphate of iron exists in the form of crystals or small crystalline masses of a pale green colour, wholly soluble in water. It is a valuable tonic and astringent in doses of from $\frac{1}{4}$ grain to 2 grains. In solution it forms a useful external application, especially in cases of rapidly spreading erysipelas. When used for this purpose, 10 grains of sulphate of iron should be dissolved in 1 ounce of spirits of wine (*not* water) and this solution should be applied with a camel-hair brush over the reddened parts of the skin and allowed to dry on. The application should be repeated once every day until the redness disappears, and between the applications the part should be covered with cotton wool so as to exclude air.

203. IXORA COCCINEA.

(*N. O.*—RUBIACEÆ.)

Sans.—Pàthalee. *Tam.*—Chetti, Cheddi. *Can.*— Kepala, Kissâr-gida. *Mal.*—Chetti, Thechhi. *Mah.* and *Kon.*—Patkali.

Habitat.—This small shrub is found growing almost everywhere in India.

Properties and Uses.—The root and the flowers are used medicinally. The root, about 30 to 40 grains, ground into pulp with a little water and long-pepper, or in the form of tincture made with four ounces of the dried root to one pint of proof-spirit, is said to be a valuable remedy in acute dysentery. Two tolas of the flowers fried in ghee are rubbed down with four *gunjas* each of cummin and *nagkessar* and made into a bolus with butter and sugarcandy and administered twice a day in cases of dysentery.

204. JASMINUM ANGUSTIFOLIUM.

(*N. O.*—JASMINACEÆ.)

Sans.—Priyá, Supoojà. *Hind.* and *Ben.*—Ban-mallica. *Guz.* and *Mah.*—Kusara. *Tel.*—Adavi-malle. *Tam.*—Kátu-mallige, Shiru-malli. *Can.*—Kádu-mallige. *Mal.*—Kattu-mallika. *Kon.*—Kusari.

Habitat.—This plant is met with generally in the forests in the sea-board districts of India.

Properties and Uses.—The bitter powdered root, mixed with the root of Acorus calamus and lime-juice, is considered a valuable external application in cases of ringworm.

205. JASMINUM GRANDIFLORUM.

(*N. O.*—JASMINACEÆ.)

Sans.—Játi. *Eng.*—The Spanish Jasmine. *Hind.*—Jàti. *Ben.*, *Guz.* and *Mah.*—Chameli. *Tel.*, *Tam.* and *Can.*—Jàji-malle. *Mal.*—Pichhakam, Málati. *Kon.*—Jayiche-mogre.

Habitat.—This plant with fragrant flowers is generally met with all over India, especially in the temperate regions, and on the temperate Himalaya.

Properties and Uses.—The leaves and fragrant flowers have long been known in Hindu medicine. From the flowers a perfumed oil or otto is prepared, which is greatly esteemed. Otto of Jasmine is used in India as a perfume. It is cooling when applied externally, in skin diseases, headache and weak eyes. The leaves are regarded as useful, administered internally in skin diseases, aphthæ, otorrhœa, etc., and the fresh juice of the leaves is a valuable application for soft corns between the toes. In ulcerations in the mouth the leaves are recommended to be chewed. An alkaloid called *Jasminine* has been isolated from the leaves.

---

206. JASMINUM PUBESCENS.

(N. O.—JASMINACEÆ.)

Hind., *Ben.*, *Guz.* and *Mah.*—Mogrà. *Tel.*—Kundamu, Gujari. *Mal.*—Kundam, Kurukutti-mulla. *Can.*—Kasturi mallige. *Kon.*—Kasturi-mogre.

Habitat.—This is common in most parts of India, especially in Bengal and on the East and West Coasts of India.

Properties and Uses.—The flowers are *lactifuge*. Two to three handfuls of the flowers bruised, unmoistened and applied to each breast and renewed once or twice a day, has the effect of arresting the secretion of milk, sometimes in 24 hours, although the period is more frequently two to three days. The dried leaves soaked in water and made into a poultice are applied to indolent ulcers to generate a healthy action. The root of the wild variety *(Kádu mallige)* is used as an emmenagogue; also useful in snake-bite and weakness of sight.

207. JASMINUM SAMBAC.

(*N. O.*—JASMINACEÆ.)

Sans.—Mallikà. *Eng.*—Arabian Jasmine. *Hind.* and *Ben.*—Bal-phul, Motiyà, Mogra. *Guz.* and *Mah.*—Mogri. *Pers.*—Zambak. *Tel.*—Malle. *Tam.*—Malligai. *Can.*—Mallige. *Mal.*—Cherupichhakam, Nallamulli.

Habitat.—This, another of the jasmine species, is cultivated in India, Burma and Ceylon.

Properties and Uses.—The flowers yield a fragrant essential oil similar to that of *J. Grandflorum.* The leaves are considered valuable as a lactifuge, the bruised leaves being applied to the breasts; the application is employed to arrest the secretion of milk in the puerperal state in cases of threatened abscess. The leaves, if boiled in oil, exude a balsam which is used for anointing the head in eye-complaints. It is said to strengthen the vision.

208. JATROPHA CURCAS.

(*N. O.*—EUPHORBIACEÆ.)

Sans.—Kànana-eranda. *Eng.*—Angular-leaved physic nut. *Hind.*—Jangli-arandi. *Ben.*—Ban-bheranda, Gabbheranda. *Guz.* and *Mah.*—Moghli-erendi, Rân-erendi. *Pers.*—Dandi-nahri. *Tel.*—Adavi-àmudamu. *Tam.*—Kattâmanakku. *Can.*—Kàdaharalu. *Mal.*—Kâtâmanak. *Kon.*—Kád-eradi. *Cing.*—Val-erandu. *Burm.*—Késugi, Simbo-kêsu.

Habitat.—This evergreen plant is common in waste places throughout India; in the southern parts it is cultivated chiefly for hedges.

Properties and Uses.—The seeds, in their native state, are acro-narcotic poison. They yield on expression about 30 per cent. of a pale yellow oil which, in doses of 12 to 15 drops, acts as a purgative equal in action to one ounce of castor oil, but is far less certain in its operation and causes more griping than castor oil. Its ill effects are corrected by lime juice as in the case of croton seeds. Externally it is an esteemed remedy for itch, herpes and eczema, and it is said to be a cleansing application for wounds and ulcers. Diluted with a bland oil (1 part to 2 or 3) it forms a useful embrocation in *chronic* rheumatism. The active principle of the oil has been named *Jatrophic acid*; but the activity of the seeds is attributed to a poisonous tox-albumen analogous to ricin and named *Curcin*. The leaves locally applied to the breasts are stated to increase the secretion of milk. For this purpose a decoction is made by boiling a handful of the plant in six or eight pints of water. With this the breasts are bathed for a quarter of an hour, and then the boiled leaves in the form of a poultice spread over them. In a few hours the effects of the application will be manifest. A simpler mode of application consists in applying layers of the fresh leaves, simply warmed before a fire, over the breasts. The leaves warmed and rubbed with castor oil and applied to boils and abscesses have the suppurative effect. The fresh juice from the stem is a reputed hæmostatic and styptic and is employed to arrest bleeding or hæmorrhage from wounds, ulcers, cuts and abrasions; it is also said to promote healing by coagulating the blood and forming an airtight film like that produced by collodion. The sticks of this plant are used as tooth-brushes, and are said to strengthen the gums and to cure spongy-gums or gum-boils.

209. JUGLANS REGIA.

(*N. O.*—JUGLANDEÆ.)

Sans.—Akshota. *Eng.*—Walnut.—*Hind.* and *Ben.*—Akhrôt. *Arab.*—Jouz. *Pers.*—Charmaghz.

Habitat.—This valuable timber tree is wild in the Himalaya and largely cultivated in Afghanistan, Kashmir and Thibet.

Properties and Uses.—The kernels of the cultivated varieties are edible. They contain about 50 per cent. of a clear fixed oil, which is used by the hill tribes, where the walnut grows, as an illuminant and lubricant. The bark of the tree is said to be used as an astringent and antheimintic.

---

210. JUNIPERUS COMMUNIS.

(*N. O.*—CONIFERÆ.)

Eng.—Juniper. *Hind.*—Aarar. *Bom.*—Abbhal-arar.

Habitat.—The juniper tree is common on the North-west of the Himalayas.

Properties and Uses.—The wood is resinous and is used as an incense. The fruit, commonly known as "juniper berries," is aromatic and terebinthinate and a volatile oil is distilled from it—"Juniper berry oil," which is used in Europe principally to flavour a spirit called Geneva. An oil is also distilled from the leaves and young twigs. The fruits also contain glucose and a bitter principle named *Juniperinc.* The fruit and oil are carminative and diuretic, useful in dropsy and renal affections. They are chiefly employed as an adjuvant to other remedies, to increase the flow of urine. The dose of the berries taken in powder is from 1 to 3 drachms. The dose of the oil is from 4 to 6 minims and of the compound spirit from 2 to 4 drachms. An infusion of juniper tops is sometimes taken; it may be prepared thus:— Fresh tops of the plant, 1 ounce and boiling water, 1 pint; infuse for two hours and strain; take a wine-glassful twice a day. It is best used as a vehicle for other diuretics. In some parts of Europe, juniper berries are roasted, ground and used as a substitute for coffee; they are also employed in Sweden and Germany as a conserve and as a culinary spice.

211. KÆMPFERIA GALANGA.

(*N. O.*—ZINGIBERACEÆ.)

Sans.—Sugandhavacha. *Tel.*—Chandramoola. *Tam.*—Kachholakilangu. *Can.* and *Kon.*—Kachhura. *Mal.*—Kachhuram.

Habitat.—This grows abundantly in gardens in the southern parts of India.

Properties and Uses.—The tubers are used generally in perfumery. The roots or rhizomes are attached to the necklaces for their perfume and also placed in the clothes. Medicinally the tubers reduced to powder and mixed with honey are given with much benefit in coughs and pectoral affections. The oil in which they are boiled is useful in applying to the stoppages of the nasal organs.

212. KÆMPFERIA ROTUNDA.

(*N. O.*—SCITAMINEÆ.)

Sans.—Bhuichampaka. *Hind.* and *Ben.*—Bhuichampa. *Tel.*—Bhûchampakamu. *Tam.*—Nèrpichan. *Can.*—Nelasampige. *Mal.*—Chenchineerkilang.

Habitat.—This plant with round leaves and fragrant flowers is found cultivated in gardens in India and Burma.

Properties and Uses.—The roots have a hot ginger-like taste. The fresh bruised tubers are in popular use in many parts of India as an application to wounds and bruises to reduce swellings; used in cancerous swellings also. The decoction is applied with much benefit to wounds with coagulated blood and with any purulent matter.

213. KALANCHOE LACINIATA.

(*N. O.*—CRASSULACEÆ.)

Sans.—Hemasägara. *Hind.* and *Ben.*—Hemsägar. *Bom.*—Zakhm hyät.

Habitat.—This succulent plant, cultivated in gardens, is wild on the hills of North-Western India.

Properties and Uses.—The bruised leaves and juice have some reputation as an application to bruises and contusions to allay inflammation and prevent discolouration and as a styptic on fresh wounds.

214. KARIYAT.

(*See also* ANDROGRAPHIS PANICULATA.)

(*N. O.*—ACANTHACEÆ.)

Sans.—Mahâtceta. *Hind.*—Kiryat. *Ben.*—Cherorta. *Guz.*—Kiryäta. *Mah.*—Chiráyita. *Cing.*—Binko hamba. *Malay.*—Charita.

Habitat.—This is the dried stalk and root of *Andrographis paniculata* which is common throughout the plains of India and cultivated in gardens in some parts. The stem with the root attached occurs in pieces of about a foot or more in length, usually sold in the bazaars. This article is often confounded with Chiretta (*Ophelia chirata*) from the similarity between their native names and sensible qualities.

Properties and Uses.—Kariyat is a valuable bitter tonic useful in general debility, in convalescence after fevers and in the advanced stages of dysentery. It is best given as follows :—Take of kariyàt bruised, ½ ounce; acorus or sweet flag root and dill seeds bruised, of each 60 grains; boiling water, ½ pint; infuse in a covered vessel for an hour and strain. Dose, from 1½ to 2 ounces twice or thrice daily. The following preparation has been highly spoken of :—Take of kariyât cut small, 6 ounces; myrrh and aloes in coarse powder, of each 1 ounce; brandy, 2 pints. Macerate for 7 days in a closed vessel, occasionally shaking it, strain, filter and add sufficient brandy to make two pints. Of this the dose is from 1 to 4 teaspoonfuls in a little water taken on an empty stomach. It acts as a gentle aperient and is said to prove very useful in many forms of dyspepsia attended with torpidity of the bowels. In the bowel complaints of children, a decoction of the fresh leaves of the *Kariyàt* plant has been well spoken of. It is prepared by boiling 2½ ounces of the fresh leaves in 1½ pints of water down to 6 ounces; of this the dose is one ounce every two or three hours. It may be used in conjunction with other remedies required.

215. LACTUCA SCARIOLA.

(*N. O.*—COMPOSITÆ.)

Eng.—The Lettuce. *Hind.* and *Ben.*—Kâhu, Sàlàd. *Bom.*—Kàhu. *Arab.*—Bazr-ul-khas. *Pers.*—Tukm-i-kahu.

Habitat.—This familiar herb is wild on the Western Himalaya. *Lactuca sativa*, the common or garden variety, is cultivated in many parts of India as a culinary vegetable.

Properties and Uses.—The inspissated juice of this plant, *Lactucarium*, also called *Thridace* or lettuce-opium, was formerly held in great repute as a sedative, anodyne and antispasmodic. It contains a crystalline principle, *Lectucerin*, besides *Lectucin* and *Lectucic acid*. *Extractum Lectucæ* of the British Pharmacopœia is a corresponding preparation made from the closely allied plant *L. virosa*.

The wild variety is believed to possess the sedative property in greater degree than the cultivated. *Hyoscyamine* is said to be found both in *L. sativa* and *L. virosa*. The seeds are obtainable in the Indian bazaars; they contain a fixed oil.

---

216. LAGENARIA VULGARIS.

(*N. O.*—CUCURBITACEÆ.)

Sans.—Alâbu. *Eng.*—The bottle-gourd, white pumpkin. *Hind.*—Lauki, Jangli-khaddu. *Ben.*—Lau, Kodu. *Guz.*—Karwa bopla. *Mah.*—Räu bhopla, Dudhya-bhopla. *Pers.*—Kaddu. *Tel.*—Surakâya. *Tam.*—Soriai-käy. *Can.*—Kahisore. *Mal.*—Kâtuchuram *Kon.*—Kädu-duddi.

Habitat.—This climbing plant is found wild and cultivated nearly all over India.

Properties and Uses.—The fruit and leaves are edible. The fruit contains a thick white pulp which, in the cultivated variety (*kodu*) is sweet and edible, while in the smaller wild variety (*tumri*) it is bitter and a drastic purgative, like colocynth. The seeds yield a clear limpid oil which is cooling and is applied to relieve headache. It is also administered internally. The pulp of the cultivated forms is occasionally employed as an adjunct to purgatives, and considered cool, diuretic and antibilious, useful in coughs, and as an antidote to certain poisons. Externally it is applied as a poultice and a cooling application to the shaved head in delirium. The leaves are purgative and recommended to be taken in the form of decoction for jaundice.

---

217. LATHYRUS SATIVUS.

(N. O.—LEGUMINOSÆ.)

Sans.—Triputi. *Hind.*—Khesäri. *Ben.*—Teora. *Pers.*—Masang.

Habitat.—This is largely cultivated as a pulse crop, chiefly on alluvial soils in the North-West and Central Provinces.

Properties and Uses.—The seed is a nutritious food, but its continued use induces paralysis, termed lathyrismus, in the lower limbs in men and animals. The toxic property has been traced to a volatile alkaloid which is readily dissipated by heat and when the pulse is properly cooked.

---

218. LAWSONIA ALBA.

(N. O.—LYTHRACEÆ.)

Sans.—Mendhi. *Eng.*—Henna, Camphire, Samphire. *Hind.*, *Duk.* and *Punj.*, Mendhi. *Ben.*—Mèhèdi. *Kash.*—Mohuz. *Guz.* and *Mah.*—Mehndi. *Cing.*—Meritondi. *Burm.*—Dämbin. *Arab.*—a Hinà. *Tam.*—Maruthonri. *Tel.*—Goeranta, Kuravamu. *Can.*—Madarangi. *Mal.*—Mailänchi. *Malay.*—Hinie.

Habitat.—This small fragrant shrub is common nearly all over India, cultivated chiefly as a hedge plant.

Properties and Uses.—The leaves are generally useful in the treatment of that troublesome and painful affection called "burning of the feet." For this purpose the fresh leaves are beaten into a paste with vinegar or lime-juice and applied as a poultice to the soles of the feet. Another plan is to use strong friction with the bruised leaves over the parts. The leaves are also similarly applied with benefit in cases of rheumatism. The leaves yield a dye which is extensively used for staining hands and finger nails; in conjunction with catechu and indigo they are also used as a hair-dye. Applied to the hair they are said to promote healthy growth. An ointment prepared from the leaves has valuable healing properties and is used in curing wounds and ulcers. Their decoction is useful as an external application in inflammations and burns; it is also an astringent gargle in ulcers of the mouth, and is an excellent injection for gonorrhœa. The leaf juice mixed with water and milk is given in spermatorrhœa. The bark in infusion is given in jaundice and enlargement of the spleen, in calculus affections and as an alterative in leprosy and obstinate skin diseases. In decoction it is applied to burns, scalds, etc. The seeds contain an oil; with honey and tragacanth they act as cephalic. The flowers yield a fragrant otto or oil. They are used in perfumery and embalming. The fragrant water distilled from the flowers was formerly employed by the Jews in baths and for perfuming the oils and ointments with which they anointed the body, and for embalming. An extract from the flowers, leaves and tender shoots is a valuable remedy in cases of lepra and other depraved conditions of the body,—half a drachm twice a day. The infusion of the flowers cures headache and is a good application to bruises.

219. LENS ESCULENTA.

(*N. O.*—LEGUMINOSÆ.)

Sans.—Masura. *Eng.*—The Lentil. *Hind.*—Masùr. *Ben.*—Masùri. *Arab.*—Adas. *Tel.*—Misur-pappu.—*Tam.* Misur-purpu.

Habitat.—The lentil is grown in various parts of India, chiefly in Behar, the Central Provinces and Madras.

Properties and Uses.—The lentil is used as a food pulse; it has the property of preventing constipation. A paste prepared from the seeds is a cleansing application to foul and indolent ulcers.

Its chemical composition (in 100 parts):—

	Husked	With Husk
Water	11·8 p. c.	11·7 p. c.
Albuminoids	25·1 ,,	24·9 ,,
Starch	58·4 ,,	56·0 ,,
Oil	1·3 ,,	1·5 ,,
Fibre	1·2 ,,	3·6 ,,
Ash	2·2 ,,	2·3 ,,

220. LEPIDIUM SATIVUM.

(*N. O.*—CRUCIFERÆ.)

Sans.—Chandra-sura. *Eng.*—The common cress. *Hind.*—Chansar, Hälim, Hurf. *Guz.*—Asáliya. *Mah.*—Ahaleeva. *Tel.*—Adityalu. *Tam.*—Alivirai.

Habitat.—This familiar shrub is cultivated as a culinary vegetable all over Asia.

Properties and Uses.—The herb and seeds contain a volatile aromatic oil. The seeds contain a fatty oil. The seeds are available in the bazaars of Western India and are used to some extent in Hindoo medicine. They are described as tonic and alterative and useful in hiccup, diarrhœa and skin diseases caused by impurity of blood. A decoction of the seeds (1 in 20) is found useful in cases of diarrhœa, the chief virtue being in its mucilaginous property.

Native Indian Preparations.—Bhâvaprakâsh recommends the following formula to be given in cases of obstinate hiccup: Macerate *Hâlim* seeds in eight times their weight of water; when the seeds are softened rub them in the water and strain the emulsion through cloth. This emulsion is recommended to be given frequently in doses of about an ounce for the relief of obstinate hiccup.

221. LINUM USITATISSIMUM.

(*N. O.*—LINEÆ.)

Sans.—Atasi. *Hind.*—Alsi, Tisi. *Ben.*—Tisi, Mosinà. *Guz.* and *Mah.*—Alashi. *Tel.* and *Can.*—Atasi. *Tam.*—Alashi-virai. *Pers.*—Zaghu.

Habitat.—The flax plant is extensively cultivated, chiefly in Bengal, Behar and the United Provinces, for its seed—linseed—which is exported from Calcutta and Bombay.

Properties and Uses.—The seed—linseed—on expression yields 25 to 30 per cent. of a fixed oil—linseed oil. The seeds also contain a considerable quantity of mucilaginous matter which is extracted by cold water as a viscid jelly-like mass. The crushed seed or the powdered seed cake after expression of the oil constitutes what is called "linseed meal." The fibres of the stem prepared and bleached are manufactured into linen cloth. The best qualities of lint are still made from the retted and finely-carded fibre. The stems are burned as fuel in India. The infusion of the seeds, known as "linseed tea," and made with or without the addition of a little liquorice root (one to three of linseed), is given internally as a demulcent drink in colds, coughs and irritations of the urinary organs. The poultice made from linseed meal is a valuable soothing application to ulcerated or inflamed surfaces. A popular remedy to alleviate the pain of burns is "carron oil," a mixture of equal parts of raw linseed oil and lime water. Linseed oil is largely used in the fine and useful arts.

222. LIQUIDAMBAR ORIENTALIS.

(*N. O.*—HAMAMELIDEÆ.)

Sans.—Silhaka. *Eng.*—Liquid storax, rose malloes. *Hind.*, *Ben.*, *Guz.*, and *Mah.*—Silāras. *Pers.*—Meih-sila. *Tel.*—Shilārasam. *Tam.*—Neri-arishippāl. *Can.*—Shilàrasa. *Mal.*—Rasamalla.

Habitat.—This forest-tree yielding liquid storax is a native of the South-Western districts of Asia Minor. The drug is well known in the bazaars of Calcutta, Bombay and Madras under the above names, and forms an article of import and export at Bombay.

Properties and Uses.—The liquid storax is an aromatic, semifluid, opaque, grey balsam, obtained by boiling the inner bark in water. It is used by the Hindus for perfuming medicinal oils. It is a stimulant expectorant, useful in chronic coughs and pulmonary (lung) affections. It is an ingredient of the compound tincture of Benzoin of the British Pharmacopoea.

223. LIPPIA NODIFLORA.

(*N. O.*—VERBENACEÆ.)

Tel.—Bokkena. *Tam.*—Poduthalai, Talaibòdam. *Can.*—Nelahippali, Karehippali. *Mal.*—Kâttu-thippali.

Habitat.—This creeper is generally found growing in moist ground, mostly in the Southern parts of India.

Properties and Uses.—The leaves and young shoots are very bitter and astringent, given to children in diarrhœa and indigestion in the form of infusion or decoction; which is also given as a demulcent drink in case of gonorrhœa; also said to be useful for women after the lying-in state.

224. LITSÆA SEBIFERA.

SYN:—TETRANTHERA ROXBURGHII: T. LAURIFOLIA.

(*N. O.*—LAURINEÆ.)

Hind.—Garbijaur. *Ben.*—Kúkùr-chhta. *Bom.*—Maida-lakri (the bark). *Tam.* Maida-lalki (the bark).

Habitat.—The bark of this tree, which is common in Upper India, especially in Bengal, is a popular native medicine well known in the bazaars of Bengal as *Maida-lakri.*

Properties and Uses.—The bark of this tree, which is known as *Maida-lakri*, is feebly balsamic, mucilaginous, and esteemed as a demulcent in diarrhœa; externally it is used as an emollient application to bruises.

225. LODOICEA SECHELLARUM.

Eng.—The sea cocoanut. *Hind.*—Daryàkà-nàriyal. *Bom.*—Jàhari-nàral. *Tam.*—Kadala-tangáy.

Habitat.—This palm is growing in the Seychelles, but its fruit is obtainable on the Bombay side.

Properties and Uses.—The fruit or nuts attain to a great size and frequently 40 to 50 lb. in weight, taking, it is said, four years to form and at least ten years to ripen. They were formerly cast ashore in India from the Indian Ocean and much esteemed in native medicine. They are now imported and used to some extent by the natives of North-Western India as food and medicine, being regarded as preservative and alexipharmic.

226. LUFFA ACUTANGULA.

(*N. O.*—CUCURBITACEÆ.)

Sans.—Koshâtaki. *Hind.*—Turai. *Ben.*—Ghoshâ latä. *Guz.* and *Mah.*—Sirola. *Tel.*—Beerakâya. *Tam.*—Peeram. *Can.*—Heere-kây. *Mal.*—Peechhakam, Cherupeeram. *Kon.*—Ghosâle.

Habitat.—This plant is cultivated in India, chiefly on the Western side.

Properties and Uses.—The fruit is a well-known culinary vegetable, demulcent, diuretic and nutritive. The seeds of this gourd, especially the ripe ones, have been found to possess emetic and purgative properties; the emetic property is believed to reside in the kernel, twenty to thirty grains of the dried kernel being administered. Dr. Warden has found in the fruit a principle soluble in alcohol, having very marked gelatinizing properties. It is named *Luffein.* The leaves are applied locally in splenitis, hæmorrhoids and leprosy. The juice of the fresh leaves is dropped into the eyes of children in granular conjunctivitis, also to prevent the lids from adhering at night on account of excessive meibomian secretion.

The fruit of *Luffa echinata* (*Hind.*—Bindál, *Mah.*—Kukadavel) has the reputation in Sindh of a remedy for jaundice.

---

227. LUFFA PLUCKETIANA (AMORA).

(*N. O.*—CUCURBITACEÆ.)

Sans.—Katuki, Raktâ-koshâtaki. *Hind.*—Karvi-turai. *Ben.*—Ghoshalatâ. *Bom.*—Kadu-sirolä, Ran-turai. *Tel.*—Verri-beera. *Tam.*—Peppirakam. *Can.*—Kahi-keera, Nágtháli.

Habitat.—This creeper is to be found growing mostly in Southern India and Bengal.

Properties and Uses.—Every part of the plant is remarkably bitter and the fruit is violently cathartic and emetic. The kernel of the seeds is said to be a safe, sure and efficient remedy for dysentery, equal to ipecacuanha. It is rubbed and mixed with water, forming a greenish-white emulsion, which is used for administration. Dose:—As emetic, 20 to 30 grains; as nauseant, 10 to 15 grains; as demulcent and expectorant, 5 to 10 grains. It contains albumin and oil. The juice of the roast fruit is applied to cure headache; the juice is also applied to different kinds of bites, and the dried fruit is used as a snuff in jaundice. The root with equal parts of *Jasud* root *(Hibiscus Rosa Sinensis)* and *Hemidesmus* is given with milk, cummin and sugar in gonorrhœa.

228. MÆRNA ARENARIA.

(*N. O.*—CAPPARIDEÆ.)

Eng.—The earth sugar root. *Tel.*—Puta-tiga. *Tam.*—Pùmi-chakarei.

Properties and Uses.—The earth sugar root of the Tamils has been known in Southern India for centuries. The root slightly resembles liquorice root in appearance and taste. It is said to be used as an alterative, tonic and stimulant. From an analysis of the drug made by Hooper it was found to contain ordinary plant constituents and a quantity of sugar.

229. MALLOTUS PHILIPPINENSIS.

SYN :—ROTTLERA TINCTORIA : CROTON PHILIPPINENSIS.

(*N. O.*—EUPHORBIACEÆ.)

Sans.—Kampilla, Rechanaka. *Eng.*—Monkey-Face tree. Kamelâ or Kamala dye. *Hind.*—Kamala, *Ben.*—Kamila-guri, Kamalà-gundi. *Mah.*—Shendri. *Arab.*—Kinbil. *Pers.*—Kanbélà. *Guz.*—Kapilo. *Tel.*—Kúnkuma. *Tam.*—Kapila.

Habitat.—This small evergreen forest tree is found all over India, from Kashmere to Ceylon, and in Burma, Singapore, and the Andamans. It is the source of the valuable dye-stuff, *Kamela,* which is met with in most bazaars in the form of a beautiful purplish red powder.

Properties and Uses.—Kamela powder is used as an orange-brown dye, especially for silk. It is quite insoluble in water but soluble in alcohol and ether; the solution in the latter medium extracting about 70 to 80 per cent. of a red resin, from which yellow crystalline substances, *Rottlerin* and *Isorottlerin,* may be isolated. The roots are said to yield a red dye. In medicine Kamela has attained considerable repute as a remedy for *Taenia* or *Tape-worm.* The dose for an adult is about two to three drachms in honey or a little aromatic water. It acts freely on the bowels, causing, in many instances, considerable nausea and griping, though not generally more than is caused by other remedies of the same class; the worm is generally expelled in a lifeless state in the third or fourth stool. Should the first trial not prove successful, it may be repeated after the interval of a week; but should this be a failure also, it will be useless to continue its use further; then other remedies may be tried. Externally it has been used in skin diseases.

Native Indian Preparations.—Take of *kampilla*, *baberang* seeds, chebulic myrobalan, *yavakshàra* (impure carbonate of potash) and rock-salt, equal parts, powder and mix. Dose: about a drachm with butter-milk (Chakradatta).

230. MALVA ROTUNDIFOLIA.

(*N. O.*—MALVACEÆ.)

Eng.—Mallow leaf. *Tam.*—Kàttu-kadalai. *Mal.*—Kàtkada-lekka. *Kon.*—Kàdu-chanyapàllo. *Can.*—Kàdu-kadle-soppu.

Habitat.—This plant is generally met with in the Deccan and Mysore Provinces.

Properties and Uses.—The leaves are mucilaginous and emollient, when applied as a poultice or paste in scurvy, piles, &c. The seeds are demulcent, and prescribed in the form of powder in cases of bronchitis, cough, inflammations and ulcerations of the bladder, and in hæmorrhoids. They are also externally applied in the form of paste in skin diseases.

231. MALVA SYLVESTRIS.

(*N. O.*—MALVACEÆ.)

Eng.—The common mallow. *Hind.*—Vilàyati-kangai. *Pers.*—Nàn-i-kulàgh (crow's bread). *Arab.* and *Bom.*—Khubazi.

Habitat.—A herbaceous plant growing on the temperate Western Himalaya.

Properties and Uses.—In common with other malvaceous species it abounds, and especially the fruit, in mucilaginous principles. The seeds are employed internally in decoction as a demulcent. The leaves are made into a poultice as an emollient external application.

232. MANGIFERA INDICA.

(*N. O.*—ANACARDIACEÆ.)

Sans.—Amra, Chùta. *Eng.*—Mango tree. *Hind.*, *Guz.*, and *Ben.*—Am. *Mah.*—Amba. *Bom.*—Thayet. *Tel.*—Māvi. *Tam.*—Màmaram. *Can.*—Màvina-mara. *Mal.*—Màvu. *Pers.*—Amba, Naghzak.

Habitat.—This tree is indigenous to India and cultivated in many varieties almost everywhere in the plains, yielding large crops annually of the familiar egg-shaped fruit, mango.

Properties and Uses.—The mango is well known and is the most delicious of Indian fruits. The ripe fruit is very wholesome, nourishing and antiscorbutic. A confection prepared out of the juice of the ripe fruit, with the addition of sugar and aromatics, is recommended as a restorative tonic. The fruit is also diaphoretic, astringent and refrigerent. The unripe fruit is made into refreshing *sherbets* and custards, into pickles and preserves, as a sour ingredient in certain curries and as the principal ingredient of the *chutnies* so popular in Indian cookery. The kernel inside the large flattened stone or seed contains tannic acid (about 10 per cent.) and turpentine, which is useful in cases of asthma, diarrhœa, chronic dysentery, leucorrhœa, &c., given in doses of about 20 to 30 grains in the form of powder; it is also used as an anthelmintic. The pulp of the ripe fruit contains a trace of gallic acid with citric acid and gum; the unripe fruit contains about 20 per cent. of the free acids, tartaric, citric and malic. The *Ām-chur*, which is very popular among native troops in India, is a valuable antiscorbutic, equal in effect to lime juice. It consists of green mangoes skinned, stoned, cut into pieces and dried in the sun; half an ounce of this is said to be equivalent to an ounce of good lime juice. Sweet mango pickle, freely eaten with the diet, is an excellent method of administering *Am-chur*.

The bark of the tree contains tannic acid, and from it exudes a pink-coloured gum partly soluble in water. A fluid extract or the infusion of the bark is used in menorrhagia and leucorrhœa, and in bleeding piles, in cases of hæmorrhage from the lungs or intestines. The juice of the fresh bark administered with white of egg or mucilage and a little opium is also similarly effective.

The smoke of the burning leaves is said to have a curative effect in some affections of the throat, in hiccup, etc. The dried flowers in decoction or powder are a useful astringent in diarrhœa, chronic dysentery and gleet. The gum of the tree is applied with benefit to cracked feet.

Chemical composition (Mango):—

Water	20·98	Alkalinity of soluble ash as potash	0·41
Watery extract	61·40		
Cellulose	4·77	Tartaric acid with a trace of citric acid	7·04
Insoluble ash	1·43		
Soluble ash	1·91	Free acid as malic acid	2·66

Native Indian Preparations.—In diarrhœa a decoction of the kernel is given alone or in combination with bela and ginger (Sharngadhara). In bleeding from the nose the juice of the kernel is recommended to be snuffed. In bleeding from internal organs a cold infusion of the barks of *Mangifera Indica*, *Eugenia Jambolana*, and *Termenalia Arjuna* is prescribed. This infusion is also administered in diarrhœa.

233. MARANTA ARUNDINACEA.

(*N. O.*—SCITAMINEÆ.)

Eng.—West Indian Arrowroot. *Hind.*—Tikhor. *Ben.* and *Bom.* —Ararut. *Tam.*—Kuâmâu. *Can.*—Kûve-hittu. *Mal.*—Kûva. *Burm.*—Pen-beva

Habitat.—This true arrowroot plant is cultivated in Eastern Bengal, the United Provinces, and in Madras.

Properties and Uses.—The arrowroot obtained from the rasped tubers of this plant is a pure starch, and is chiefly included as a light food in invalid diet. It is manufactured and largely consumed in India. The arrowroot obtained in the bazaars is frequently adulterated with potato starch, which may be detected by the microscope, the granules of potato starch being larger.

---

234. MELALEUCA LEUCADENDRON (Minor).

(*N. O.*—MYRTACEÆ.)

Eng.—The Cajuput Tree. *Hind.*—Kayaputi. *Ben.*—Cajuputi, Ilachi. *Bom.*—Kayakuti. *Tam.*—Kijaputè.

Habitat.—This large, evergreen tree is indigenous to the islands of the Indian Archipelago. The oil distilled from the leaves is imported from Java, Manilla, the Celebes and other islands where the oil is prepared.

Properties and Uses.—Kayaputi-ka-tel, as it is called in the Calcutta bazaar, is a transparent, limpid, volatile oil of a pale, bluish-green colour, pungent odour and bitter aromatic taste. It consists largely of a body which has been named *Cajuputol*. The oil may be used internally, although it is very seldom employed, as a stimulant, carminative, antispasmodic and sudorific, in hysteria, flatulence and colic, rheumatism and low fevers; the dose is from two to five minims or half to two fluid drachms of the official spirit. Externally it is largely used in India as a rubefacient in rheumatism, either alone or as an ingredient of croton liniment or combined with other stimulating applications. It is a domestic remedy for all muscular pains. The following makes a good and useful liniment: cajeput oil, half a drachm; castor oil, one drachm; olive oil, $4\frac{1}{2}$ drachms. If a stronger stimulant for rheumatism is required use this: soap liniment, camphor liniment and cajeput oil, of each an ounce; mix and rub well in.

235. MELANORRHŒA USITATA.

(*N. O.*—ANACARDIACEÆ.)

Eng.—The Black Varnish Tree. *Burm.*—Thitsi. *Karen.*—Kiahong.

Habitat.—This is a forest tree allied to the *Diptero-carpus* species, found at Prome and neighbouring districts in Burma.

Properties and Uses.—This tree is the source of an oleo-resin known as the black varnish *(thitsi)* of the Burmese, and extensively used as a natural varnish or lacquer and to some extent as a medicine. The oleo-resin is used in Burma in combination with honey as an anthelmintic.

236. MELIA AZADIRACHTA.

(*N. O.*—MELIACEÆ.)

Sans.—Mahânimba, Ravipriya, Vembaka, Vranashodhakari. *Eng.*—The Neem or Margosa Tree, Indian Lilac. *Hind.*, *Duk.*, *Punj.* and *Ben.*—Nim. *Guz.*—Limba. *Mah.*—Nimba. *Tel.*—Vèpa. *Tam.*—Vêmbu. *Can.*—Bèvina-mara. *Mal.*—Vèppu. *Kon.*—Bèvâ-rooku. *Cing.*—Kohumba. *Burm.*—Tamàbin, Kamàkha. *Malay.*—Dawoon Nambu, Baypay.

Habitat.—A large ornamental tree, indigenous to India and cultivated nearly all over the Peninsula and in Burma. It thrives best in the drier climate of the United Provinces.

Properties and Uses.—This tree is believed in many places to be advantageous to health when planted around villages, as a prophylactic against malaria. Almost every part of the tree is useful medicinally. The root-bark, bark and young fruit are astringent, tonic and antiperiodic; the bark is also a general vermifuge. The bark is used in the form of powder or fluid extract, in one-drachm doses, or decoction, in doses of one to two ounces, in cases of intermittent fevers, general debility, convalescence after fevers, and loss of appetite. The bark contains a bitter principle of a resinous nature, believed to reside in the inner bark or liber, so that the alcoholic tincture or fluid extract is the most efficient preparation of the bark. Another important product of the tree is the yellow fixed oil contained to the extent of about 10 per cent. in the seeds and extracted by pressure. It consists, according to the research by Dr. Warden, of the fixed fatty acids—stearic, oleic and a small amount of lauric—with butyric and a trace of valeric acids as the volatile fatty principles. The oil has markedly antiseptic properties and may be used like carbolic oil as a dressing for foul ulcers, also as an external stimulant application in leprosy, urticaria, eczema, erysipelas, scrofula and similar skin diseases. For leprosy it may either be used alone or combined with chaulmoogra oil or gurjun balsam. It is also used internally in doses of 30 minims to one drachm, as anthelmintic. As insecticide it is applied for the destruction of lice.

The dry seeds possess the same properties as the oil when bruised and mixed with water or some other fluid. The leaves are useful as stimulant in the form of paste or poultice made with a little tepid water and applied on a rag to boils and ulcers. In hot decoction or infusion, they form a valuable antiseptic and healing lotion like a weak solution of carbolic acid, and an anodyne fomentation to unhealthy ulcers, swollen glands, bruises and sprains. The fruit is purgative, emollient and anthelmintic. The gum which exudes from the bark is regarded as a stimulant and demulcent tonic, useful in catarrhal and other affections. The flowers are stimulant, tonic and stomachic, given in infusion in cases of atonic dyspepsia and general debility. The toddy or the fermented sap of the tree acts as a refrigerent nutrient and alterative tonic, said to be valuable in consumption, chronic leprosy and other skin diseases. The tender twigs of the tree are used as tooth-brushes, which are believed to keep the system healthy and the breath and mouth clean and sweet.

---

237. MELIA AZEDARACH.

(*N. O.*—MELIACEÆ.)

Sans.—Mahànimba. *Eng.*—The Persian Lilac, Common Bead tree. *Hind.*—Drek, Bakayan. *Ben.*—Ghorâ-nim. *Bom.*—Vilayati-nim. *Tel.*—Konda-vepa. *Tam.*—Malai-vémbu. *Arab.*—Hab-ul-ban. *Pers.*—Tàk. *Can.*—Turaka-bèvu, Hucha bèvu.

Habitat.—This large tree is found wild in Persia and the Western Himalaya, cultivated in some parts of India as an ornamental tree.

Properties and Uses.—The root-bark, fruit, flowers and leaves have deobstruent, resolvent properties. The bark is recommended as an anthelmintic, a fluid extract being a suitable preparation. The bark has been found to contain resinous principles of an alkaloidal nature which reside in the inner bark. The fruits or berries are poisonous in large doses, *i. e.*, six to eight; but they are used in leprosy and scrofula. The dried berries immersed in whisky have been employed against ascarides, tape-worm, etc., and the pulp of the berries stewed in lard is useful in scald head. The seeds are used in rheumatism.

238. MENISPERMUM FENESTRATUM.

(*N. O.*—MENISPERMACEÆ.)

Eng.—Tree Turmeric. *Tel.*—Mànu-pasupu. *Tam.* and *Mal.*—Mara-manjal. *Can.*—Daddamaradarasina.

Properties and Uses.—The wood and bark have valuable stomachic properties. The root is used as an efficient bitter tonic like calumba. Good results are obtained when given in the form of tincture or infusion. It has also antipyretic, antiperiodic and stomachic properties, useful in slight cases of continued and intermittent fevers, in debility and in certain forms of dyspepsia. It contains "berberine." It is also useful in diabetes and in cases of suppression of lochia. Externally employed it acts as antiseptic, useful for dressing wounds and ulcers.

239. MENTHA ARVENSIS.

(*N. O.*—LABIATÆ.)

Eng.—The Marsh Mint. *Hind.*, *Ben.*, *Pers.*, *Bom.*, *Tel.* and *Tam.*—Pudinà. *Arab.*—Naanai-hindi.

Habitat.—This fragrant herb is a native of the temperate Western Himalaya.

Properties and Uses.—*M. Arvensis* yields by distillation an aromatic essential oil similar to that obtained from peppermint, but inferior in quality and aroma. The herbs of mint are much esteemed in India as aromatic, carminative, stimulant, antispasmodic and stomachic, They are used in *chutneys*. The oil and menthol have the same properties. The latter is an invaluable anti-neuralgic applied externally in alcoholic solution or in the form of the popular "menthol cone."

240. MESUA FERREA.

(*N. O.*—GUTTIFERÆ.)

Sans.—Nâgkesara, Nâgpushpa. *Hind.* and *Tel.*—Nágakésara. *Ben.*—Nágèsar. *Mah.* and *Kon.*—Nâgchámpe. *Tam.*—Veilutta-champakam, Nâgapû. *Can.*—Nâgasampige. *Mal.*—Nâgacham-pakam, Veila.

Habitat.—This tree is common on the mountains of Eastern Bengal, the Eastern Himalaya, Burma and the Andamans; it is cultivated in gardens in Bengal.

Properties and Uses.—The bark, root and other parts of the plant exude an aromatic oleo-resin which has demulcent properties. The pericarp of the fruit is very astringent. The bark is mildly astringent and feebly aromatic. A fixed oil is expressed from the seeds which has been used as an application for cutaneous affections, such as sores, etc., and an embrocation in rheumatism. The dried flowers are much used as a fragrant adjunct to decoctions and oils. They are regarded as astringent and stomachic and useful in thirst, irritability of the stomach, excessive perspiration, etc.

Native Indian Preparations.—A paste of the flowers with the addition of butter and sugar is recommended to be taken in bleeding piles. The powdered flowers mixed with old clarified butter that has been washed a hundred times in water are said to be an effectual application in burning of the feet (Chakradatta).

---

241. MICHELIA CHAMPACA.

(*N. O.*—MAGNOLIACEÆ.)

Sans.—Champaka, Kusuma. *Hind.*, *Ben.* and *Mah.*—Champà, Champak. *Tel.*—Sampagni-puvvu. *Tam.*—Shampang. *Can.*—Sampige. *Mal.*—Champakam. *Kon.*—Chàmpe.

Habitat.—A tall evergreen tree growing wild in Nepal, Bengal, Assam and Burma and commonly cultivated for its yellow, sweetly-scented flowers, which are given as an offering to the gods.

Properties and Uses.—An infusion of the flowers has been advocated as a stimulant tonic and carminative, in cases of dyspepsia, nausea and fevers. Of the flowers an otto somewhat resembling that of the *ilang* is prepared. The flowers beaten up with, or macerated in, oil form excellent application to fœtid discharges from the nostrils; also in sub-acute rheumatism and in vertigo, ophthalmia and gout, and the oil of the seeds rubbed over the abdomen relieves flatulence. The bark is bitter and aromatic and regarded as antiperiodic in doses of 10 to 30 grains or as decoction in two to three-ounce doses; and the bark of the root in infusion, is an emmenagogue, also purgative; the bark is said to be an excellent substitute for guaiacum. The dried root and root bark mixed with curdled milk makes a useful application to abscesses. The juice of the leaves acts as vermifuge. It is given with honey to relieve colic. The young leaves contused and macerated in water and instilled into the eyes are said to relieve the vision.

242. MIMOSA PUDICA.

(*N. O.*—LEGUMINOSÆ.)

Sans.—Ajàlikalika, Namaskâri. *Eng.*—Sensitive Plant, Humble Plant. *Hind.*—Lajàlü. *Ben.* and *Bom.*—Lajjâbati. *Tel.*—Munugudâ-maramu. Muttavapulagamu-chettu. *Tam.*—Thottál-pádi, Thottalshurungi. *Can.*—Náchike-gida. *Mal.*—Thôttamvâti, Théndârmani.

Habitat.—This familiar plant, which is a native of Brazil, has long been naturalized and is plentiful in the hotter regions.

Properties and Uses.—The root of the plant contains a peculiar tannin. In the form of decoction it is considered useful in gravel and other similar complaints. It is also considered as resolvent and alterative, useful in diseases arising from corrupt blood and bile. The leaves and root in the powdered state are given in milk in cases of piles and fistula. The juice is applied externally to fistulous sores. The leaves rubbed into a paste are applied to hydrocele. Their juice with an equal quantity of horse's urine is made into an *anjan* which is used to remove films of the cornea by setting up an artificial inflammation. The juice of the leaves is used to impregnate cotton wool for a dressing in any form of sinus.

243. MIMUSOPS ELENGI.

(*N. O.*—SAPOTACEÆ.)

Sans.—Bakula. *Hind.*—Mulsári. *Ben.*—Bakul. *Mah.*—Ránjanasál. *Tel.*—Pogada. *Tam.*—Vakulam. *Can.*—Bakula, Ranjë. Pagade-mara. *Mal.*—Makura. *Kon.*—Vovali-ruku. *Burm.*—Khaya.

Habitat.—A large ornamental evergreen tree cultivated in India and found wild in the forests of Southern India and Burma, and generally reared in gardens for the sake of its fragrant flowers.

Properties and Uses.—The star-shaped fragrant flowers of this tree contain a volatile oil from which a sweet-scented water is distilled, which is useful as a stimulant medicine and as a perfume. From the seeds a fixed oil is obtained by expression, which is used for culinary purposes, for burning and for medicine. The seeds bruised into a paste and mixed with oil or ghee are made to form suppositories in cases of obstinate constipation, especially in children. The unripe fruit is astringent and a useful masticatory. It is therefore recommended to be chewed for fixing loose teeth. The bark is similarly useful as a gargle in diseases of the gums and teeth; also used in discharges from the mucous membranes of the bladder and urethra. The bark is also a tonic and febrifuge. The bark is said to be much sought after in the Punjaub as a medicine for increasing fertility in women. The pulp of the ripe fruit is edible and contains a large amount of sugar. It is applied to relieve headache.

244. MIRABILIS JALAPPA.

(*N. O.*—NYCTAGINACEÆ.)

Sans.—Sandhya-ràga. *Eng.*—Four-o'clock flower. *Tel.*—Chandra Kàntha. *Tam.*—Patharâshu. *Can.*—Madhyanha mallige. *Mal.*—Anthimalari. *Kon.*—Akàshamugri.

Habitat.—This small shrub is generally found cultivated in gardens for the sake of its beautiful flowers of variegated colours.

Properties and Uses.—The dried root of this plant is said to possess some nutrient qualities. Powdered and fried in ghee with spices it is given in milk as a *paushtik* (nourishing or strengthening medicine). Rubbed with water it is applied as *lep* in contusions. The leaves bruised and heated and applied as poultice to boils and abscesses hasten the suppurative process.

---

245. MOLLUGO CERVIANA.

(*N. O.*—CARYOPHYLLACEÆ.)

Sans.—Grishmasundara, Parpàtaka. *Hind.*—Taph-Jhâd. *Ben.*—Ghimashak. *Tel.*, *Tam.*, *Mal.*, *Can.*, and *Kon.*—Parpâtaka.

Properties and Uses.—The roots of this well-known common plant have an aromatic smell; the oil in which the roots are boiled has been used with much benefit in gouty and rheumatic complaints. The flowers and tender shoots, in the form of infusion or decoction, have a diaphoretic effect and are useful in fevers.

---

246. MOMORDICA CHARANTIA.

(*N. O.*—CUCURBITACEÆ.)

Sans.—Kàravetta. *Hind.*—Kareli. *Ben.*, *Guz.*, and *Mah.*—Karalâ. *Tel.*—Kâkara. *Tam.*—Pâvakka. *Can.*—Hágala-kayi. *Mal.*—Päval, Kaipavalli. *Kon.*—Kàrâthi. *Arab.*—Quisaul-barri.

Habitat.—This climbing plant is cultivated in gardens everywhere in India for its fruit.

Properties and Uses.—The fruit is bitter, but wholesome and, therefore, eaten as a vegetable. There are two varieties, one with a small roundish or ovoid fruit and the other longer and more cucumber-like. The fruit is tonic, stomachic, antibilious and laxative, useful in gout, rheumatism and diseases of the spleen and liver. It is supposed to purify the blood and dissipate melancholia and gross humours. The fruit also acts as an anthelmintic. The juice of the fresh leaves is given to children as a mild purgative, but is not unattended with danger. The fruit and leaves are both administered internally in leprosy, piles, jaundice, etc. The leaves act as galactagogue. The juice of the leaves is applied round the orbit as a cure for night-blindness. The root is applied externally to piles. The whole plant mixed with cinnamon, long-pepper, rice and marothy oil forms a good ointment in psora, scabies and other skin affections. The expressed juice together with chalk is used in aphthæ and also as an emmenagogue in dysmenorrhœa. Externally it is applied to the scalp in pustular eruptions, burns, boils, etc.

247. MOMORDICA DIOICA.

(*N. O.*—CUCURBITACEÆ.)

Tel.—Kárkotaki. *Tam.*—Aegâravalli. *Can.*—Mádahàgalakayi, Kàrchi-balli. *Mal.*—Vempàval. *Kon.*—Phägil.

Habitat.—This climbing creeper is generally met with in the forests of Southern India.

Properties and Uses.—The fruits are generally used as vegetable and they are very wholesome and grateful when cooked and eaten with food. The mucilaginous tubers, especially those of the female plant, which is larger than that of the male, are used medicinally in the form of electuary in cases of bleeding piles and in similar bowel affections. Dose is two drachms or more twice daily. The plant or the juice of the leaves, mixed with cocoanut, pepper, red sandalwood, etc., in order to form an ointment, and applied to the head is said to relieve pain in the head.

248. MORINDA CITRIFOLIA.

(*N. O.*—RUBIACEÆ.)

Sans.—Áchhuka. *Eng.*—Indian Mulberry. *Hind.*—Al, Achhi. *Ben.*—Ach. *Bom.*—Aal. *Tel.*—Maddi-chettu. *Tam.*—Nùna, Tunavu. *Can.*—Haladi-pavaté, Tagache-mara. *Mal.*—Kadappilävu.

Habitat.—This small tree or bush is found wild and cultivated nearly all over India.

Properties and Uses.—The root and root-bark yield a red dye somewhat resembling that imparted by madder. This is used for colouring the red *kharua* cloth which is universally used for covering account books by the people of India, as it is not attacked by white ants. A crystalline principle has been isolated from the root-bark and named *Morindin.* The leaves and fruit have been regarded as deobstruent and emmenagogue. The leaves are administered internally, also as tonic and febrifuge. The charred leaves made into a decoction with mustard are said to be a remedy for infantile diarrhœa. The leaves applied to wounds and ulcers have a healing effect. The unripe berries charred and mixed with salt are applied successfully to spongy gums.

249. MORINGA PTERYGOSPERMA.

(*N. O.*—MORINGEÆ.)

Sans.—Shobhânjana, Dvishigru. *Eng.*—Horse-radish tree. *Hind.*—Shäjna. *Duk.*—Munge-ka-jhad. *Punj.*—Sohánjna. *Ben.*—Sojna. *Tel.*—Munaga. *Guz.*—Saragava. *Mah.*—Shegut, Munagacha-jhad. *Tam.*—Murungai. *Can.*—Nugge. *Mal.*—Murina. *Kon.*—Mashinga-jhàd. *Cing.*—Murungà. *Burm.*—Dandalon-bin. *Malay.*—Kaylor, Ramoongie.

Habitat.—A beautiful tree, wild in the sub-Himalayan range and commonly cultivated in India and Burma for its leaves, flowers and immature capsules which are eaten in curries.

Properties and Uses.—The fresh root of this tree closely resembles in taste, smell and general appearance the common horse-radish of Europe. Distilled with water it yields an essential oil more pungent and offensive in odour than those of mustard or garlic. The seeds yield a fine fixed oil (*Ben* oil) which does not turn rancid, and hence is highly esteemed by perfumers for extracting the odours of flowers and by watch-makers as a lubricant. It is used to relieve the pain of gout and acute rheumatism. It is considered aperient. The root is regarded as an acrid, pungent stimulant, also as diuretic, given in infusion in 1½ ounce doses thrice a day. Take fresh moringa root and mustard seed, of each well bruised, one ounce; boiling water, one pint. Infuse for two hours in a covered vessel and strain. Of this the dose is about 11 ounces thrice daily. It may also be used as a vehicle for nitre and other more active remedies. In doses of 20 grains it is given in intermittent fevers. In hoarseness and relaxed sore-throat, a decoction of moringa root (or the above infusion) has been found serviceable as a gargle. The juice of the root with milk is regarded as diuretic, antilithic and digestive, useful for administration in asthma, gout, rheumatism, enlarged spleen or liver, internal and deep-seated inflammations and calculus affections. The decoction of the root-bark is also recommended and used for much the same purpose. The fresh juice of the root-bark is poured into the ears to relieve otalgia, while the gum which exudes on incision is used for the same purpose and also for dental caries. Externally the fresh root has been used as a vesicant, and considered a good remedy in bites of rabid animals, epilepsy and hysteria. It is also reckoned a useful rubefacient in palsy and chronic rheumatism. In the preparation of mustard poultices when it is desired to make them act more speedily or energetically, the addition of the expressed juice of the fresh root, or the scraped root answers these purposes effectually. The pods are esteemed as a vegetable and act as a preventive against intestinal worms. The leaves ground into a paste with a few pods of garlic, a bit of turmeric, salt and pepper are given internally in cases of dog-bite and applied externally over the bite. In 5 or 6 days the wound is said to heal, the inflammation and the febrile symptoms subsiding.

Native Indian Preparations.—In ascites and enlarged spleen, a decoction of the root-bark of *Moringa-pterygosperma* and the leaves of *Rumex vesicarius (Amlalonikâ)* is given with the addition of long-pepper, black-pepper and rock-salt in powder. In the enlargement of spleen and liver, a decoction of the root-bark is recommended to be given with the addition of plumbago root, rock-salt and long-pepper, or of the ashes of *butea frondosa* (*palása*) or of *yavakshára* (impure carbonate of potash). In internal and deep-seated inflammation and abscess a decoction of the root-bark is recommended to be given with the addition of asafœtida and rock-salt. The expressed juice of the root-bark is also given in these cases with the addition of honey or rock-salt. The root-bark is used externally in the shape of plaster and the inflamed part is fomented with its decoction. In calculous affections the decoction of the root-bark is administered internally (Chakradatta).

The seeds of *Moringa pterygosperma* enter into the composition of some stimulant applications, of which the following is an illustration :—Take of the seeds of *Moringa pterygosperma*, rock-salt, mustard seeds and *putchuk* root, equal parts, and reduce them to a paste with goat's urine. When dried this is used as a snuff for rousing comatose or drowsy persons.

---

250. MORUS ALBA or M. INDICA.

(*N. O.*—URTICACEÆ).

Sans.—Toola, Tooda. *Eng.*—White Mulberry. *Hind.*, *Pers.* and *Ben.*—Tút. *Duk.* and *Guz.*—Tutri. *Tam.*—Kambilipuch.

Habitat.—The Indian white mulbery is found wild on the temperate Himalaya and cultivated in Kashmir, the Punjab, Bengal and Burma for its leaves.

Properties and Uses.—The leaves of this plant are chiefly used as food for the silkworm. They are also eaten by cattle. It yields a pleasant acidulous fruit which is eaten fresh, or made into a preserve or syrup which is useful as a refrigerent in fevers and as an expectorant in coughs and sore throat. It is also slightly laxative and keeps best as a syrup.

251. MOSCHUS MOSCHIFERUS.

(*N. O.*—RUMINANTIA. *Fam.*, MOSCHIDÆ.)

Sans., *Hind.*, *Ben.*, *Can.* and *Mah.*—Kasturi. *Eng.*—Musk. *Pers.*—Musk. *Tel.*, *Tam.* and *Mal.*—Kasturi.

Habitat.—The musk deer lives at altitudes above 8,000 feet throughout the whole range of the Himalaya and in Tibet and Assam.

Properties and Uses.—The musk is an odoriferous secretion obtained from the preputial follicles contained in a globular sac, about 1½ inch in diameter, known as the "musk pod," of the male of the musk-deer. Each animal yields one pod, weighing on an average one ounce, which costs on an average from Rs. 30 to 40, in the markets of Northern India. The characteristic constituent of musk is a volatile oil which it contains in addition to ammonia. stearin and cholesterin. The musk has been regarded as a stimulant and aphrodisiac, useful in general debility and impotence, in low fevers, chronic coughs, and spasmodic diseases such as hysteria and epilepsy; frequently prescribed in tincture or powders in combination with other restoratives and antispasmodics. It is sometimes combined with ammonia carbonate or the aromatic spirit; sometimes with ether and camphor.

Native Indian Preparations.—In low fevers with prostration, two grains of musk with two of *Makaradhwaja* are given every three hours with the addition of honey.

Svalpa Kasturi Bhairava Rasa:—Take of cinnabar, aconite, borax, nutmeg, mace, long-pepper, black-pepper and musk equal parts and make into four-grain pills. These are given in remittent fever of low type (Rasendrasârasangraha).

Mriganábhyádirava leha:—Take of musk, cardamoms, cloves, cinnamon and dates equal parts and make into a linctus with honey and clarified butter. This is given in hoarseness and loss of speech. (Bhâvaprakâsh).

Vasantatilaka Rasa:—Take of prepared gold one part, talc and tin two parts each, iron three parts, the preparation of mercury called *rasasindura* and calcined pearls and coral four parts each; mix them together, soak for seven days in the juice of sugar-cane, of the fruits *Tribulus terrestris*(*gokshura*) and of other strenghtening vegetables. Enclose the mass in a covered crucible and roast it in a sand-bath for three hours. Lastly add to it four parts of camphor and four of musk and make into four-grain pills. These are given as an alterative tonic in a variety of diseases, but more especially in chronic affections of the lungs supposed to be caused by deranged phlegm.

---

252. MUCUNA PRURIANS.

(*N. O.* LEGUMINOSÆ).

Sans.—Atmaguptä, Kapikachchhu. *Eng.*—The Cowhage Plant. *Ben.*—Alkushi. *Duk.*—Kanch Kooric. *Mah.*—Kuhili. *Tel.*—Pilliadagu. *Tam.*—Poonaikkali. *Can.*—Nasuganni, Turachêe, Kàdavare. Näyisonagu-balli. *Mal.*—Nàyikuruna, Chorivalli. *Kon.*—Khavalyàvâli.

Habitat.—An annual climbing shrub wild in Bengal and common in the forests throughout the plains; it is also cultivated in some parts for the sake of its golden-brown velvety legumes, which are cooked and eaten as a vegetable.

Properties and Uses.—The pods are covered with stiff hairs which produce an intense irritation of the skin if incautiously handled. The hairs covering the seed pods mixed with honey have been used as a vermifuge, the action being purely mechanical. The seeds have been regarded as a nervine tonic and prescribed in the form of powder in doses of 20 to 40 grains in leucorrhœa, spermatorrhœa, etc., and in cases requiring an aphrodisiac action; and the root is considered useful in diseases of the nervous system, such as facial paralysis, hemiplegia, etc. A strong infusion of the root sweetened with honey is given in cholera morbus. The root is also useful for delirium in fevers, and when powdered and made into a paste it is applied in dropsy, a piece being also applied to the wrist and ankle. The seed is said to absorb scorpion poison when applied to the part stung. In Europe the drug is used chiefly as a vermifuge in the form of electuary or confection with honey or treacle.

Native Indian Preparations.—Take of the seeds of *Mucuna Pruriens* and the fruits *Tribulus Terrestris* (*gokshura*) equal parts and administer in doses of about a drachm with sugar and tepid milk (Shushruta).

Vánaree Vatika: Take of the seeds of *Mucuna Pruriens* 32 tolas, boil them in 4 seers of cow's milk till the latter becomes thick. The seeds are then decorticated, pounded and fried in clarified butter and made into a confection with double their weight of sugar. The mass is then divided into balls, which are kept steeped in honey. Dose—about a tola. This preparation is said to be the best of aphrodisiacs.—(Bhavaprakash).

253. MUSA SAPIENTUM *or* M. PARADISIACA.

(*N. O.*—SCITAMINEÆ).

Sans.—Kadali, Rambha. *Eng.*—The Plantain, Banana. *Hind. Mah.* and *Guz.*—Kela. *Duk.*—Maoz. *Ben.*—Kalà. *Tel.*—Kadalamu, Arati. *Tam.*—Kadali, Välei. *Can.*—Bäle. *Mal.*—Vàla, *Kon.*—Keli. *Cing.*—Kehal-gahà. *Burm.*—Napiya-bin.

Habitat.—This indigenous, perennial, herbaceous plant, usually 10 to 12 feet high, is cultivated universally in many varieties throughout India for its nutritious and delicious fruit.

Properties and Uses.—The plantain is one of the safest and most nourishing foods. The unripe fruit is considered cooling and astringent, and useful as a valuable article of diet, especially for those suffering from hæmoptysis and diabetes, and, in the dried state, it is antiscorbutic. Flour made of green plantains dried in the sun, is used as *chappaties* in cases of dyspepsia with flatulence and acidity. The ripe fruit contains about 20 per cent. of sugar. It is esteemed as a valuable food in chronic dysentery and diarrhœa, when it is usually combined with tamarinds and common salt in the following proportions:—Plantain, 1 ounce; tamarind pulp, ½ an ounce; common salt, 1 drachm. The ingredients to be mixed immediately before they are consumed. Raw plantains are also made into a soup for the same purpose. When used for children, sugar or sugarcandy, instead of salt, may be used. The fully ripe fruit is laxative if taken regularly in the early mornings. A syrup of bananas is popular in America for producing a refreshing beverage and as an effectual remedy in relieving bronchitis. The leaves and leaf stalks when burnt yield alkaline ashes which can be used instead of country-soap or Fuller's earth in washing clothes. The old leaves are collected, dried and burnt to ashes. The ashes are placed on a cloth supported on four posts, water is made to percolate through them into an earthen vessel. The alkaline water thus obtained is used for steeping clothes intended to be washed. The ashes produced by burning the plant contain potash salts and are, therefore, useful in acidity, heart-burn and colic. The plantain leaves are used in India for many domestic purposes, chiefly for serving food on at feasts and public dinners. The young tender leaves are useful as a cool dressing for inflamed and blistered surfaces; the blister having been removed, a piece of plantain leaf of the required size, smeared with any bland oil, is applied to the denuded surface and kept in place by means of a bandage. The dressing should be changed twice daily with fresh leaves, or oftener if required. The blistered surface generally heals satisfactorily in four or five days. The tender leaves are also useful as a substitute for oiled silk and gutta-percha in the water dressing of wounds and ulcers to retain the moisture, provided the piece used is sufficiently large to cover or envelop the whole part, and is kept in its place by bandages, etc. As a shade for the eyes in ophthalmia and other diseases of the eye no manufactured shade is superior to plantain-leaf; the older and greener leaves answer best for this purpose. The root is antibilious and, in powder, it is used in anæmia and cachexia. The juice of the tender roots contain, much of tannin and is used with mucilage for checking hæmorrhages from the genital and air passages. The root juice in which burnt borax and nitre are dissolved is given in retention of urine; mixed with ghee and sugar it is given in gonorrhœa. The juice of flowers mixed with curds is administered in dysmenorrhœa and menorrhagia. The cooked flowers are used in diabetes. The juice of the plant is styptic in effect. The juice of the bark and leaf is given to children suffering from an overdose of opium: one ounce with one ounce of ghee is a brisk purgative. A mucilage prepared from the seeds has been found of great service in the catarrhal and mild inflammatory form of diarrhœa.

Native Indian Preparations.—The unripe fruit called *mochaka* in Sanskrit is much used in diabetes in the form of a *ghrita*, prepared as follows:—

Kadalyâdi Ghrita:—Take of plantain flowers 12½ seers, watery juice of the root-stock of the plantain tree 64 seers; boil them together till reduced to one-fourth, and strain. To the strained decoction add four seers of prepared clarified butter and the following substances in the form of a paste, namely unripe plantains, cloves, cardamoms, red sandalwood, wood of *Pinus longifolia* (*sarala*), *jatâmànsi* root, the three myrobalans, *Raphanus Sativus* (*mulaka*), and the fruit of *Feronia Elephantum* (*Kapittha*) in equal parts, one seer in all, and prepare a *ghrita* in the usual way. This medicine is generally given along with some preparation of tin or other metallic medicine in diabetes. The dose is about two tolas.

254. MUSSAENDA FRONDOSA.

(*N. O.*—RUBIACEÆ).

Can.—Belloti-gida. *Mal.*—Vellil. *Kon.*—Belloti.

Habitat.—This plant grows abundantly on the Malabar Coast.

Properties and Uses.—The root is used medicinally. Half a tola is given rubbed with cow's urine in white leprosy. The root rubbed in water and applied as a paste to relieve the burning of sore-eyes, and the juice of the leaves and fruit is applied with much benefit in cases of weakness of eyesight. The infusion or weak decoction of the dried shoots is given to children to relieve the cough due to cold and catarrh. In cases of jaundice two tolas of the white calycine leaves are given in milk.

---

255. MYLABRIS CHICORII.

(*Species.*—COLEOPTERA.)

Eng.—Telini Fly. *Hind.*—Telni, Telni-makhi. *Ben.*—Telini-poka. *Duk.*—Zirangi. *Tel.*—Igelu. *Tam.*—Pinstlarin-i.

Several species of insects of the *Coleoptera* or beetle order, with vesicant properties when dried, similar to those of the blistering or Spanish fly (*Cantharis Vesicatoria*), are common in India. The most important is the *M. Chicorii*, which exists plentifully in many parts of India, quite common in the Hyderabad district and Deccan.

Properties and Uses.—This insect has been found to yield a fatty acid believed to be *Cantharidin*, which is apparently a complete substitute for the European article as a vesicant, provided that due care is taken in its preparation, etc. The best season for collecting the insects is just previous to the setting in of the monsoon, in the early morning or evening; they should be killed by the steam of boiling vinegar, thoroughly dried in the sun and preserved in well-stoppered bottles. Its principal use is as a blistering agent, and for this purpose it is used in the form of plaster, prepared as follows: Take Telini Fly finely powdered; White or Black Dammer, Beeswax, and Suet (mutton or goat) of each two ounces; liquify the three latter with a gentle heat, then remove from the fire and sprinkle in the Telini; mix the whole thoroughly and continue to stir the mixture while it is allowed to cool.

256. MYRICA NAGI or M. SAPIDA.

(*N. O.*—MYRICACEÆ).

Sans.—Katphala. *Eng.*—The Box-Myrtle. *Hind.*, *Ben.*, and *Bom.*—Kaiphal. *Tel.*—Kaidaryamu. *Tam.*—Marudam-pattai.

Habitat.—An evergreen tree of the sub-tropical Himalaya, found also in the Khasia mountains and the hills of Burma. The bark is exported from the bazaars of Northern India and is usually to be found in the drug markets of the large cities.

Properties and Uses.—The bark is said to contain an alkaloidal principle and 11 to 14 per cent of tannin. It is aromatic and astringent. The powder of the bark is recommended as a snuff in catarrh with headache, and combined with ginger as a stimulant application in cholera.

257. MYRISTICA FRAGRANS.

Syn:—M. OFFICINALIS; M. MOSCHATA; M. AROMATICA.

(*N. O.*—MYRISTICACEÆ).

(Nutmegs):—*Sans.*—Jàti-phalam. *Hind.*, *Duk.*, and *Ben.*—Jaèphal. *Kash.*—Zâfal. *Bom.*, *Punj.*, *Guz.*, and *Mah.*—Jäyiphal. *Tel.*—Jäjikaya. *Tam.*—Jàdikày. *Can.*—Jajikai. *Mal.*—Jätikä. *Cing*—Jàdikà. *Burm.*—Zadi-phu. Malay—Buah-pala.

(Mace):—*Sans.*—Jätipatri. *Hind.*, *Can.*, *Tel.*, *Mah.*, and *Guz.*—Jäepatri. *Ben.*—Jotri. *Punj.*—Jäuntari. *Kash.*—Jow-watir. *Bom.*—Jäwantri. *Tam.* and *Mal.*—Jadi-pattiri. *Cing.*—Vasäväsi. *Burm.*—Zadi-phu apoen. *Malay.*—Bunga-pala.

Habitat.—The nutmeg tree is indigenous to the Malay Peninsula and Penang. It has been successfully cultivated in Madras and Southern India. The seeds are the nutmegs of commerce, and the *arillus* surrounding the seed within the outer shell constitute, when dried, the product known as mace.

Properties and Uses.—Nutmegs are aromatic, stimulant and carminative, closely allied to cloves and cinnamon, for which they may be substituted. In large doses they are narcotic. They are largely employed as a flavouring agent and condiment. They yield an essential oil and a fixed oil; mace also contains a peculiar essential oil. The fixed oil or, as it is called, "butter of nutmeg," is obtained by expression, the powdered nuts being steamed and pressed while hot. It consists essentially of *myristin* and *myristic acid* and retains a certain proportion of the essential oil. The essential oil is obtained by distillation and is water-white in colour, with the fragrant spicy odour of the nutmeg. Its constituents have been named *myristicene* and *myristicol*. The essential oil of mace is of a yellowish colour with the odour of mace and consists of *Macene.* These volatile oils are used to a large extent in perfumery. The concrete oil of nutmeg is used as a rubefacient and as an ingredient in ointments and plasters. The essential oil is stimulant and carminative and is administered in atonic diarrhœa and dysentery to relieve pain, and is used in combination with other stimulating oils as an external application in rheumatism. The dose of powdered nutmeg or mace, which possesses the same properties, is from 5 to 15 grains; of the oil from 1 to 3 drops; of the spirit, ½ to 2 drachms. Mace is useful in low stages of fever, in consumptive complaints, humoral asthma, and with aromatics in wasting and long-continued bowel complaints. It is also aphrodisiac and carminative in effect. When roasted it is useful in choleraic diarrhœa and in obstructions of the liver and spleen. Nutmeg is useful in atonic diarrhœa, flatulent colic and some forms of dyspepsia. Its infusion is said to be useful in quenching the thirst of cholera patients.

---

258. MYRISTICA MALABARICA.

(*N. O.*—MYRISTICACEÆ.)

Sans.—Kamuk, Malati. *Eng.*—Bombay Mace or Country Nutmeg. *Bom.*—(The nut) Jangli, Jaiphal (mace), Rampatri.

Habitat.—This tree is indigenous to the Koncans, Canara and Malabar.

Properties and Uses.—The seed, which this tree yields, is larger and more oblong than the true nutmeg; it possesses little of its fragrance or its aromatic taste and is inferior as an internal remedy. Bruised and subjected to boiling it yields a considerable quantity of a yellowish concrete oil which, when melted down with a small quantity of any bland oil is regarded as an excellent application to indolent and ill-conditioned ulcers, allaying pain, cleansing the surface and establishing healthy action. It is also serviceable as an embrocation in chronic rheumatism. The oil in which the seed is boiled is a useful instillation in cases of earache. The *Arillus Rampatri* is considered to be a nervine tonic; it is used in stopping vomiting, also as a substitute for the true mace, from which it differs in being destitute of aroma.

259. MYRSINE AFRICANA.

(*N. O.*—MYRSINEÆ).

Punj., *Kash.* and *Hind.*—Bebrang, Bahbarang, Baibarang.

Habitat.—A small shrub found in the Himalaya from Kashmir to Nepal. The fruit is common in the Punjab bazaars.

Properties and Uses.—The fruit is regarded to be a powerful cathartic vermifuge. The plant yields a gum which is prescribed for dysmenorrhœa.

260. MYRTUS COMMUNIS.

Eng.—The Myrtle. *Hind.*—Habulas, Vilayati Mehndi.

Habitat.—This shrub is cultivated in many parts of India.

Properties and Uses.—The fragrant volatile oil distilled from the leaves has antiseptic and rubefacient properties. It is generally employed in perfumery. A fixed oil is obtained from the berries; it strengthens and promotes the growth of hair. The fruit, myrtle berry, is carminative and given in diarrhœa and dysentery; also useful in hæmorrhages, internal ulcerations and rheumatism. The decoction is useful as a mouth-wash in aphthæ.

261. NARDOSTACHYS JATAMANSI.

(*N. O.*—VALERIANEÆ.)

Sans., *Can.*, *Duk.*, *Tel.* and *Ben.*—Jatamansi. *Eng.*—Indian Spikenard. *Hind.* and *Punj.*—Jatamashi, Bal-chir. *Kash.*—Bhut-jatt Kukilipot. *Arab.*—Sumbul-hind. *Pers.*—Sunbulut-tib. *Bom.*—Sumbul. *Tam.*—Jatamashi. *Mah.*—Jatamavshi. *Mal.*—Jatamanchi. *Cing.*—Jaramanshi.

Habitat.—This herb is growing at great elevations on the Alpine Himalaya, in Nepal, Butan and Sikkim, ascending in some places to 17,000 feet. The drug, which consists of coarse, dark, hair-like fibres, resembling a "shock" head of hair, (the Sanskrit and other names, indeed, have a reference to the resemblance) is met with in most bazaars in India.

Properties and Uses.—Jatamansi has been held in high repute in Hindu medicine from very old days as an antispasmodic, and trials made with it by Europeans tend to show that, in this character, it is a good substitute for the official Valerian. It is also regarded as tonic and nervous stimulant, and employed in the treatment of hysterical affections, especially palpitation of the heart, chorea, flatulence, etc., it is also used with much success in epilepsy and similar nervous and convulsive ailments. The dose is from 30 to 40 grains in powder. It has been also recommended as deobstruent, diuretic and emmenagogue, and used in very many diseases of the digestive and respiratory organs. It is useful in jaundice. It is generally used as an aromatic adjunct in the preparation of medicinal oils and in perfumery. It is said to promote the growth and blackness of hair. A fluid extract prepared with an ammoniacal menstruum or a tincture (5 ounces of bruised *Jatamansi* in 2 pints of proof spirit) is a suitable preparation for administration, the dose is from 1 to 2 drachms. In all cases it may be advantageously combined with camphor, ammonia and other remedies of the same class. It may also be given in infusion (2 drachms of the bruised root in half a pint of boiling water) in doses of a wine-glassful twice or thrice daily.

Native Indian Preparations.—Take of the pulse of *Phaseolus Roxburghii* (*Kuláttha*), barley, jujube fruit, seeds of *Crotolaria juncea* (*Sana*), bdellium, *jatamansi* root, the ten drugs collectively called *dasamula* and chebulic myrobalan, equal parts and prepare a decoction in the usual way. This decoction is to be administered with the addition of clarified butter and goat's urine (Sushruta).

---

262. NAREGAMIA ALATA.

(*N. O.*—MELIACEÆ.)

Eng.—Goanese Ipecacuanha. *Mah.*—Tinpani, Pittvel. *Goa.*—Trifolio. *Can.*—Nela-naringa. *Mal.*—Nilanarakam. *Kon.*—Bhui-naringa.

Habitat.—This small woody shrub is growing in Western and Southern India. It is known as "country ipecacuanha" at Goa and Calicut where it is collected.

Properties and Uses.—The drug, consisting of the creeping roots and slender stems divested of leaves, has a pungent aromatic odour and little taste. Emetic properties, like those of ipecacuanha, have been attributed to the root, which is used in same doses as a remedy in acute dysentery. The drug has recently been tried with considerable success as an expectorant, in chronic forms of bronchitis, where there is a thick, scanty and tenacious expectoration, and in bronchial catarrh with asthmatic tendencies and heart difficulty. The preparation recommended is a fluid extract in doses of 2 to 10 minims. The juice of the plant mixed with cocoanut oil is used in cases of psora.

263. NELUMBIUM SPECIOSUM.

(*N. O.*—NYMPHÆCEÆ.)

Sans. and *Ben.*—Padma. *Eng.*—Sacred Lotus. *Hind.*—Kanwal. *Arab.* and *Pers.*—Nilufer. *Mah. Can.* and *Kon.*—Kamala. *Tel.*—Tamara. *Tam.*—Tamarai, Ambal. *Mal.*—Aravindam, Tamara.

Habitat.—This large aquatic herb with its elegant sweet-scented white or red flowers is generally met with in tanks and ponds in most parts of India.

Properties and Uses.—This is held in great regard by the Hindus on account of its flowers, called *Padma* or *Kamala*, which are sacred to Laksmi the goddess of wealth and prosperity. Of this species of Nymphæceæ there are 3 varieties, N. Lotus, N. Stellata and N. Rubra. Medicinally, the entire plant, the root, flower, stalks and leaves are all useful. The flowers, filaments and juice of the flower stalks are regarded as refrigerent and astringent, useful in fevers; are also recommended as cardiac tonic. The honey formed in the flowers by the bees feeding upon the *padma* is called *padmamadhu* or *makaranda*. This is very useful in eye diseases. The tubers boiled in gingelly oil are rubbed on the head to cool the head and eyes. The expressed juice is also employed instead of pieces of the tuber. The root is mucilaginous and demulcent, given in piles. The seeds are used as an application in skin affections. The pistils are used with black-pepper externally and internally as an antidote in snake poisoning. The large leaves are used as cool bed-sheets in high fever with much burning of the skin.

Native Indian Preparations.—In bleeding piles the filaments of the lotus are given with honey and fresh butter or with sugar (Bhâvaprakâsh). In menorhagia the filaments are given with the addition of *sonchal* salt, nigella seeds, liquorice powder, curdled milk and honey (Chakradatta).

Utpalâdi Sritam:—Take of the filaments of *Nymphæa Lotus, N. Stellata* and *N. Rubra*, and liquorice root equal parts, in all two tolas, and prepare a decoction in the usual way. This decoction is said be useful in thirst, burning of the body, fainting, vomiting, hæmorrhage from the internal organs and bleeding from the womb during gestation (Bhâvaprâkash).

A cooling application for external use is prepared as follows:—Take of the filaments and leaf-stalks of *Nelumbium Speciosum, Nymphae Lotus* and *Nymphae Stellata* and of red sandal-wood equal parts, and rub them together into a thin paste with cold water. This is applied to the forehead in cephalalgia. A paste made of emblic myrobalans and the filaments of the lotus is also used for the same purpose. Similar compositions are recommended for external inflammations, erysipelas, etc. (Chakradatta).

264. NERIUM ODORUM.

(*N. O.*—APOCYNACEÆ).

Sans.—Karavira. *Eng.*—Sweet-scented Oleander. *Hind.*—Kaner, Kanel. *Ben.*—Karabi. *Mah.*—Kanera. *Tel.*—Ganneru, Karaviramu, Kasturipatte. *Tam.*—Kanaveeram, Alari. *Can.*—Kanagilu, Paddale. *Mah.*—Kanaviram.

Habitat.—This small evergreen shrub is wild in Western Afghanistan and in several other parts of Northern India and cultivated in gardens for its flowers which are given as an offering to the gods.

Properties and Uses.—There are two varieties of this plant, namely the white and the red-flowered. The fresh roots of the white variety, known in Bengal as *Sheth-Karabi*, are intensely poisonous as are also the leaves, bark and flowers. The bark has been found to contain two resinous bitter principles which are named *Neriodorin* and *Neriodorein*, both of which are powerful heart poisons, and it has been shown that the physiological action of oleander is analogous to that of digitalis. It is not, however, used internally in any form. The leaves have been found to contain two principles named *Oleandrine* and *Pseudocurarine*, and three glucosides have been isolated from the leaves and named *Neriine Neriantine* and *Rosaginine*, the first being believed to be identical with *digitaleine*. The root is used externally, made into paste with water, as an external application in cancers and ulcerations and the paste is also applied in leprosy. The drug is a powerful resolvent and attenuant, but serviceable only for external application. The decoction of the leaves is applied externally to reduce swelling. Criminal records show that the root is used to procure abortion.

Native Indian Preparations.—*Karavirádya Taila:* Take of sesamum oil 4 seers, decoction of the root of *Nerium Odorum* 8 seers, cow's urine 8 seers, *Plumbago rosea* root and *Baberang* seeds, each half a seer in the form of a paste; boil them together and prepare an oil in the usual way. This oil is used in eczema, impetigo, and other skin diseases. The fresh juice of the young leaves is dropped into the eyes in ophthalmia with copious lachrymation—(Chakradatta).

265. NICOTIANA TABACUM.

(*N. O.*—SOLANACEÆ.)

Sans.—Támrakúta. *Eng.*—Tobacco. *Hind.*, *Pers.*, and *Mah.* —Tambâku. *Arab.*—Tanbak. *Tel.*—Pogàku. *Tam.*—Púgaielai. *Can.*—Hogesoppu. *Mal.*—Púkayil. *Kon.*—Dhurápàn. *Tulu.*—Pugere.

Habitat.—The tobacco plant is originally a native of America. It is now quite common in India, being cultivated to a large extent in many parts of Bengal, Bombay and Burma and in Madras and Travancore. N. Rustica is cultivated and prepared in some parts of Upper India, Bengal and Punjab. It is known as East Indian tobacco.

Properties and Uses.—Tobacco is used in India as an article of luxury by all classes of the people, chiefly for smoking and some classes in powder as snuff and by others with lime and *pán* for chewing, while Burma and Trichinopoly cheroots of Indian manufacture are popular with Europeans. The preparation made by Indians for smoking is as follows:—The coarsely-powdered tobacco is mixed with unrefined sugar (*gúr*) and aromatic and fragrant substances, sometimes with sandal-wood oil, patchouli leaves, otto of roses, musk and other perfumes into the form of a black-looking conserve known as *gurákù*. A portion of this is placed with live charcoal in the *chilam* of the universal *hookah*, made commonly of a cocoanut shell or of metal, and which, as is well known, contains water through which the vapour is passed in smoking. The practice, in some parts of India, is equally common with women and children as with men. Medicinally tobacco is little used on account of its poisonous properties. The dried leaves are powerfully sedative, affecting the heart, frequently causing great depression, antispasmodic, emetic and narcotic and unfit for internal administration. A decoction has been used as a local application to relieve pain and irritation in rheumatic swellings, syphilitic nodes and skin diseases, and as a means of inducing muscular relaxation, thus aiding in the reduction of strangulated hernia and dislocations. Tobacco-smoking is resorted to with excellent effect in many cases of asthma, nervous irritability and sleeplessness. The tobacco leaves when distilled with water at a temperature above that of the boiling water, afford an empyreumatic oil—*nicotianine* or tobacco-camphor—a most virulent poison containing *nicotine*. Nicotine has been recommended in tetanus and as an antidote to strychnine. Its internal use is attended, however, with the greatest danger. The water from the *hookah* is diuretic and the black oil which collects in the pipe stem is used on tents to heal up sinuses and is dropped into the eye to cure night blindness and purulent conjunctivitis. A paste made with snuff, lime and the powdered bark of *Calophyllum Inophyllum (Undi)* is applied in orchitis.

266. NIGELLA SATIVA.

(*N. O.*—RANUNCULACEÆ.)

Sans.—**Krishna-jiraka, Upakunchikà.** *Eng.*—**Small Fennel or Black Cumin.** *Hind.*—**Kálajira, Kulanji.** *Ben.*—**Mugrela.** *Bom.*, or *Mah.*—**Krishnajira.** *Pers.*—**Siyáhdánah.** *Tel.*—**Nallajilakara.** *Tam.*—**Karunjiragam.** *Can.*—**Kari-jirige.** *Mal.*—**Karinchirakam.** *Kon.*—**Karijire.**

Habitat.—This plant is cultivated in some parts of India for its seeds.

Properties and Uses.—The seeds are used as a condiment in curries. The small triangular seeds which resemble coarse gun powder, contain two kinds of oil—one a fixed and yellowish volatile oil of disagreeable odour, and specific gravity 0·875; and the other of the consistence of castor oil. The seeds are found to contain *Melanthin*, a substance allied to helleborin, and like saponin possessing emulsifying powers. The seeds are aromatic, carminative, stomachic and digestive; they are employed as a corrective of purgatives and other medicines and are believed to possess diuretic, anthelmintic and emmenagogue properties, useful in indigestion, loss of appetite, fever, diarrhœa, dropsy, puerperal diseases, etc. They have a decided action as a galactagogue, and are therefore given to recently-delivered females in combination with a few other medicines. In doses of 10 to 20 grains, they have a well-marked emmenagogue effect, useful in dysmenorrhœa and in large doses cause abortion. The seeds scattered between layers of woollen clothes, shawls, etc., preserve them from the ravage of insects. This use of the seeds is common all over India. For this purpose they are mixed with powdered camphor. The seeds have also antibilious property and are administered internally to arrest vomiting. The seeds fried, bruised, tied in muslin bag and smelt relieve cold and catarrh of the nose by constant inhalation.

Native Indian Preparations.—In intermittent fever nigella seeds slightly roasted are recommended to be given in two-drachm doses with the addition of an equal quantity of treacle (Chakradatta). In loss of appetite and distaste for food, a confection made of nigella seeds, cumin seeds, black pepper, raisins, tamarind pulp, pomegranate juice and *sonchal* salt with treacle and honey is said to be very useful (Chakradatta). In the after-pains of puerperal women, Chakradatta recommends the administration of nigella seeds with the addition of long-pepper, *sonchal* salt and wine.

In puerperal diseases such as fever, loss of appetite and disordered secretions after delivery, the following preparation called *Pancha jiraka páka* is used:—Take of nigella seeds, cumin seeds, aniseeds, *ajowan*, seeds of *Carum sativum (ajanodá)*, *Anethum sowa* (*sulpha*) and *Trigonella Fœnum-græcum* (*methi*), coriander, ginger, long-pepper, long-pepper root, plumbago root, *habushá* (an aromatic substance), dried pulp of the fruit *Ziziphus jujuba (vadariphala)*, root of *Aplotaxis auriculata* (*Kushtha*) and *Kamala* powder each one tola, treacle 100 tolas, milk one seer, clarified butter 4 tolas. Boil them together and prepare a confection. Dose is about a drachm every morning.

267. NYCTANTHES ARBOR-TRISTIS.

(*N. O.*—OLEACEÆ.)

Sans.—Pàrijàta, Siphàlikà. *Eng.*—Night Jasmine, Weeping Nyctanthes. *Hind.*—Har, Har-singhár. *Ben.*—Seoli, Singhar. *Bom.*—Harsingara. *Tel.*—Pagadamalle, Shwétasurasa, *Tam.*—Manjapu, Pavala-Malligai. *Can.*—Pârijâta. *Mal.*—Manpumaram.

Habitat.—This small tree with its fragrant flowers is found wild in the forests of Central India and Sub-Himalayan regions and commonly cultivated in gardens in many parts of India for its flowers.

Properties and Uses.—The fragrant flowers are given as votive offerings. They contain an essential oil similar to that of jasmine and which is utilised in perfumery. The leaves are found to contain an alkaloidal principle named *Nyctanthine*. The leaves are regarded as anti-bilious and expectorant, useful in bilious fevers. The juice of the fresh leaves is a safe purgative for infants. It is given with honey in chronic fever. As anthelmintic it is given with honey mixed with common salt. In the form of infusion in doses of 2 ounces it is useful in fever in children as diaphoretic and diuretic. A decoction of the leaves prepared over a gentle fire is a specific for obstinate sciatica. Six or seven young leaves rubbed up with water and a little fresh ginger are administered in obstinate fevers of the intermittent type. The powdered seeds are employed to cure scurvy, affections of the scalp, etc.

268. NYMPHÆA LOTUS.

(*N. O.*—NYMPHÆACEÆ.)

Sans.—Kamala. *Eng.*—Water-Lily. *Hind.*—Nilofar, Chota Kanval. *Ben.*—Säluka, Nàl. *Bom.* and *Mah.*—Kamalaphul. *Tel.*—Allikâda, Tellakaluva, *Tam.*—Vellâmbal, Indiravácham. *Can.*—Bilè-Naidile, Bilè-Tavare. *Mal.*—Vellânpal, Neerampal. *Kon.*—Dhuve Sälaka.

Habitat.—The water-lily, which exists in three varieties, the white, red and blue, is found to grow in tanks and marshes throughout the warmer parts of India.

Properties and Uses.—The water-lily is regarded as the queen of Indian flowers, beloved of the poets and sacred to the gods and only second in estimation to the lotus. The medicinal uses are the same as those of the corresponding parts of *Nelumbium speciosum* already described. The roots and seeds are edible, the latter forming the diet known as *Dhapar-koki*. The tubers of the red variety when boiled form a very beneficial diet in cases of piles.

---

269. OCIMUM ALBUM.

(*N. O.*—LABIATÆ.)

Sans.—Ajaka, Gambhèram, Gandhapanirjaka. *Bom.* and *Mah.*—Ran-tulasi. *Tel.*—Kukka-tulasi. *Tam.*—Ganjànkorai. *Can.*—Nayi-tulasi. *Mal.*—Kattarâma-tulasi. *Kon.*—Ram-tulasi.

Properties and Uses.—The plant has aromatic and stimulant properties. During fever when the extremities are cold the leaves made into a paste are applied to the finger and toe-nails. The same preparation is used as a cure for parasitical diseases of the skin, such as ringworm, etc.

---

270. OCIMUM BASILICUM.

(*N. O.*—LABIATÆ).

Sans.—Varvara. Manjàriki. *Eng.*—Sweet Basil. *Hind.*—Bäbul. *Duk.*—Sabza. *Ben.*—Bàbui-tulasi. *Pers.*—Pharanjamushk. *Tel.*—Bhu-tulasi, Vebùdipatri. *Tam.*—Tirunìrupachhai, Karandai. *Can.* and *Kon.*—Kàm kasturi. *Mal.*—Ràm-tulasi.

Habitat.—This small shrub, indigenous to Persia and Sindh, is cultivated in gardens in India.

Properties and Uses.—The whole plant is aromatic with an odour slightly resembling that of cloves. On distillation with water, the leaves yield an essential oil which, being kept, solidifies into a crystalline camphor allied to menthol and called *Basil-camphor.* The seeds are mucilaginous and are demulcent and diuretic in effect. They are useful in internal piles and constipation, which they relieve; they have an aphrodisiac property and the dose is from 1 to 3 drachms; steeped in water they swell into a mucilaginous jelly which is taken with the addition of sugar in dysentery, gonorrhœa and cough; also in diarrhœa and kidney affections. The cold infusion of the seeds is useful in after-pains of parturition. The juice of the leaves is dropped into the ear in earache and dullness of hearing. When mixed with ginger and black pepper they are given during the cold stages of ague. The leaves dried and powdered and used like snuff are said to dislodge maggots from the nose. A 12 per cent decoction of the plant used as irrigation in nasal myosis produces anaesthesia and acts as a parasiticide and antiseptic, so that the larvæ which cause the disease are rendered inactive and expelled. It has long been in use in Bengal with like effect for a similar affection known as *Pinàsh.*

271. OCIMUM SANCTUM.

(*N. O.*– LABIATÆ.)

Sans.—Tulasi, Divya, Bhârati, Krishnamûl, *Eng.*—Holy Basil. *Hind.*—Käla-tulasi. *Ben.*—Tulasi? *Bom.*, *Tel.*, *Tam.* and *Mah.*—Tulasi. *Can.*—Kari-tulasi. *Mal.*—Krishna-tulasi, Shiva-tulasi. *Kon.*—Kàli-tulasi.

Habitat.—This small herb is found throughout India and universally cultivated for ceremonial purposes.

Properties and Uses.—The holy basil is the most sacred plant of the Hindus, being dedicated to Vishnu, the Preserver of the World. It may be seen everywhere near Hindu houses. Medicinally the *tulasi* plant is useful in a variety of diseases. An infusion of the leaves is given in malaria and as a stomachic in gastric diseases of children; also used as a protection against mosquitoes, which it undoubtedly drives away. The dried plant has expectorant and stomachic properties. It is a domestic remedy for croup, catarrh and bronchitis. It is applied externally to the skin in ringworm and other cutaneous diseases; poured into the ear it is said to be a first-rate remedy for earache. The infusion of the leaves is administered as stomachic in the gastric disorders of children and in hepatic affections. The juice of the leaves mixed with ginger is given for colic in children, and mixed with black pepper it is given in the cold stages of intermittent fever. With honey, ginger and onion juice it forms a good expectorant remedy, useful in cough and bronchitis. The juice of the fresh leaves and the flower tops and the slender roots are used as an antidote in snake poisoning. The dried leaves are powdered and employed as a snuff in ozæna. The wood or the stems of the plant are made into beads or rosaries used by Hindus for counting the recitations of their prayers.

Native Indian Preparations.—The following is a compound decoction recommended by Chakradatta in cough and affections of the chest:—Take of the leaves of *Ocimum sanctum*, *gulancha*, ginger, root of *Clerodendron siphonanthus* (*bhargi*) and *Solanum jacquinii* (*kontakàri*), equal parts and prepare a decoction in the usual way. An oil which is prepared with a paste of the leaves of *Ocimum sanctum*, roots of *Solanum jacquinii*, *Baliospermum montanum* (*danti*), *Acorus Calamus* (*Vacha*), *Moringa pterygosperma* (*sigru*), long-pepper, black-pepper and ginger, is recommended for application in ozæna—(Chakradatta).

272. OLDENLANDIA CORYMBOSA.

(*N. O.*—RUBIACEÆ.)

Sans.—Parpata. *Hind.*—Daman-papar. *Ben.*—Khetpapra.

Habitat.—This plant is common as a weed throughout India.

Properties and Uses.—It is considered useful as an alterative in low forms of fever administered in decoction.

273. OLDENLANDIA UMBELLATA.

(*N. O.*—RUBIACEÆ.)

Eng.—Indian Madder, Chay-root. *Tel.*—Chirivèr. *Tam.* and *Mal.*—Chày-vèr. *Can.*—Chây-bèru.

Habitat.—This plant is found generally growing in the districts bordering on the sea-coasts.

Properties and Uses.—The root-bark of this plant is generally used as a dyeing material. The leaves are useful as expectorant in asthma and consumption.

274. OPHIORRHIZA MUNGOS.

(*N. O.*—RUBIACEÆ.)

Sans.—Sârpâkshi, Pàtalabhèdi. *Eng.*—The Mongoose Plant. *Hind.*—Sarahati. *Ben.*—Gandhanâkuli. *Bom.*, and *Mah.*—Nagavelli. *Tel.*—Sarpàshi-chettu. *Tam.*—Keerippùndu. *Can.*—Pàtàla-garuda, Garuda-pâtâla. *Mal.*—Avilpòri. *Kon.*—Garda-pátáli.

Habitat.—This herb is found in the mountains of Assam, Burma, the Western Peninsula and Ceylon.

Properties and Uses.—The roots are sold to ignorant people in some places as a charm against snake-bite, a notion derived from the fact that the plant is supposed to furnish the mongoose with an antidote to the bites of poisonous snakes. In Ceylon it has a high reputation as a remedy for snake-bite. It is also used as an antidote against the bites of mad dogs. Medicinally the root is an agreeable bitter tonic. The parts used are the leaves, root and bark made into decoction and administered in doses of half ounce as a stomachic.

275. OPUNTIA DILLENII.

Syn:—CACTUS INDICUS.

(*N. O.*—CACTEÆ.)

Eng.—The Prickly-pear. *Hind.* and *Ben.*—Phani-manasa, Nàgphana. *Tel.*—Nâgajamudu. *Tam.*—Nagatali, Palakai Kalli. *Can.*—Shivaràm Kalli, Mullugalli. *Mal.*—Nágtali, Palakalli. *Kon.*—Kântya nivali.

Habitat.—It is a native of America. now naturalised in India, growing in great tracts in Rajputana, and in Madras, and Mysore and other places.

Properties and Uses.—The fruit is refrigerent and, when baked or made into a syrup, it acts as an expectorant and is a good remedy in asthma and whooping cough. The dose of the syrup is about a teaspoonful, three or four times a day. It has the effect of increasing the secretion of bile. The fruit contains malic acid and manganese. The ripe fruit when eaten has the power of dyeing the urine red, said to be useful in gonorrhœa as a demulcent. The juice and the fruit are both useful in gonorrhœa. The milky juice is given as a purgative in doses of 10 drops, mixed with a little sugar. The leaves made into a pulp are used as a poultice to allay heat and inflammation in scorbutic ulcers; also applied with much benefit to the eyes in ophthalmia. Hot leaf applied to boils is said to hasten suppuration.

276. ORCHIS MASCULA.

(*N. O.*—ORCHIDEÆ.)

Eng.—The Salep Orchid. *Hind.*, *Pers.*, and *Ben.*—Salabmisri. *Mah.*, *Kon.*, *Tel.*, *Can.*, *Mal.* and *Tam.*—Sàlâmisri.

Habitat.—The salep of Indian Bazaars is principally imported from Persia and Afghanistan *viá* Bombay, some of it being probably of European origin. For, the salep of commerce is obtained not only from *Mascula* but also from some other allied species found in Europe and Northern Asia. The tubers of *Eulophia Campestris* found in Northern India are often sold as a substitute for the true salep. A bitter variety known in India as Royal Salep (*Badshah Salab*) is derived from *Allium Mecleani* (*Liliaceae*).

Properties and Uses.—The salep met with in the bazaars is found in several forms—palmate and in more or less ovoid or rounded tubers, sometimes strung together. It yields a large quantity of mucilage to water and, on boiling even with 40 parts of water, forms a thick jelly which is regarded as highly nutritious and wholesome.

When carefully prepared, it is one of the best articles of diet for a weakly or convalescent person. For this purpose it is best to purchase the salep ready powdered from the chemist. It consists almost entirely of a peculiar gummy substance called bassorin and starch and is considered to be more nutritious than either sago or arrowroot. It is usually cooked with milk in the proportion of one tea-spoonful of salep to a tea-cupful of milk. It is given in all forms of wasting diseases such as phthisis, diabetes, etc., and in cases of chronic diarrhœa and dysentery. Salep has long been esteemed in India as possessing great restorative and invigorating virtues and therefore recommended as a tonic aphrodisiac in diseases characterised by weakness or loss of sexual powers. It is also much prescribed in paralytic affections.

277. ORIGANUM VULGARE.

(*N. O.*—LABIATÆ).

Hind.—Sàthra.

Habitat.—This is a common herb of the temperate Himalaya.

Properties and Uses.—It is used in some parts of the Punjab as a pot herb like mint. It yields a volatile oil which is used as an aromatic stimulant in colic and locally in rheumatism and earache.

278. OROXYLUM INDICUM.

(*N. O.*—BIGNONIACEÆ.)

Sans.—Shyonàka, Aralu. *Hind.*—Arlù. *Ben.*—Sonà, Nàsonà. *Bom.*—Tetu, Sauna assar. *Tel.*—Dundillum. *Tam.*—Va ıga-maram.

Habitat.—This small tree is growing all over India and Ceylon.

Properties and Uses.—The root-bark is well known and much esteemed, being an ingredient of the *Dasamula* of Hindu Medicine. It is found to contain a crystalline body named *Oroxylin*, in addition to acrid, pectinous and astringent principles and citric acid. The root-bark is regarded as astringent and tonic, useful in diarrhœa and dysentery. It is said to be used by the Gonds as a discutient application to rheumatic swellings and in powder (5 to 15 grains) as a diaphoretic. The tender fruits are described as grateful, carminative and stomachic.

Native Indian Preparations.—The root-bark is enclosed with some leaves and a layer of clay and roasted. The juice expressed from this roasted bark is given in diarrhœa and dysentery with the addition of *mocharasa* (gum of *Bombax Malabaricum*)—(Saranghadhara). In otorrhœa, Sarangadhara recommends the use of an oil prepared by boiling, over a gentle fire, sesamum oil with a paste made of the root-bark of *Calosanthes Indica*, or *Oroxylum Indicum.*

---

279. ORYZA SATIVA.

(*N. O.*—GRAMINEÆ.)

Sans.—Vrihi, Tandula. *Eng.*—Rice (the husked seed). *Hind.*, *Duk.*, and *Punj.*—Châval. *Ben.*—Chául, Dhán (unhusked). *Kash.*—Thomûl. *Guz.*—Chôkha. *Mah.*—Tàndul, Bhât (unhusked) *Arab.*—Arruz. *Pers.*—Biranj. *Tel.*—Biyyam. *Tam.*—Arshi. *Can.*—Akki. *Mal.*—Ari. *Cing.*—Hál. *Burm.*—Sân, Chân. *Malay.*—Bras.

Habitat.—This well known cereal occupies the foremost place among the food crops of India and forms the staple food of the people of Bengal, Assam, Burma, and several parts of Madras and Bombay Presidencies. The plant producing it and scientifically termed as *Oryza* *sativa* is one that is spread over the tropical and sub-tropical regions of both hemispheres.

Properties and Uses.—No grain not even wheat is more valuable to the human kind than this, which affords sustenance to about three-fourths of the inhabitants of the globe. The seed of the plant deprived of its husk is the rice of commerce, which is exported very largely from Burma; before it is husked it is called paddy. As an article of food rice is nutritious, easy of digestion and therefore suited for weak stomachs; having no laxative properties it suits those in whom there is a tendency to diarrhœa. Its nutritive value, however, is comparatively small, containing, as it does, only about 5 per cent. of nitrogenous matter, while the proportion of mineral matters is very small. According to an analysis it contains 83·20 of starch, 5·00 of gluten or nitrogenous matter, ·80 of fatty matter, 10 of watery matters and ·5 of nutritive salts. The small quantity of gluten which this grain contains prevents its being made into bread; it rapidly swells and softens under the influence of heat and moisture and thus it is easily prepared for food, no grinding or baking process being required. It is, therefore, the best suited for the peoples of tropical climates, not only because so little labour is required in preparing it but also because it is easy of digestion, and is not heating or stimulating. For young persons and invalids nothing is so good in the way of puddings as those made of rice. When intended to correct a diarrhœic tendency it should be used ground. At all times care should be taken to have it well cooked, as it is indigestible if not so. Where there is an irritable or inflammatory state of the stomach, bowels or kidneys rice water (the decoction) is good taken as a drink. It is a pleasant, demulcent and refrigerent drink in fevers. A little lemon peel or lemon juice may be added to improve the flavour. It forms an excellent drink not only in ordinary fevers, but also in small-pox, measles, scarlet fever, and inflammations of all kinds, also in gonorrhœa and other cases where there is pain and difficulty in passing urine. The decoction or "*conjee* water" as it is commonly called, is prepared by boiling one ounce of cleansed rice in a quart of water for about 20 minutes, straining and flavouring with sugar and with lime-juice, if desired, to taste. Plain rice water is used also as an enema in bowel affections. Rice may be utilised in medicine, also in the form of powder and poultice. In the form of powder or rice-flour dusted thickly over the surface it forms a very cooling and soothing application in small-pox, measles, erysipelas, prickly heat and other inflammatory affections of the skin. It is pleasant to the patients' feelings and allays heat and irritation. To burns and scalds rice flour is an excellent application; it should be used as soon as possible after the occurrence of the injury and it should be dusted thickly over the whole of the burnt surface, so as to absorb any discharge that may be present and at the same time exclude the air as far as possible. If, in a few days, this becomes hardened and irritating, a warm rice poultice should be applied, so as to soften it and allow its easy removal; the surface should then be dressed with lime liniment (composed of equal parts of lime water and a bland oil such as olive oil, linseed oil or sesamum oil) or resin ointment.

Rice poultice is used also as a substitute for linseed meal. To prepare this place a sufficiency of rice flour in an open vessel over the fire, gradually add water and stir until the mass has the required consistence. A more ready method is to place the rice flour in a basin and then gradually to add boiling water, constantly stirring it as above. A piece of cloth of the required size being ready at hand, the poultice should be smoothly spread on it, to the thickness of from a quarter to half an inch, and applied over the affected part. In most cases it is advisable, before applying it, to smear the surface of the poultice with a bland oil; this renders it more soothing and keeps it longer soft and moist. A rice poultice requires changing twice or even thrice daily. It is an excellent application to abscesses, boils, buboes, ulcers and other local inflammatory affections, inflamed piles, etc. In chronic bronchitis and other chronic coughs considerable relief often results from the application of a large soft rice poultice placed over the chest at bed-time and allowed to remain on all night; another may also be advantageously placed on the back between the shoulder blades. The efficacy of these poultices is, in many cases, increased by the addition of a little mustard flour (1 part to 3 or 4 of rice flour), so as to produce a slight redness of the skin, or the surface of the poultice may be smeared over with oil of turpentine.

Native Indian Preparations.—The preparations of rice used in sick diet and described in Sanskrit medical works are as follows:—(1) Yavàgu or powdered rice boiled with water for the use of the sick or convalescent. It is made of 3 strengths, namely, with nine, eleven and nineteen parts of water called respectively *Vilepi*, *Peyá* and *Manda*. Sometimes instead of water, a decoction of medicinal herbs is used in preparing *Yavágu*. Thus, for example, if it is ordered to give the patient *Yavágu* made with ginger and long-pepper, take of dry ginger and long-pepper one tola each, boil in 4 seers of water till reduced to two, and strain. Now take 9, 11 or 19 parts of this strained decoction and 1 part of powdered rice for making *Yavágu* of the strength ordered. (2) *Lájá* (*Khai*) is paddy fried in a sand bath. The husks open out and the rice swells into a light spongy body. It is considered a light article of diet suited to invalids and dyspeptics. (3) *Bhrishta tandula* (*Muri*) is rice fried in a sand bath. This is also a light preparation of rice and is given to sick persons as a substitute for boiled rice. It is also much used by the poorer classes for tiffin and early breakfast. (4) *Prithuka* (*Churá*).—To prepare this, paddy is moistened and lightly fried. It is then flattened and husked. This preparation of rice is given with curdled milk *(dadhi)* in dysentery. It is well washed and softened in water or boiled before use. (5) *Páyasa* is a preparation of rice with nine parts of milk. (6) *Tandulámbu* is water in which unboiled rice has been steeped. This sort of rice water is sometimes prescribed as a vehicle for some powders and confections.

A common kind of alcoholic liquor known as rice beer (*pachwai*), prepared in a very simple manner by half boiling the grain in water and allowing it to ferment slightly, is in almost universal use by the lower classes in many parts of India. A raw spirit is prepared from this liquor to a considerable extent by a rude process of distillation.

280. OXALIS CORNICULATA.

(*N. O.*—GERANIACEÆ.)

Sans.—Amlalonikä, Chängeri. *Eng.*—The Indian Sorrel. *Hind.*—Amrul. *Ben.*—Amrulsäk. *Bom.*—Bhui-sarpati. *Duk.*—Umbuti. *Tel.*—Puli chintaku. *Tam.*—Puli-yärai. *Can.*—Huli-huniche-gida. *Mal.*—Pullampurachi. *Kon.*—Teltuppi.

Habitat.—This is a common garden weed found throughout India.

Properties and Uses.—The plant has an acid taste, due to the presence of acid oxalate of potassium to which is due its property in domestic use of removing ink-spots or iron-stains from linen. The leaves have long been considered cooling, refrigerent and antiscorbutic. They have also been used for removing corns, warts and other excrescences on the skin. Bruised with or without water and formed into a poultice and applied over inflamed parts they relieve pain and other inflammatory symptoms. The fresh leaves are made into a curry, which improves the appetite and digestion of dyspeptic patients. The fresh juice is believed to relieve the intoxication, produced by datura; it is also believed, on application, to remove fibres over the cornea or opacities of the cornea. The expressed juice of the leaves made into a sherbet with a little sugar is often prescribed in dysentery to allay thirst. The plant is rubbed down with water, boiled and the juice of white onions added; the mixture is applied to the head in bilious headaches. Various preparations in which this plant forms a chief ingredient are much esteemed in the treatment of fevers, dysentery and scurvy.

Native Indian Preparations.—*Chāngeri Ghrita:*—Take of clarified butter 4 seers, the fresh juice of *Oxalis Corniculata* 4 seers, curdied milk called *dadhi* 16 seers and the leaves of *Oxalis Corniculata* reduced to a paste 1 seer. Boil them together in the usual way and prepare a *ghrita*. This preparation is useful in diarrhœa, dysentery, prolapsus of the rectum, tympanites, piles and difficult micturition—(Chakradatta). The Bhavaprâsha gives the following process for preparing a compound *ghrita*. Take of the fresh juice of *Oxalis Corniculata*, decoction of jujube fruits and ginger, alkaline water and curdled milk each 4 seers, clarified butter 4 seers and prepare a *ghrita* in the usual way. It is recommended for use in prolapse of the rectum.

281. OXYSTELMA ESCULENTUM.

(*N. O.*—ASCLEPIADEÆ.)

Sans.—Tiktadugdha. *Hind.* and *Ben.*—Dudhlata.

Habitat.—This climbing plant is found wild in the plains.

Properties and Uses.—The fruits are edible. A decoction of the plant is used as a gargle in aphthous ulcerations of the mouth and in sore throat. The fresh roots are said to be used in Orissa as a specific for jaundice.

282. PÆDERIA FŒTIDA.

(*N. O.*—RUBIACEÆ)

Sans.—Prasārini. *Hind.*—Gandhāli, Khip. *Ben.*—Gandhabhaduli. *Bom.*—Prasāram. *Tel.*—Savirela.

Habitat.—A twining plant found in the Central and Eastern Himalaya, Western India and Bengal and Assam.

Properties and Uses.—The plant gives off, when bruised, a marked odour of carbon disulphide. By distillation of the plant with water a volatile oil is obtained, which has the highly offensive odour of the fresh drug. Evidence of the presence of at least two alkaloids has also been obtained. The leaves and root are considered wholesome and tonic and are used to a considerable extent in Bengal as a constituent of a food given to the sick and the convalescent. The leaves are boiled and made into a soup. The offensive odour is removed in the process of cooking. The entire plant, including stem, leaves and root, is used both internally and externally in rheumatic affections, for which it is regarded as a specific.

Native Indian Preparations.—*Prasárini Leha*, or electuary of *Paederia Fœtida:*—Take of the leaves, root and stem of *Paederia Fœtida*, two seers, water 32 seers, boil till reduced to one-fourth. To the strained decoction add two seers of treacle, and again boil till reduced to the consistence of a thick syrup. Lastly add powdered ginger, long pepper, black pepper, plumbago root and the root of *Piper chabá* (*chaviká*) equal parts, in half a seer. Dose, about 1 tola in acute rheumatism—(Bhâvaprakasa).

Several oils or liniments for external application are prepared with this plant. The following called *Kubja Prasárini Taila* is largely used by Hindu Vaidyans:—Take of the entire plant of *Paederia Fœtida* 800 tolas, boil in 64 seers of water till reduced to 16 seers, and strain. To the strained decoction, add sesamum oil 16 seers, milk 32 seers, whey and fermented paddy water (*Kânjika*) each 16 seers and the following substances, namely, root of *Paederia Fœtida*, plumbago root, long pepper root, liquorice, rock-salt, *Acorus calamus* root, dill seeds, bark of *Cedrus Deodara*, root of *Vanda Roxburghii* (*Rásná*), *Scindapsus officinalis* (*gajapippali*), *jatamansi* root and marking nuts, each two tolas in the form of a paste. First boil the oil with the decoction of *Paederia Fœtida* till the water is nearly evaporated, then boil the oil successively with the addition of milk, whey and *Kánjika*, adding the aromatic paste during the last process of boiling. This oil is used externally in rheumatism with contraction and stiffness of the joints. After the application of the oil, the affected parts should be fomented with dry heat—(Chakradatta.)

283. PÆONIA EMODI.

(*N. O.*—Ranunculaceæ.)

Eng.—The Pæoney Rose. *Hind.*—Ud-sälap, Mamekh. *Bom.*—Ud-salam.

Habitat.—Tubers of this plant are imported from Turkey.

Properties and Uses.—The tubers of this plant have some reputation in uterine disorders, epilepsy, bilious obstructions, convulsions and hysteria. It was once a common belief, among the peasantry of Europe, that the pæony root worn round the necks of children had the effect of preventing and curing epileptic attacks.

284. PANDANUS ODORATISSIMUS.

(*N. O.*—Pandaneæ.)

Sans.—Ketaki, *Eng.*—Fragrant Screw-pine, Caldera Bush. *Hind.*—Keora. *Ben.*—Keora, Keya. *Bom.*, and *Mah.*—Kevda. *Tel.*—Mogili, Gâjangi, Ketaki. *Tam.*—Tälamchedi, Kedagai. *Can.*—Kedage, Mundige. *Mal.*—Kaitha, Ketaki. *Kon.*—Kedagi, Bondayi.

Habitat.—This shrub with fragrant flowers is found wild in Southern India, Burma and the Andamans; cultivated in gardens in Bengal.

Properties and Uses.—A perfumed oil called *Kevda* Oil is extracted from the floral bracts, by means of sesamum oil, and a fragrant otto and water, *Keora-ka-arak*, are also prepared from the bracts. Both are employed medicinally. The oil and the otto obtained from the bracts are considered stimulant and antispasmodic and are used in headache and rheumatism. The oil is also useful in ear-ache. A medicinal oil is prepared from the roots.

285. PANICUM ITALICUM.

(*N. O.*—GRAMINACEÆ.)

Sans.—Kanku, Shyama. *Eng.*—Italian Millet. *Hind.*—Kangni. *Ben.*—Kora, Kangu. *Tel.*—Korralu. *Tam.*—Tinnai. *Can.*—Navane-akki, Kungo-gida. *Mal.*—Tina. *Kon.*—Varayi.

Properties and Uses.—This seed is much esteemed in some parts of India as an article of food; but it has heating properties and when taken as the sole food it is apt to produce diarrhœa. It acts as a diuretic and astringent and is of use externally in rheumatism. It is a popular domestic remedy for alleviating the pains of parturition.

286. PAPAVER SOMNIFERUM.

(*N. O.*—PAPAVERACEÆ.)

(The Capsules)—*Sans.*—Khäs khas. *Eng.*—Opium-Poppy. *Bën.*—Postodheri. *Tel.*—Gasagasalu. *Tam.*—Gasagasa. *Can.* and *Kon.*—Kasakase. *Mal.*—Kashakasha.

(Opium, the inspissated juice)—*Sans.*—Ahiphena. *Eng.*—Opium. *Hind.*, *Duk.*, *Ben.*, *Punj.*, and *Kash.*—Afim. *Bom.*, *Guz.*, and *Mah.*—Aphim, Appo. *Tel.*—Abhini. *Tam.*—Abini. *Can.*—Affini. *Arab.* and *Pers.*—Affimu. *Cing.*—Abin. *Burm.*—Bhin, Bhain. *Mclay.*—Affiun.

Habitat.—The opium-poppy with white flowers and white seeds is very extensively grown in India for the manufacture of opium, embracing great tracts in Behar, producing what is known as Patna opium, in Benares and the United Provinces, producing Benares opium, and in Central and Western India and Rajputana, the source of what is known as Malwa opium. Opium is also grown and produced in Nepal, Assam and Burma.

Properties and Uses.—The poppy seeds yield a bland oil which is used for culinary purposes and in lamps. The seeds themselves are innocuous and used as food. They are boiled, mixed with a little oil and salt and taken as curry with rice, or they are made into balls and formed with tamarind into an acid curry. Poppy seeds are sprinkled over some parts of native sweetmeats.

Poppy seeds are described as demulcent and nutritive and useful in cough and asthma. The capsules of the poppy are regarded as light, astringent and narcotic. They promote talkativeness and destroy or diminish the sexual power. Bruised poppy-heads are used as a sedative fomentation and poultice. They contain a trace of opium. For fomentations, they should be broken up and boiled in water; and the liquor only is used. Into this, when quite hot, a flannel should be dipped and wrung out and then laid on the part affected, dipping it afresh as it begins to cool.

Opium, one of the most valuable medicines we possess when properly employed, is very powerful in its operation and therefore great caution is necessary in its employment. Primarly and, in small doses, its action is stimulating, secondarily it is narcotic, anodyne and antispasmodic. Under its influence the pupil of the eye becomes contracted; in overdoses it is a powerful poison. The opium procurable in the bazaars is always more or less adulterated, and hence the uncertainty which attends the operation of bazaar opium. Of the several kinds of opium met with in India the chief are:—(1) Patna Garden opium; (2) Malwa opium. The former, prepared exclusively for medicinal purposes, occurs in square packages of from 2 to 4 pounds' weight, covered with layers of talc. It is solid, brittle in the cold season, of a brown colour and fine smell. It yields a large proportion (7 to 8 or even 10 per cent.) of morphia. Of Malwa opium there are many varieties; of these the two principles are, first, that in flat circular cakes of about 1½ pounds in weight without any exterior covering, dull opaque, blackish brown, externally and internally somewhat darker and soft; it yields only from 3 to 5 per cent of morphia. The other, a superior kind of Malwa opium, occurs in balls or cakes of smaller size, about 10 ounces in weight, covered with a coarse dust composed of broken poppy petals; it yields from 7 to 8 per cent of morphia. The other varieties of Indian opium, the Himalayan or "Hill opium," the Kandeish, the Cutch, etc., are less applicable than the preceding for medicinal purposes, on account of their varying strength.

There are some points connected with opium which should always be borne in mind:—

(1) Some persons are very intolerant to the action of opium; in these even the smallest dose produces great

nervous excitement, violent headache and vomiting. In such cases the drug should be avoided.

(2) Infants and young children bear opium badly; cases are on record in which 3 drops of laudanum have proved fatal to infants. Still, there are diseases of childhood in which it proves valuable, but in these it should not be given except under professional advice or superintendence.

(3) It should be avoided as far as possible during pregnancy, as it seems to exercise a prejudicial effect on the fœtus.

(4) The previous habits of the patient materially influence the effects of this medicine. A confirmed opium-taker requires a far larger dose to produce a given effect than one not habituated to it.

(5) When the use of opium is clearly indicated and the patient from any cause is unable to swallow it may be given in an enema; in this case a larger dose, a third of even a half larger is required than when given by mouth.

(6) Whenever in doubt as to the advisability of giving opium, take the safer course and avoid it.

(7) Never prescribe opium for a person whom you have reason to believe to be suffering from disease of the kidneys, especially if there be a tendency to dropsy.

As an anodyne and narcotic opium is invaluable and is used in many diseases such as rheumatism, tumours, cancer, carbuncles, abscesses, and ulcers, connected either with leprosy, syphilis or scrofula in which the pain, especially at night, effectually banishes sleep. An adult may commence with one grain pill or fifteen drops of laudanum, taken about an hour before the usual bed-time; if this succeeds in procuring sleep it may safely be repeated nightly; if not the dose may be doubled the second night and trebled the third night, but it is not advisable to go beyond this quantity except under professional advice. Even these quantities after being used for a week or two lose much of their power, and may require to be cautiously increased. When the pains are lessened and the patient is improving the quantity of opium should be decreased gradually, rather than the whole supply left off at once. To control the sleeplessness and restlessness of delirium tremens opium given as above may be necessary, but each dose should be combined with 4 or 5 grains of camphor in the form of pill; in fact camphor alone in doses of 2 to 3 grains every 3 or 4 hours, exercises a most soothing influence, and when this treatment is adopted, the opium at bed-time may be given alone.

The antispasmodic action of opium is made use of in cases of spasmodic affections of the bowels, violent colic and the passage of all stones, and when the pain is violent a full dose, *i.e.*, 20 to 25 drops of laudanum in a wine-glassful of omum water or infusion of sweet-flag root often affords speedy relief; should it not do so, however, in half an hour the dose may be repeated and a third dose after an hour should the pain continue unabated. For relieving the pain and irritation of the bladder caused by the presence of stone in the bladder, gravel, etc., no medicine gives more relief than opium in full doses. It proves, however, even more effectual if introduced into the rectum either in the form of suppository (2 grains of opium with 4 grains of soap), or in enema (30 to 40 drops of laudanum in 2 ounces of thin *conjee* water). It may also be given with great benefit in irritable states and painful affections of the kidneys. In retention of urine due to spasmodic stricture of the urethra a hot-bath and a full dose of opium (25 to 30 drops of laudanum), followed by a dose of castor oil will often suffice to give relief in recent cases of no great severity following a debauch, exposure to wet, etc. The opium given in an enema of two or three ounces of rice *conjee* sometimes succeeds when it fails if given by mouth.

In diabetes opium occasionally produces the most beneficial results, especially in old cases occurring in the aged. It requires to be given in full doses and to be persevered in, the effects being carefully watched; the dose diminished or the remedy left off altogether, if it gives rise to headache or other bad symptoms. It is worthy of remark, however, that persons suffering from this disease will take large doses with impunity.

In many affections of the uterus opium is of the greatest service. Besides being employed in the form of suppository or enema, as mentioned above, camphorated opium liniment warmed, may likewise be rubbed into the loins or a hot rice poultice sprinkled with laudanum applied over the lower part of the abdomen. When given internally in these cases it requires to be given in full doses and it may be advantageously combined with camphor. For the relief of after-pains 15 to 20 drops of laudanum in a wine-glassful of camphor julep or omum water or a little simple *conjee* generally affords speedy relief. In threatened abortion from a fall, over-exertion, etc., in dysentery, a full dose of laudanum, and for the relief of the local pain, bearing down and straining in this disease (dysentery) a small enema (30 to 40 drops of laudanum in two ounces of *conjee*) affords relief. Opium is a valuable adjunct to catechu and other astringents in the treatment of diarrhœa. Vomiting is sometimes speedily relieved by a few drops of laudanum (5 to 10 drops) in an effervescing draught, or a little omum-water.

A simple opium liniment, readily made by rubbing down a drachm of bazaar opium in two ounces of cocoanut, sessamum or other bland oil proves very useful in many external or local diseases, including chronic rheumatism, lumbago and other muscular and neuralgic pains, spasms and bruises, enlarged glands, mumps, etc. Its efficacy, however, is greatly increased by conjoining it with an equal quantity of camphor liniment. This, which may be called camphorated opium liniment, is an excellent application in many painful external affections. It should be well shaken before being used. Care should be taken not to apply it to an abraded or sore surface; it is only adapted for the sound skin, and not even then if the pain is attended with much heat and redness. This camphorated liniment well rubbed in along the course of the spine is occasionally very useful in whooping cough. For stiff neck, warm laudanum rubbed in over the part answers better.

In ophthalmia attended with great intolerance of light great relief may be obtained by fumigating the eye with the vapour of boiling water to which has been added a tea-spoonful of laudanum, or a couple of grains of opium. An excellent eye-wash in these cases is composed of laudanum, vinegar and brandy each one part and water four parts. Toothache depending upon a decayed tooth is often relieved by a grain of opium put into the hollow of the tooth; the saliva should not be swallowed. Ear-ache also frequently yields to a mixture of equal parts of laudanum and any bland oil inserted into the outer passage of the ear on a piece of cotton wool; care should be taken not to push it in too far. To painful piles where there is much swelling and heat, a very soothing application is a soft rice poultice sprinkled over with laudanum or smeared over with simple opium liniment.

Native Indian Preparations.—*Grahani Kapàta Rasa*, which is recommended in chronic diarrhœa and dysentery, is prepared thus;—Take of nutmeg, borax, prepared taic and *datura* seeds, each one part, opium two parts and make into two-grain pills with the juice of *Pæderia Fœtida* (*prasârâni*)—Rasendra-sarsangraha.

Dugdhavati, which is much used by Kavirajas in cases of diarrhœa with anasarca, is prepared as follows:—Take of opium and aconite, 24 grains each; prepared iron, 10 grains; prepared talc, 12 grains. Beat them into a mass with milk and make into four-grain pills. One pill is to be given every morning with milk. The diet is restricted to milk alone, water and salt being prohibited.—Bhaishajyaratnavali.

Sambunâtha Rasa:—Take of orpiment, realgar, cinnabar, white arsenic, borax, aconite and alum each one part, mercury, sulphur and opium each seven parts. Soak them for seven days in each of the following fluids, namely juice of the leaves of *cannabis sativa, vitex negundo, datura* and *nim*. Make into two-grain pills.

These are given with ginger juice in diarrhœa with high fever—Bhashajya tantra.

Akarádi Churna :—Take of pellitory root, ginger, seeds called *kakkola*, saffron, long-pepper, nutmegs, cloves, and red sandalwood, each two tolas, opium eight tolas. Rub together and pass the powder through a cloth. Then add sugar, equal in quantity to all the above ingredients. Dose :—grains 6 to 12 with honey. This medicine is used as an aphrodisiac.

The Amritasagar recommends the following preparation of opium in diabetes :—Take of camphor and musk, each one part, opium and mace, each four parts. Make into two-grain pills. They are administered with the juice of betel leaves.

---

287. PARMELIA PERLATA.

Hind.—Charela, Phathar-ke-phul.

The above and several other species of the lichen order are sold in the bazaars under vernacular names meaning "stone-flowers."

Properties and Uses.—These lichens have long been regarded in India as astringent and resolvent. They were formerly considered useful as a diuretic, applied in the form of a poultice to the renal and lumbar region.

---

288. PAVETTA INDICA.

(*N. O.*—RUBIACEÆ).

Sans.—Pappäna, Käkachhadi. *Hind.*—Papari, Kankra. *Ben.*—Kukura-chura. *Tel.*—Päputtä-vayru. *Tam.*—Pàvattai-vayr. *Can.*—Pâvate, Sùle-bottu-gida. *Mal.*—Pàtta, Pàvata kodi.

Habitat.—This is a common shrub found throughout India.

Properties and Uses.—The bitter root is frequently prescribed by Vaidyans in visceral obstructions. It has a purgative action. The root, together with dried ginger, is rubbed and given in *conjee* water in cases of ascites, renal dropsy, etc. The local fomentation with the leaves is useful in relieving the pain in case of piles.

289. PAVONIA ODORATA.

(N. O.—MALVACEÆ.)

Sans. and *Ben.*—Bàla. *Hind.*—Sugandha-vàla. *Bom.*—Kàlà-vàlà. *Tel.*—Muttupalàgamu. *Tam.*—Perámuttai, Avibattam. *Can.*—Bala rakkasi-gida.

Habitat. This herb is wild in the North-West Provinces, the Western Peninsula, Sind and Burma.

Properties and Uses.—The herb has a musk-like odour. The roots also have that odour; they are regarded as cooling and stomachic, ; they enter into the composition of a well-known fever drink called *Sadanga Pániya.* The carminative action of the root is believed to be due to the aromatic odorous principle. The fragrant root is also used in combination with other medicines of the sort in inflammation, hæmorrhage from internal organs, etc.

290. PEARLS.

Sans.—Muktà. *Hind.*, *Ben.*, *Guz.*, *Mah.*, and *Kon.*—Moti. *Tel.*—Mutiamu. *Tam.* and *Can.*—Muthu.

The Indian pearl fisheries have been notable from time immemorial. Off the coast of Ceylon and the South-eastern Coast of India near Tinnevelly and Madura, fishing is being held every year on a grand scale, for the "pearl-oyster."

Properties and Uses.—Pearls have been used in Indian Medicine from a very ancient period and are mentioned by Susruta. They form an ingredient in several of the complex prescriptions peculiar to Sanskrit *Materia Medica*. Pearls are prepared for medicinal use by being calcined in covered crucibles and then reduced to powder. Pearl in the calcined state as an alkaline ash, chiefly carbonate and oxide of lime, acts as an antacid in heart-burn and bilious affections. It is esteemed by the Hindus to be of much value in urinary diseases and consumption and is believed to increase the strength, nutrition and energy of weak patients. Corals are also similarly prepared, and used in combination with pearls in the above diseases, as the properties of both these articles are said to be alike.

Native Indian Preparations:—*Pittántaka rasa:*—Take of nutmegs, mace, *Jatamansi* root, root of *Aplotaxis auriculata* (*Kushtha*), leaves of *Abies Webbiana* (*Talis-patra*), aconite, iron pyrites, iron, talc and realgar, one part each, prepared pearls equal in quantity to all, the above ingredients. Beat them together into a paste with the aid of water and make into four-grain pills. This medicine is useful in diseases caused by deranged bile, such as dyspepsia, jaundice, biliousness, vomiting of bile, etc.

Vasanta Kusumákara Rasa:—Take of prepared gold and camphor each two parts, of prepared tin, lead and iron three parts each, prepared talc, pearls and coral four parts each. Rub these ingredients together in a mortar and soak the powder seven times successively in each of the following fluids, namely milk, sugar-cane juice, juice of *Adhatoda vasica* (*vásaka*), decoction of *lac* and of *Pavonia Odorata* (*bálá*), juice of the flowers and root-stock of the plantain tree, of the root-stock of *Nelumbium speciosum* (*padma*) and of the flowers of *Aganosma Caryophyllata* (*málati puspa*). Lastly, soak in an infusion of musk prepared by macerating one part of musk in eight parts of warm water for twelve hours. Divide this mass into four-grain pills. They are given with sugar, honey and ghee in urinary diseases, impotence, gleet, diabetes, consumption and general debility. This medicine is regarded as a valuable alterative tonic in chronic gonorrhœa and spermatorrhœa and is much prescribed in these complaints in combination with an extract called *Kusávalehá*.

291. PEDALIUM MUREX.

(*N. O.*—PEDALINEÆ.)

Sans.—Gaja daunstree. *Hind.*, *Duk.*, and *Ben.*—Barà-gokhru. *Bom.*, and *Mah.*—Motto-gokhru. *Tel.*—Pedda pallèru, Eenuga pallëru. *Tam.*—Peru-neranji. *Can.*—Aneneggilu. Doddaneggilu. *Mal.*—Kâka mulla. *Cing.*—Ati naranchi. *Burm.*—Sulegi.

Habitat.—This succulent herb is common in the Deccan, Southern India and Ceylon.

Properties and Uses.—The four-angled spiny fruit, easily obtained in the bazaars, has the property, in common with the leaves and stems, of rendering water or milk mucilaginous when agitated with, or steeped in them without imparting any colour or taste. The infusion thus prepared is an effctive demulcent and diuretic, useful in disorders of the urinary system such as the ardor urinæ, gonorrhœa, dysuria, spermatorrhœa and incontinence of urine. It is said to relieve strangury and to dissolve calculi. It is of considerable value as a speedy diuretic. In gonorrhœa half a pint of the above infusion taken every morning for ten days successively, relieves the scalding, and, in many cases, a cure is effected. One of its principal effects is to increase the flow of urine; hence it might prove very useful in some forms of dropsy. The seeds have also gained some reputation as remedies for spermatorrhœa and incontinence of urine in cold infusion of one ounce to a pint, this quantity being administered daily. Water rendered mucilaginous by this plant soon regains its original fluidity; hence the infusion should be freshly prepared each time it is to be administered. The juice of the leaves is a local application to aphthæ. The leaves are used very largely as a healing application to ulcers. Also as an emmenagogue the juice is used in puerperal diseases and to promote the lochial discharge. *A paushtik* taken with milk is made of the powdered root with ghee, sugar and spices.

---

292. PEGANUM HARMALA.

(*N. O.*—RUTACEÆ.)

Eng.—Syrian Rue. *Hind.*—Harmal. *Ben.*—Isband. *Bom.*—Hurmal. *Pers.*—Ispand. *Tel.*—Shimagorantivittulu. *Tam.*—Shimai-azha-vanai-virai.

Habitat.—This shrub is found in North-Western India, the Punjab, Sind and Persia and the Western Deccan. The seeds are imported from Persia and are easily obtainable.

Properties and Uses.—The seeds yield a red dye. They also contain two alkaloids, *Harmaline* and *Harmine*, and a soft red-coloured resin with a narcotic odour resembling that of *Cannabis Indica.* The seeds may be regarded as narcotic, anodyne, emetic and emmenagogue. The powder in doses of ½ to 2 drachms is a good anodyne in asthma, colic and jaundice, and the watery infusion is similarly useful. A tincture is said to have mild emmenagogue properties resembling those of ergot. Wounds are fumigated by burning the seeds, the smoke being believed to have antiseptic properties.

293. PERICAMPYLUS INCANUS.

(*N. O.*—MENISPERMACEÆ.)

Ben. and *Hind.*—Bàrak-kanta.

Properties and Uses.—The roots of this plant are held in great repute by snake-charmers in India as an antidote to the bites of poisonous snakes. Dr. Cunningham's research has proved that a fluid extract of the roots, when injected into the bitten place, possesses decided remedial power though it has no general action. It acts by precipitating the poison and thus rendering it inert when brought into direct relation with it prior to the absorption of the venom into the system generally.

294. PETROSELINUM SATIVUM.

(*N. O.*—UMBELLIFERÆ.)

Syn:—Apium Petroselinum. The Parsley.

Habitat.—This culinary herb is cultivated in gardens in India.

Properties and Uses.—This herb is interesting as being the source of *apiol,* a green oily liquid which is distilled from the root. The name is also applied to a crystalline stearoptene contained in parsley oil distilled from the seed. Apiol has been much recommended in amenorrhœa and in dysmenorrhœa in doses of 2 to 3 minims administered in capsules.

295. PEUCEDANUM GRAVEOLENS.

(*N. O.*—UMBELLIFERÆ.)

Sans.—Satapushpi. *Eng.*—The Dill. Anethum sowa. *Hind.* and *Punj.*—Sòyà, Suvä. *Duk.*—Sòvi. *Kash.*—Sòl biòl. *Ben.*—Sowa, Sùlpha. *Guz.*—Suvà-nu-bi. *Tel.*—Shatakupivittulu. *Tam.*—Shatakupi-virai. *Can.*—Sabbasige. *Mal.*—Chatukuppa. *Cing.*—Sadakuppa. *Burm.*—Samin. *Malay.*—Adaspudus.

Habitat.—This herb is cultivated in Indian gardens for culinary purposes. The seeds are obtained in every Indian bazaar.

Properties and Uses.—The seeds yield an essential oil which is largely used for its valuable carminative action. This oil, essence and the distilled water of dill are much esteemed in India as carminatives for flatulence, colic and abdominal pain in children and in adults. An infusion of the bruised seeds, three drachms to half a pint of hot water, is also very useful in the absence of the distilled water; of this, when strained and cold, the dose for an infant is a dessertspoonful or more sweetened with a little sugar. Its efficacy is much increased by the addition of a teaspoonful of lime water. The seeds bruised and boiled in water and mixed with the roots are applied externally in rheumatic and other swellings of the joints. The leaves are moistened with a little oil and warmed and applied to boils and abscesses to hasten suppuration.

296. PHASEOLUS MUNGO.

(*N. O.*—LEGUMINOSÆ).

Sans.—Mada, Mudga. *Eng.*—Green gram. *Hind.*—Moong. *Ben.*—Mug. *Bom.*, *Mah.*—Mùg. *Tel.*—Pachhai-pesulu. *Tam.*—Pachhai-payaru. *Can.*—Hesaru. *Mal.*—Cherupayar. *Kon.*—Mùgu.

Habitat.—This pulse is grown and cultivated commonly all over India.

Properties and Uses.—This pulse forms a very nutritious article of diet but is rather difficult to digest. It is considered cool and astringent. The green variety is regarded as most wholesome and suited to sick persons. The soup made of it is often the first article of diet prescribed after recovery from acute illness. It is said to be useful in relieving the heat or burning of the eyes, when applied in the form of powder.

CHEMICAL COMPOSITION (PROFESSOR CHURCH):—

Water	10·8 to 11·4 p.c.	Oil	2·7 to 2·0 p.c.
Albuminoids	22·2 to 23·8 „	Fibre	5·8 to 4·2 „
Starch	54·1 to 54·8 „	Ash	4·4 to 3·8 „

The former figures are for typical green seeded variety, the latter for typical yellow seeded. In husked beans the fibre is reduced to 1.1 per cent, all the other constituents being proportionately increased.

---

297. PHASEOLUS ROXBURGHII.

(*N. O.*—LEGUMINOSÆ.)

Sans.—Masha. *Hind.*, and *Mah.*—Udid. *Ben.*—Mash Kulay. *Tel.*—Minumu. *Tam.*—Ulundu. *Can.*—Uddu. *Mal.*—Ulunnu *Kon.*—Udidu.

Habitat.—A common pulse found cultivated everywhere in India.

Properties and Uses.—This is a highly-valued article of diet as well as of Hindu Medicine. It is prescribed both internally and externally, especially in paralysis and rheumatism and affections of the nervous system, used in the form of decoction. Oils for external application containing this pulse as their basis are useful in rheumatism, contracted knee, stiff shoulder, etc. It is useful in piles, paralysis and liver affection. The root is said to be narcotic and is a remedy for aching bones. It is used as a poultice for abscesses and inflammations; as a lactagogue in the form of ordinary cooked *dal.*

CHEMICAL COMPOSITION (PROFESSOR CHURCH):—

Water	10·1 p.c.	Oil	2·2 p.c.
Albuminoids	22·7 ,,	Fibre	4·8 ,,
Starch	55·8 ,,	Ash (Phosphoric acid)	4·4 ,,

It resembles the typical spices very closely in all its constituents, but has a larger proportion of starch, oil and ash than the yellow-seeded form of *P. Mungo.*

Native Indian Preparations.—Take of the pulse of *Phaseolus Roxburghii*, root of castor oil plant, of *Mucuna pruriens* (*âtma gupta*) and *Sida Cordifolia* (*balâ*) half a tola each and prepare a decoction in the usual way. This decoction is given with the addition of rock-salt and asafœtida—(Chakradatta).

Svalpa Masha taila :—Take of the pulse of *Phaseolus Roxburghii* 8 seers, water 64 seers, boil down to 16 seers and strain. Boil the strained decoction with 4 seers of sesamum oil and one of rock salt till the water is evaporated. This oil is said to be useful in rheumatism. contracted knee joint, stiff shoulder joint, etc—(Chakradatta).

298. PHOENIX DACTYLIFERA.

(*N. O.*—PALMÆ.)

Sans.—Kharjjura. *Eng.*—The Edible Date. *Hind.* and *Bom.*—Khurmâ, Chhuhàra. *Ben.*—Gharar-khejur. *Punj.*—Khajúr. *Pers.*—Khurmal-khushk. *Arab.*—Khurmàl-yàbis. *Tel.*—Karjúra-káya. *Tam.*—Perich chankay. *Can.*—Gijjira-hannu, Kharjùra.

Habitat.—This tall date-palm is cultivated in Sind and in Southern and Western Punjab, chiefly in the Multan District.

Properties and Uses.—The fruit has long been valued in India and in some parts used as a food although it is much inferior to that imported from Arabia and Egypt. The seeds have been roasted and ground and used as coffee—"date coffee." The sweet pulpy fruit is demulcent, expectorant, laxative and nutrient. The fruit pounded and mixed with almonds, quince seeds, pistachia nuts, spices and sugar forms a *paushtik* much in vogue. A paste made of the ground seeds is said to be applied in Southern India for opacity of the cornea. A gum, ***kukm chil***, obtained from the tree is used as a demulcent in genito-urinary affections.

---

299. PHOENIX FARINIFERA.

(*N. O.*—PALMÆ.)

Eng.—Small Date. *Tel.*—Eechakoyya. *Tam.*—Eechamaram. *Can.*—Sanna-eechale-mara. *Mal.*—Chitteenth.

Habitat.—This palm is met with mostly in Malabar and Travancore.

Properties and Uses.—These are generally the same as those of the above variety. The edible dates are prescribed in cough, asthma, also in fever and gonorrhœa. The gum is esteemed as a useful remedy in diarrhœa and diseases of the genito-urinary system. The seeds, like those of the above species, are made into a paste by trituration with water and applied over the eyelids in ophthalmia, keratitis and for opacity of the cornea. The fruit is used in fœtid breath. The fresh juice is cooling and laxative.

300. PHŒNIX SYLVESTRIS.

Sans.—Kharjjùri. *Eng.*—The Wild Date Palm; the Date Sugar Palm. *Hind.*—Khajùr, Sendhi, Thalma. *Ben.*—Khejur. *Tel.*—Eetha, Indu, Ishan-chedi. *Tam.*—Paerichhu. *Can.*—Eechala-mara. *Mal.*—Kâténth.

Habitat.—This is indigenous to India and is widely cultivated for the sake of its sweet sap.

Properties and Uses.—The sweet sap is manufactured into *gur* or *jagari*. This date sugar is made by evaporating the sap obtained by notches cut in the tree; this soft yellowish sugar is more nutritious and agreeable than cane-sugar and a good substitute for maltine and its various preparations. The juice is also fermented and used as an intoxicating drink for toddy (*tari*). The fresh juice is a cooling beverage. The central tender part of the palm is useful in gonorrhœa and gleet. The root is used in tooth-ache and is also good in nervous debility.

301. PHYLLANTHUS MULTIFLORUS.

(*N. O.*—EUPHORBIACEÆ.)

Hind.—Kàmuni. *Tel.*—Nalla puru gudu. *Tam.*—Neerpoola. *Can.*—Sanna-kâge-soppu. *Mal.*—Kâtu nìrùrì. *Kon.*—Kákesappu.

Habitat.—This plant is met with generally on the East and West Coasts of India.

Properties and Uses.—The root-bark has alterative and attenuant properties and is given in the form of decoction in 4-ounce doses twice daily or as pill made with other alteratives and aromatics. The leaves are employed as a diuretic and cooling medicine, especially their juice; it is made into a pill with camphor and cubebs which is allowed to dissolve in the mouth in cases of bleeding from the gums.

---

302. PHYLLANTHUS NIRURI.

(*N. O.*—EUPHORBIACEÆ.)

Sans.—Bhùmyamlaki, Bhùta-dhâtri. *Hind.*—Jaràmlà. *Ben.*—Bhuiámlá. *Duk.*—Bhùnounlâ. *Bom.*, and *Mah.*—Bhúiàvalà. *Tel.*—Nèla usirika. *Tam.*—Kizhkày-nelli. *Can.*—Kirunelli. *Mal.*—Kilänelli. *Kon.*—Bhúyávàli.

Habitat.—This herb is common in Central and Southern India, extending to Ceylon.

Properties and Uses.—The plant is considered deobstruent, diuretic, astringent and cooling. It is administered in jaundice, half ounce rubbed up in a cup of milk is given morning and evening; or the root or the dried small bitter leaves in powder, are used in teaspoonful doses. The young tender shoots are administered in the form of infusion for chronic dysentery. The whole plant is employed in native Indian practice for some forms of dropsy, gonorrhœa and other genito-urinary affections of a similar type. A bitter neutral principle named *Phyllanthin* has been isolated from the plant.

---

303. PHYSALIS FLEXUOSA or P. SOMNIFERA.

(*N. O.*—SOLANACEÆ.)

Sans.—Ashvaganda. *Hind.*—Asgandh. *Ben.*—Ashvagandi. *Bom.*—Asgand. *Tel.*—Ashvagandi. *Tam.*—Achuvagandi. *Can.*—Sogadà bæru. *Mal.*—Amukiram, Pivate.

Habitat.—This small shrub is common in Bombay and Western India, occasionally met with in Bengal.

Properties and Uses.—The leaves and root are reputed to have narcotic properties; the latter is also regarded as diuretic and deobstruent. As tonic and alterative it is used in consumption, emaciation of children. debility from old age, rheumatism, etc., etc. In consumption a decoction of the root and long pepper is given with the addition of clarified butter and honey. For improving the nutrition of weak children, the root reduced to a paste, is given with milk and clarified butter for about a fortnight.

Native Indian Preparations.—*Asvagandha Ghrita.*—Take of the decoction of *Asvagandha* root 1 part, milk 10 parts, clarified butter 1 part; boil them together and prepare a *ghrita*. It is said to promote the nutrition and strength of children.—(Chakradatta.)

About half a drachm of *Asvagandha* root taken with milk or clarified butter is said to act as an aphrodisiac and restorative to old men.

304. PHYSALIS INDICA.

(*N. O.*—SOLANACEÆ.)

Eng.—Winter Cherry. *Can.*—Bondula-gida. *Mal.*—Ottampuli.

Properties and Uses.—The fruit is sometimes used in nephritis, dysuria, ascites, etc. The juice of the leaves is administered in cases of colic due to worms in children.

305. PIMPINELLA ANISUM.

(*N. O.*—UMBELLIFERÆ.)

Eng.—Anise. *Hind.*—Saurif. Arab.—Anisún. *Ben.*—Muhúri, Mithi-jirá. *Bom.*—Ervados. *Tel.*—Kuppi ; Sompu. *Tam.*—Sombú. *Can.*—Sàpu-gida.

Habitat.—This well-known herb is cultivated in Persia and in Northern India.

Properties and Uses.—The fruit yields an essential oil which is known as the oil of anise-seed and consists mainly of *anethol* or *anise* camphor. The fruit and essential oil are much valued as being aromatic, stomachic and carminative. Anise water—*Arak Badian*—is also much used for the same purposes, *i.e.*, for flatulency, indigestion and colic, particularly in children. Dose of the powdered seeds is from 10 to 30 grains; of the infusion or distilled water, 1 to 2 ounces; of the essential oil, 4 to 20 drops on sugar.

---

306. PINUS LONGIFOLIA.

(*N. O.*—CONIFERÆ.)

Sans.—Sarala. *Eng.*—The Long-leaved Pine. *Hind.*—Saral, Chír, Chil, (for the oleo-resin), Gandha biroza, Chirkagond. *Sans.*—Sarala-drava, Srivasa, Kshira.

Habitat.—This tree is very common on the Himalayas. It covers great areas in Upper and North-Western India from Afghanistan to Kashmir.

Properties and Uses.—The wood of *Pinus longifolia* is aromatic and is employed in Hindu medicine as stimulant, diaphoretic, useful to cool the burning sensation of the body, in cough, in fainting and as an application in ulcerations. It is generally used in combination with other medicines. It yields on incision an oleo-resin or turpentine, which is the source of the resin which is usually employed, in common with the oleo-resin, as an external stimulating application for ulcers and abscesses, and as a basis for plasters and an ingredient in ointments. Internally they are used to some extent and with some success as a stimulant diuretic in gleet and in similar affections. The purified oleo-resin might be given in doses of one to two drachms in emulsion. The tar is employed in chronic bronchitis and phthisis and is a favourite application in skin diseases.

---

307. PIPER BETLE.

(*N. O.*—PIPERACEÆ.)

Sans.—Támbula, Nàgavalli. *Eng.*—Betel-leaf Pepper. *Hind.*, *Ben.*, *Punj.*, *Guz.*, *Mah.*, and *Kon.*—Pân, Tàmbola. *Pers.*—Tâmbol. *Tel.*—Nâgavalli, Tamalapâku. *Tam.*—Vettilac. *Can.*—Villyadele. *Mal.*—Vettila, Tâmbúlam. *Cing.*—Balät. *Burm.*—Kun-yœ. *Malay.*—Seereh.

Habitat.—This twining plant is cultivated very extensively in the warm and moist parts of India, in Bengal and Orissa, Madras, United Provinces, Central Provinces, Bombay and Burma, for its leaves, which are in almost universal use as a masticatory in conjunction with lime and areca-nut.

Properties and Uses.—The leaves of this creeper are generally used for chewing by almost all classes and castes. The poorer classes make their packet of betel with the addition of lime, catechu and betelnuts. The rich, who can afford, add cardamoms, nutmegs, cloves, camphor and other aromatics. The betel leaf thus chewed acts as a gentle stimulant, tonic and digestive. It increases the salivary secretion. It is taken generally early in the morning, after meals and at bed-time. It sweetens the breath, removing all foulness from the mouth. According to some writers it acts as an aphrodisiac. The betel leaf contains an aromatic essential oil which can be isolated, and which, on being treated with caustic potash, yields a phenol called *Chavicol* which is a powerful antiseptic, five times more powerful than carbolic acid and twice as strong as eugenol. To this "betel-phenol" is due the characteristic odour of the leaves and oil. Medicinally the fresh leaves and the fresh juice of the leaves and the oil have aromatic, carminative and astringent properties. The warm leaves smeared with oil form a valuable application to the chest in cases of difficulty of breathing and in coughs, especially those of infancy and childhood. The same application has been recommended in congestion and other affections of the liver. Instead of the leaves, some apply a warm poultice consisting of two parts of the *juice* of the leaf and one part of the hydrated slaked lime. This is very useful as an application for sore-throat and over-enlarged glands. The betel leaves warmed by the fire and placed in layers over the breast (the *mammæ*) act as anti-galactagogue, and check the secretion of milk. Thus employed they are also said to be useful as resolvent to glandular swellings. The juice of the leaves is dropped into the ear to relieve earache; dropped into the eye for painful eye-affections. Internally the juice of the leaves with honey is a good expectorant and useful in coughs of children. It is a valuable stomachic and febrifuge in one drachm doses twice daily; given with milk in hysteria. The leaves administered in the form of syrup with spices in doses of an ounce three times a day are useful in general debility. The slender roots with black-pepper are used to produce sterility in women as they are said to produce paralysis and subsequent atropy of the ovaries. The root is chewed by public singers to improve their voice.

It is a common practice among Indian mothers to introduce the tender stalk of the leaf previously dipped in castor oil into the rectum of the child suffering from simple constipation.

308. PIPER CHABA, P. OFFICINARUM.

(*N. O.*—PIPERACEÆ).

Sans.—Chavikà. *Hind.*—Chát, Chair. *Ben.*—Chair. *Bom.*—Kankala, chavak.

Habitat.—This plant is a native of the Indian Archipelago (Java and Sumatra). Its fruit is the long-pepper of European commerce and is imported into Calcutta *viá* Singapore.

Properties and Uses.—The fruit is considered aromatic, stimulant and carminative occasionally used in medicines for coughs and throat affections. It is obtainable in the bazaars but is not much used in Hindu medicine.

309. PIPER LONGUM.

(*N. O.*—PIPERACEÆ).

Sans.—Pippali, Trikanà, Krishnà. *Eng.*—Long peper. *Hind.*—and *Ben.*—Pipul, Pipli. *Bom.*—Pipli. *Mah.*—Mothi, Pimpli. *Arab.*—Dàr-filfil. *Pers.*—Maghz-pipal. *Tel.*—Pippali katte. *Tam.*—Tippàli. *Can.*—Hippali. *Kon.*—Hipli.

Habitat.—This plant is indigenous to Eastern and Southern India from Nepal and Assam to Ceylon and is cultivated in Eastern Bengal for its fruit which is exported from India to some extent as long pepper as well as that of *P. Chaba* the true long pepper.

Properties and Uses—It is stimulant, carminative, and alterative tonic, more powerful than black pepper. It is useful in cough, hoarseness, asthma, dyspepsia, paralysis etc. Powdered long pepper administered with honey is said to relieve cough, asthma, hoarseness and hiccup. A mixture of long pepper, long pepper root, black pepper and ginger in equal parts is a useful combination in catarrh and hoarseness. As a valuable alterative tonic it is used thus:—An infusion of three long peppers is to be taken with honey on the first day, then for ten successive days the dose is to be increased by 3 peppers every day, so that on the tenth day the patient will take thirty at one dose. Then the dose is to be gradually reduced by three daily and finally the medicine is to be omitted. Thus administered it is said to act as a valuable alterative tonic in paraplegia, chronic cough, enlargements of the spleen and other abdominal viscera, etc. With black pepper, it is also used in the preparation of several irritating snuffs for using as a snuff in coma and drowsiness. As rubefacient, oil containing it and ginger is applied in sciatica and paraplegia. The drug has also aphrodisiac, diuretic and emmenagogue properties. Both the fruit and the root are much prescribed in palsy, gout, rheumatism, lumbago, etc. The fruit is given to women after parturition to check hæmorrhage and to ward off fever. As vermifuge it is one of the best remedies for colic in children. The fruit is used to some extent as a spice. The root is much used as a stimulant remedy and spice.

Native Indian Preparations.—Take of black pepper, long pepper, seeds of *Moringa pterygosperma*, *(sveta maricha)* and ginger equal parts, powder the ingredients and rub them together with the juice of the root of *Agati grandiflora* (*vaka*). This preparation is used as a snuff in coma and drowsiness.

Astakatvara Taila: Take of ginger and long pepper each 16 tolas, mustard oil 4 seers, butter milk 32 seers, curdled milk 4 seers, and boil them together in the usual way. This oil is rubbed externally in sciatica and paraplegia.

310. PIPER NIGRUM.

(*N. O.*—PIPERACEÆ.)

Sans.—Maricham. *Eng.*—Black pepper. *Hind.*, *Punj.* and *Ben.*—Kàli-mirich, Gol-mirich. Kàlà morich. *Duk.*—Káli-mirchi. *Bom.*, and *Mah.*—Kàla-miri, Miri. *Guz.*—Kalomirich, Miri. *Kast.*—Martz. *Tel.*—Miryálu. *Tam.*—Milagu. *Can.*—Volle-menasu. *Mal.*—Kuru-mulaka, Milaku. *Cing.*—Kalu-miris. *Burm.*—Nâyukon. *Malay.*—Ladahitam.

Habitat.—This perennial, climbing shrub is indigenous to the Malabar and Travancore coasts. It is extensively cultivated in south-western India.

Properties and Uses.—From the use of black-pepper as a culinary spice, it is well-known in almost all countries of the world. Medicinally also it has held an important place in Hindu Medicine for many centuries, being used in combination with long pepper and ginger under the name of *trikatu* or the three acrids. Black pepper is described as acrid, pungent, hot, carminative, useful in dyspepsia and flatulence, in doses of 10 to 15 grains of the powder and, in hæmorrhoids, in the form of confection; it is occasionally employed as antiperiodic in obstinate fevers. With calumba and bismuth it is used in dyspepsia and with asafœtida and camphor in flatulency. It is largely used in cholera pills. It is a useful ingredient in tooth powder. Externally it is rubefacient and stimulant to the skin. It is locally applied as resolvent to boils in the form of a paste; also in cases of relaxed sore-throat, piles, alopecia and other skin diseases.

In cholera the following pills were formerly held in high repute in Bengal: Take of black pepper, asafœtida and opium, each 20 grains; beat them well together and divide into 12 pills; of these one was the dose, repeated in an hour if required. On account of the quantity of opium they contain they should not be continued too long. They are chiefly indicated at the very outset of the attack. For piles in aged and debilitated persons the following confection is often of great service: Take of black pepper in fine powder 1 ounce; caraway fruit in fine powder $1\frac{1}{2}$ ounce; honey $7\frac{1}{2}$ ounces. Rub them well together in a mortar and give from one to two drachms twice or thrice daily. It proves useful also in the case of old and weak people suffering from descent of the rectum. An infusion of black pepper (2 drachms of bruised pepper to 1 pint of boiling water) forms a useful stimulant gargle in relaxed sore-throat and hoarseness dependent thereon.

Native Indian Preparations.—In intermittent fever black pepper, in doses of about a drachm, is recommended to be given with the juice of the leaves of *Ocimum Sanctum* (*tulasi*) or *Leucas linifolia* (*dronapuspi*)—(Bhâvaprakash.)

Pranadâ gudika:—Take of black pepper 32 tolas, ginger 24 tolas, long pepper 16 tolas, *Piper Chaba* (*chavya*) 8 tolas, leaves of *Abies Webbiana* (*talisa*) 8 tolas, flowers of *Mesua Ferrea* (*Nâgakesara*) 4 '

...ne mucous

...ctional obstructions of

long pepper root 16 tolas, leaves called *tejapatra* and cinnamon 1 tola each, cardamoms and the root of *Andropogon muricatus* (*usira*) 2 tolas each, old treacle 240 tolas; rub them together. Dose is about 2 drachms. This confection is given in hæmorrhoids. When there is costiveness and a sense of heat, chebulic myrobalan is substituted for the ginger in the above prescription.

311. PISTACIA INTEGERRIMA.

(*N. O.*—ANACARDIACEÆ.)

Sans.—Kàrkata sringi. *Eng.*—Galls. *Hind.* and *Mah.*—Kàkrasingi. *Ben.*—Kakrasringi. *Tel.*—Kâkara-shingi *Tam.*—Kakkata shingi.

Habitat.—This drug sold in the bazaars of Northern India under the above names consists of the gall-like excrescences formed by insects on the leaves and petioles of this tree found on the mountain ranges of the North-west from Peshawar to Simla.

Properties and Uses.—The galls are hard, hollow, irregular, greyish externally and yellow internally, usually 1 to 1½ inches long, sometimes much larger and shaped like a horn, hence the name *singi*. The galls are found to contain 75 per cent. of tannin. Powdered galls are given as an expectorant in coughs and phthisis in doses of 20 grains combined with demulcents and in diarrhœa with other astringents.

312. PISTACIA LENTISCUS.

(*N. O.*—ANACARDIACEÆ.)

Eng.—The Mastiche Tree. *Hind.*—Rùmi Mastiki. *Pers.*—Mastika-i-rumi.

Habitat.—This tree grows in the countries bordering Mediterranean, and its resin, called the mastiche and obtained by incisions made in the bark, is imported into India from Asia Minor through Persia and Afghanistan.

Properties and Uses.—The mastiche besides being employed in the manufacture of varnish, is used as a masticatory in tooth affections. It is used by dentists for filling carious teeth. It has the effect of preserving the teeth and sweetening the breath, when used as a tooth-paste. It forms an ingredient in stimulating tinctures applied to the mouth and gums, such as the compound tincture of Ammoniacum.

313. PISTACIA TEREBINTHUS.

(*N. O.*—ANACARDIACEÆ.)

Eng.—The Terebinth or Chian Turpentine Tree, Bombay Mastiche. *Hind.*—Mastâki, Kabuli Mastâki, Khinjak.

Habitat.—This tree, which exists in 3 varieties, *viz.*, *P. Mutica*, *P. Cabulica* and P. *Khinjuk*, is generally regarded as one species.

Properties and Uses.—The three varieties of this tree yield oleo-resins allied more or less to that of true mastiche and used in India as substitutes for it. This drug is known as Bombay or East Indian Mástiche.

314. PISTACIA VERA.

(*N. O.*—ANACARDIACEÆ.)

Eng.—The Pistachio-nut Tree. *Hind.* and *Ben.*—Pistà. *Pers.*—Pisteh.

Habitat.—The tree grows in the forests of Syria and Persia and is cultivated to some extent in Afghanistan. The plant is also extensively cultivated in Spain, Italy, France, etc. The fruit or nuts are brought to India in considerable quantities by the Kabul traders along with asafœtida and other drugs.

Properties and Uses.—The pistachio nuts are used as food by some high-class Indians and regarded as very wholesome and nourishing. They are sweet and agreeable. They enter into the composition of certain confections, and are used for flavouring ices and creams. They yield an oil by expression which is used for making an electuary for diseases of the stomach. The fruit somewhat resembles that of the olive, ovoid and reddish externally, astringent and terebinthinate, with a kernel which yields a sweet, aromatic oil. Galls are formed on the leaves which have been found to contain 45 per cent. of tannin allied to gallo-tannic acid, besides gallic acid and 7 per cent. of a resin or oleo-resin to which their terebinthinous odour is due. They are known as *Gul-i-pisteh* or *Baz-ghanj* and are also imported into India. Medicinally the nut has been regarded as tonic and useful in debility. The oil expressed from it is used as a demulcent. The galls are useful as an astringent.

---

315. PISTIA STRATIOTES.

(*N. O.*—ARIODEÆ).

Sans.—Kumbhika. *Hind.*—Jal-kunbhi. *Ben.*—Tokàpànà. *Bom.*—Prashni. *Tel.*—Antara tämara. *Tam.*—Agasa-tamaré.

Habitat.—This aquatic stemless plant grows on the surface of the water in tanks and stagnant pools in Bengal and is also found on the sea-shore.

Properties and Uses.—The ash of the plant, known as *pana* salt, has some repute in some parts of India as an application for ringworm. It has been found by Dr. Warden to consist chiefly of potassium chloride and sulphate.

---

316. PLANTAGO ISPAGULA.

(*N. O.* - PLANTAGINEÆ).

Eng.—Ispaghúl or Spogel Seeds. *Hind.*—Isapghúl, Issufgùl. *Ben. Pers. Bom., Guz.* and *Mah.*—Isapghol. *Duk.* and *Punj.*—Isapgól. *Kash.*—Is-mogul. *Tel.*—Isapagálavittulu. *Tam.*—Ishappukolvirai. *Can.*—Issabagolu.

Habitat.—This Persian herb is found also in North-West India, the Punjab and Sind ; cultivated to a small extent in Bengal.

Properties and Uses.—Ispaghul seeds are procurable in most bazaars, and are a highly useful demulcent medicine. They are of a cooling nature and used in catarrh, blenorrhoea and affections of the kidneys. Dose of the seeds is ½ to 2 drachms in powder, sometimes mixed with sugar or (better) in decoction (1 in 40) which forms a cooling demulcent drink. Steeped or boiled in water they become coated with an abundant, adherent, bland mucilage, which they also yield to water and render it mucilaginous. The decoction is very beneficial in gonorrhoea, dysentery and diarrhoea and as a demulcent in coughs and colds and other pharyngeal disorders, particularly for children. In the chronic diarrhoea of Europeans who have been long resident in India, 2½ drachms of the seeds mixed with half a drachm of powdered sugarcandy is said to be an excellent remedy ; or a drachm or two of the seeds are steeped in water for about 15 or 20 minutes and then given in spoonful doses of the whole seed. Many of the swollen seeds pass out whole with the motions, and this action is said to be mechanical as well as astringent to the intestinal ulcers. It is said that a slight degree of astringency and some tonic property may be imparted to the seeds by exposing them to a moderate degree of heat so that they shall be dried and slightly browned. This remedy sometimes cures the protracted diarrhœa of European and Indian children after many other remedies have failed. It has a beneficial action in other inflammatory affections of the mucous membrane of the alimentary canal as in gastric catarrh. In many affections of the kidneys and bladder, in gonorrhœa etc., attended with pain, local irritation and scalding or difficulty in passing urine the decoction made by boiling 2 drachms of Ispaghul seeds (bruised) in one pint of water for 10 minutes in a covered vessel, and strained and given in 2-to 4-ounce doses three or four times a day or oftener, is very serviceable. Or it may be administered as sherbet prepared with sugarcandy, either alone or combined with alkalies and diuretics. It is also a very beneficial remedy in piles. Combined with ipecac it is administered in dysentery; with cubebs and nitrate of potash in gonorrhœa. In rheumatic and gouty affections, swellings &c., the crushed seeds moistened with water form a good, soothing and emollient poultice.

---

317. PLUMBAGO ROSEA.

(*N. O.*—PLUMBAGINEÆ.)

Sans.—Raktachitraka. *Eng.*—Rose-coloured Leadwort. *Hind.*—Läl-chitarak, Lâl-chitra. *Ben.*—Rakto-chitra, Läl chitá. *Punj.*—Chitra. *Kash.*—Shitranj. *Duk.*—Lâl-Chiturmül. *Mah.*—Lál-Chitraka. *Tel.*—Yerra-chitramülam. *Tam.*—Kodimuli Shivappu Chittramülam. *Can.*—Kempu Chitramula. *Mal.*—Chekkikotuveri. *Cing.*—Ratnitul. *Burm.*—Kin-khenni. *Malay.*—Chirakamerah.

Habitat.—This plant is commonly cultivated in gardens throughout India.

Properties and Uses.—The root, which contains a crystalline principle called *Plumbagin*, has vesicant properties, and enters into the composition of caustic pastes and rubefacient applications. The bruised root mixed with oil is used as a rubefacient application in rheumatism. Taken internally it is a powerful acro-narcotic poison; it is employed to procure criminal abortion as it will expel the fœtus from the womb whether dead or alive. Externally it has been sometimes used as a substitute for cantharides, for raising a blister. The fresh bark of the root is rubbed into a paste with water and a little rice flour; it is then spread on a piece of rag and applied to the surface. In about 5 minutes a pain is felt, which increases in severity for about half an hour, when it may be removed; a rice poultice may then be applied over the part, and within 12 or 18 hours a large uniform blister will be found to have formed. The fluid having been let out, it may be dressed with plantain leaf in the usual way. The chief objection to the use of plumbago blister is the great pain it causes, hence it should only be used when other blistering agents are not at hand and a blister is an immediate necessity.

---

318. PLUMBAGO ZEYLANICA.

(*N. O.* – PLUMBAGINEÆ.)

Sans.—Chitraka. *Eng.*—Ceylon Leadwort. *Hind.* and *Ben.*—Chitrâ. *Guz.*, *Mah.* and *Kon.*—Chitramûla. *Tel.*—Agnimâtha, Chitra-mùlamu. *Tam.*—Chittira. *Mal.*—Vellakotu-véri. *Can.*—Bilë chitramûla.

Habitat.—This plant, closely allied to the preceding, is growing wild and cultivated as a hedge plant in Bengal and Southern India.

Properties and Uses.—The root contains the same active principle as the *P. rosea* and has similar properties although in a smaller degree. It also is powerfully poisonous and its internal use is said to be attended with great danger. It enters into the composition of several native Indian preparations used as caustics. The root reduced to a paste is applied to abscesses with the object of opening them. According to Hindu Vaidya Shastras, the root is said to increase the digestive power, to promote the appetite and to be useful in dyspepsia, piles, anasarca, diarrhœa, skin diseases, etc. It is much used as a stimulant adjunct to other preparations in the form of a combination called *trimada,* consisting of plumbago root, *baberang* seeds and the tubers of *Cyperus rotundus* (*mustaka*).

Native Indian Preparations.—A favourite medicine for flatulence is an old prescription of Susruta called *Shaddharana yogà.* It is a powder composed of equal parts of plumbago root, *Indrayana seeds*, root of *Stephania hernandifolia* (*pâtha*), of *Picrorrhiza Kurroa* (*katuki*), *atis* and chebulic myrobalan. The dose is about a drachm.

Externally as caustic, it is used thus:—Take of plumbago root, root of *Baliospermum Montanum* (*danti*), the milky juice of *Euphorbia nerifolia* (*snuhi*) and of *Calotropis procera* or *Hamiltonia* (*arka*), marking nut, sulphate of iron, treacle and rock salt, equal parts; mix them together and make into a paste.

319. PLUMERIA ACUMINATA.

(*N. O.*—APOCYNACEÆ.)

Sans.—Champakam. *Hind.*—Gùlchin. *Tel.*—Adavi-gannéru. *Tam.*—Eelathalari, Perungalli. *Can.*—Kâdusampige. *Mal.*—Velutharali.

Habitat.—This tree is met with generally on the sea-coast districts of Southern India.

Properties and Uses.—The bark is recommended as a cure for gonorrhœa. The leaves made into a poultice are used to dispel swellings, the milky juice is employed as a rubefacient in rheumatism. Internally the bark is given with cocoanut, ghee and rice as a remedy for diarrhœa. The flower-heads are eaten with betel leaves in ague. The milky juice, in *minute doses*, acts as an effectual purgative. The dose is as much as a grain of parched rice will absorb, the grain being administered as a pill. Externally the juice with sandal wood oil and camphor is employed as a cure for itch.

---

320. PODOPHYLLUM EMODI.

(*N. O.*—BERBERIDEÆ).

Eng.—Indian Podophyllum. *Hind.*—Pâpra, Pâpri, Bhavanbakra, Bakra-chimyaka.

Habitat.—This herbaceous plant, indigenous to the temperate Himalaya from Sikkim to Kashmir, is plentiful near Simla, usually at altitudes above 9000 feet. It is more plentiful on the Western Himalaya than on the Eastern ranges.

Properties and Uses.—The plant is closely allied in botanical characters to the American species, *P. Peltatum*, the source of the Resin of Podophyllin of the *British Pharmacopœia*. The lobed leaves have the same appearance; the scarlet red pulpy fruit of the size and shape of a pigeon's egg, is eaten by the hill tribes as the "May-apple" (fruit of *P. Peltatum*) is in America, and the rhizome or underground stem and rootlets contain similar medicinal principles. The resinous constituents of both species, called collectively *Podophyllin*, are obtained by re-percolation of the dried and powdered rhizomes, precipitation by acidulated water and drying at a low temperature. Podophyllin is an amorphous powder, usually of a bright brownish—yellow colour, soluble in rectified spirit and in aqueous ammonia. Podophyllin resin is a powerful biliary purgative, its action somewhat corresponding to that of mercury, hence the name "vegetable calomel." It is an active cholagogue and aperient in doses of $\frac{1}{8}$ to 1 grain, usually in pills alone or combined with other hepatics and purgatives or in solution in alcohol (*Tinctura Podophylli*, B. P.) The rhizome itself is not employed in medicine.

---

321. PONGAMIA GLABRA.

(*N. O.*—LEGUMINOSÆ)

Sans.—**Karanja, Naktamâla.** *Eng.*—**Indian Beech.** *Hind.*—**Korang, Kiramäl.** *Ben.*—**Karanja, Karmuj.** *Bom.* **and** *Mah.*—**Karanjala.** *Tel.*—**Känagu.** *Tam.*—**Ponga, Pungam-maram.** *Can.*—**Honge, Karanja-mara.** *Mal.*—Pongam. *Kon.*—**Karinje-rooku.**

Habitat.—This tree is common all over India, from the temperate Himalaya to Central and Southern India and Ceylon.

Properties and Uses.—The seeds yield, on expression, about 25 per cent of a thick, yellowish-brown bitter oil which is used for illuminative purposes. Medicinally, it has marked antiseptic, cleansing and healing properties when applied to skin diseases, in sçabies, herpes and the like. An embrocation made of equal parts of the oil and lime or lemon juice is useful in rheumatism, and as an application in psoriasis and pityriasis. The juice of the stem, leaves and root appear to possess similar properties. The juice with cocoanut milk and lime water is a remedy for gonorrhœa, and the juice of the leaves is useful in flatulency, dyspepsia and diarrhœa. A poultice of the leaves is applied to ulcers infested with worms. The young leaves are applied to bleeding piles. The pulp of the seeds is said to be a good application in leprosy. The flowers are used as a remedy for diabetes.

Native Indian Preparations.—The seeds of *Pongamia glabra, Cassia Tora*, and the root of *Aplotaxis Auriculata* are rubbed into a paste with cow's urine, and applied to eruptive skin diseases—(Chakradatta).

Prithvisára Taila :—Take of the expressed oil of the seeds of *Pongamia glabra*, 1 seer, *Kânjika* 8 tolas, roots of *Plumbago Zeylanica, Nerium Odorum, Vitex Negundo*, Aconite and the seeds of *Corchorus Olitorius* (*Nâdika*) 8 tolas each, in the form of a paste made with *Kânjika*. Mix them together and warm in the sun. This oil is said to be useful in various sorts of skin diseases, ulcers etc.—(Chakradatta).

Tiktädya Ghrita :—Take the leaves and fruits of *Pongamia glabra*, root of *Pi rhiza Kurroa* (*Katuki*), wax, turmeric, liquorice roc eaves of *Trichosanthes dioica* (*patala*). *Aganosma Caryophyllata* (*Màlati*) and *Azadirachta Indica* (*nim*) equal parts. in all one seer. Beat them into a paste and boil with 4 seers of clarified butter and 16 seers of water in the usual manner. This preparation is used as an ointment in unhealthy ulcerations and wounds.—(Chakradatta).

---

322. POTASSII NITRAS.

Eng.—Nitrate of Potassium, Nitre, Saltpetre. *Hind.*, *Duk.* and *Punj.*—Shorà. *Ben.*—Sorà. *Kash.*—Safed Shorâ. *Bom.* and *Guz.*—Soràkhàr. *Mah.*—Shorà mîtha. *Tel.*—Shúrâ karam, Petiluppu. *Tam.*—Potluppu. *Can.*—Petluppu. *Mal.*—Vetiuppa. *Cing.*—Vedilunu, Potlunu. *Burm.*—Yan-zin. *Malay.*—Sun-dawa.

Habitat.—This salt is obtainable in most of the bazaars in India. It is produced very largely as a natural efflorescence on the surface of the soil in many parts of India. The efflorescence or the saline earth is collected after the rains from the land inundated during the rains, and from mud heaps, mud buildings and other places on which it is formed, and then subjected to a process of solution and filtration through a crude mud filter. The solution which is thus freed of earthy matters contains a certain proportion of nitrate of lime which is removed by passing the solution through layers of wood ashes and ashes of plants (impure carbonate of potassium); carbonate of lime is thus deposited and the nitrate of potassium solution is evaporated and crystallized. The impure nitre is known as *dhoah* and contains about 45 to 75 per cent of the actual , the remainder being sulphate and chloride of sodium a insoluble matter. It is again dissolved and crystalliz before it is sent, under the name of *shora kalmi* (refined) to the bazaars for sale, while it is further re-crystallized in Calcutta and elsewhere before being sold for use.

Properties and Uses.—Potassium nitrate is an efficient diuretic and diaphoretic in action. It is generally used in solution. Given in the solid form or in concentrated solution it acts as irritant. In weak solutions, 1 to 2 drachms in a quart of thin warm rice *conjee*, it is an excellent refrigerent drink in fevers when the skin is hot and dry, the tongue parched, the thirst great and the urine scanty and high-coloured. It may also be sweetened with honey or sugarcandy; or tamarind or lime juice may be added to improve the flavour if desired. It may also be employed usefully in the early stages of dropsy, in cases of small-pox, measles, influenza, catarrh, in gonorrhœa, in acute rheumatism, in bleeding from the lungs, stomach, uterus or other internal organs attended by fever. In the early stages of inflammatory sore-throat, a small piece of nitre allowed to dissolve slowly in the mouth is a successful popular remedy. In asthma, in chronic bronchitis and other spasmodic coughs, inhalation of the fumes of burning nitre gives great relief. For this purpose, pieces of moderately thick blotting paper are kept immersed for a few minutes in a solution of the salt, made by dissolving four ounces of the salt in half a pint of boiling water in an open vessel; they are then dried and kept ready for use. Whenever an attack threatens, one or, if necessary, two pieces of this paper, are burnt so that the fumes may be freely inhaled; but it should not be held too near the face or the fumes may prove too irritating, and increase rather than diminish the symptoms. It is better to burn one or two pieces of this nitre paper in the bed room before retiring to rest at bed time, care being taken to prevent the too ready escape of the fumes. Locally nitre is employed for the relief of headache and delirium occurring in the course of fever, in the form of a cold and agreeable lotion for the head, made by dissolving two ounces of nitre and an equal quantity of sal ammoniac in a great bottle full of water; this should be applied by constant relays of freshly-wetted clothes. In acute rheumatism, a strong solution of nitre (three ounces to a pint of water) forms a most soothing application to the swollen and painful joints; cloths saturated with it should be kept constantly applied; the ease which it affords is often very great.

323. PRUNUS AMYGDALUS.

(*N. O.*—ROSACEÆ.)

Sans.—Bâdàma. *Eng.*—Almond. *Pers.*—Bádám. *Hind.*—Badàm. *Ben.*—Bilati-badám. *Bom.*—Bâdam. *Tel.*—Bàdam vittulu. *Tam.*—Vâdam kottai. *Can.*—Badámu.

Habitat.—The almond tree is a native of Western Asia, and has now become naturalised in the Mediterranean countries of Europe and Africa. It is cultivated in the Punjab, Kashmir and Afghanistan, whence the fruit (almond in shell) is exported in large quantities to India.

Properties and Uses.—Two varieties of the tree are recognised—*dulcis and amara*—yielding respectively sweet and bitter almonds. Both varieties yield to expression about 50 per cent of a fine, clear, fixed oil contained in the kernel; it has an agreeable flavour but no odour. The kernels of the bitter variety contain a crystalline glucoside called *Amygdalin*, besides a neutral principle called *emulsin* which is also contained in the sweet variety. In the presence of water the emulsion acts as a ferment on the amygdalin, producing benzoic aldehyde (essential oil of bitter almonds) hydrocyanic or prussic acid and glucose. The essential oil of bitter almonds is much used for flavouring custards, etc., but great caution is necessary in its employment on account of its poisonous nature due to the presence of prussic acid. The almond tree yields a gum known as *Badam-i-gond* which is exported from Bombay and occasionally used in place of tragacanth. Medicinally sweet almonds are emollient and demulcent, and an emulsion produced from them by triturating the powdered kernels with water is useful in bronchial diseases, in dysentery, and several affections of the urinary organs, frequently lessening the acrimony of the secretions in quite a remarkable manner. Almond meal has been recommended as a suitable diet for diabetic patients as it contains no starch. The burnt shell (almond shell charcoal) is used as a tooth-powder.

324. PRUNUS COMMUNIS.

(*N. O.*—ROSACEÆ).

Eng.—The Bokhara Plum. *Hind.* and *Ben.*—Alú, Alúbokhära, Alúcha.

Habitat.—This tree grows on the Western Himalaya.

Properties and Uses.—The fruit of this tree is common in the Indian markets, being brought down by the Afghan traders. It is largely consumed by the rich in various forms of *chatni*. It ac[illegible]s a cooling laxative and is regarded as suitable for all [illegible] purposes to which the English plum is put, as in t[illegible] reparation of confection of Senna.

325. PSIDIUM GUYAVA.

(*N. O.*—MYRTACEÆ).

Varieties :—P. PYRIFERUM (white) and P. POMIFERUM (red).

Sans.—Pérâlâ. *Eng.*—The Guava. *Hind.*—Läl sufrium (red), Amrút. *Ben.*—Läl peyara (red), Goächhi-phal. *Bom.*—Perala. *Tel.*—Jäm-pandu, Goyyä pandu. *Tam.*—Koyyapalam. *Can.*—Pérala, Jäma-phala. *Mal.*—Palampér. *Kon.*—Pæra.

Habitat.—This tree is cultivated nearly all over India and is common in Bengal.

Properties and Uses.—This tree is much valued on account of its pleasant fruit, which forms, when stewed, the well known guava jelly. The ripe fruit is a good aperient. But the unripe one is employed in diarrhœa. The stem bark is astringent and contains about 25% of tannic acid. The root-bark is also astringent and is successfully employed in chronic infantile diarrhœa in the form of decoction, half ounce of the bark in six ounces of water boiled down to three ounces and given in teaspoonful doses. Locally the decoction is applied with much benefit to the prolapsus ani of children. It is also successfully employed in scurvy and for unhealthy ulcers, and as a mouth-wash for swollen gums, and administered internally in cholera for arresting vomiting and diarrhœaic symptoms. The leaves when ground make excellent poultice.

---

326. PSORALEA CORYLIFOLIA.

(*N. O.*—LEGUMINOSÆ.)

Syn:—TRIFOLIUM UNIFOLIUM.

Sans.—Vakûchi. *Eng.*—Babchi Seeds. *Hind.*—Babachi, Bhävanj. *Ben.*—Latakasturi, Kakùchi. *Bom.*—Bawachi. *Mah.*—Bävanchi. *Tel.*—Bhavanchi Vittulu. *Tam.*—Karpokarishi.

Habitat.—This plant is common in Bengal and all over the plains of India.

Properties and Uses.—The seeds are laxative, stimulant and aphrodisiac. The seeds are used to make a perfumed oil. They yield a colourless, essential oil, lighter than water, and possessing in a marked degree the odour of the drug and a crystalline colouring matter. These constituents are partly soluble in water, alcohol and ether. The oleo-resinous extract of the seeds diluted with chaulmügra oil and with simple ointment is recommended as an application in cases of leucoderma or white leprosy. The ointment may be prepared by combining one part of an alcoholic extract of the seeds with two parts of chaulmügra oil and two parts of lanoline. The proportion of the active ingredient may be increased if the action is delayed.

327. PTEROCARPUS MARSUPIUM.

(N. O.—LEGUMINOSÆ.)

Sans.—Pitasala. *Eng.*—The Indian Kino, Malabar Kino. *Hind.*—Bija, Bijasâr. *Ben.*—Pit-sal. *Bom.*, and *Mah.*—Bibla, Honnè. *Tel.*—Peddagi. *Tam.*—Vengai-maram. *Can.*—Hanemara.

Habitat—This large tree is common in Central and Southern India and Ceylon. This tree is the source of the kino of the European Pharmacopœias and that of the United States.

Properties and Uses.—Kino is a natural exudation obtained by incisions in the trunk inspissated without artificial heat. The principal constituent of kino is a peculiar tannin *kino-tannic acid*, usually believed to be identical with catechu-tannic acid and distinct from gallo-tannic acid. By boiling an aqueous solution of kino-tannic acid a precipitate of *kino-red* is obtained; treated with dilute acid a similar precipitate occurs and crystals of *kinoin* separate. Kino is a simple astringent, administered in diarrhœa, somewhat milder in action than catechu.

328. PTEROCARPUS SANTALINUS.

(N. O.—LEGUMINOSÆ.)

Sans., *Ben.*, *Mah.* and *Can.*—Rakta chandana. *Eng.*—Red Sanders or Sandalwood. *Hind.*—Làlchandana. *Pers.*—Sandale-surkh. *Bom.*—Ratänjli. *Tel.*—Rakta gandhamu. Erragandamu. *Tam.*—Shen-chandanam. *Mal.*—Chenchandanam. *Kon.*—Rachandana.

Habitat.—This small tree is generally met with in the forests of Madras and Mysore and the Coromandel and Malabar Coasts of Southern India.

Properties and Uses.—Red sanders wood has faint astringent properties, probably due to traces of tannic acid which it contains. It also contains a red crystalline, resinoid, colouring matter insoluble in water, soluble in alcohol and named *Santalin* or *Santalic acid*. From the wood has also been isolated a colourless principle called *Santal*, which is capable of being converted into what is believed to be resorcin. Another crystalline body, *Pterocarpin*, has also been isolated.

The wood enters into the composition of numerous prescriptions of an astringent character used in complaints like bleeding piles, hæmorrhages, etc. Powdered and mixed with milk it is taken for bleeding piles. It is also employed as an ingredient of cooling external applications for inflammations, piles, headaches etc. Powdered or beaten up into a paste, it is applied to eyes in ophthalmia and to sore eyes; rubbed with honey or with oil it is applied to boils and abscesses. The wood rubbed on a piece of stone with water forms an excellent cooling application and purifier of skin after bathing, like white sandalwood (*Santalum aloum*). In British Pharmacy the wood is generally employed as a colouring agent in the compound tincture of lavender and, in native preparations, as an ingredient of several medicated oils.

---

329. PTYCHOTIS AJOWAN.

(See also *Carum Copticum.*)

(*N. O.*—UMBELLIFERÆ.)

Syn :—CARUM AJOWAN, AMMI COPTICUM, PTYCHOTIS COPTICA.

Sans.—Yavânikà, Ajamada, Agniverdhana, Deepyaka. *Eng.*—Bishop's weed, Omum seeds. *Hind.*, and *Duk.*—Ajawän. *Ben.*—Jowan. *Punj.*—Ajwain. *Kash.*—Jàwind. *Mah.*, and *Kon.*—Ovä, Vóvó. *Guz.*—Ajwán. *Tel.*—Omamu, Ajamoda. *Tam.*—Omum. *Can.*—Oma, Vóma. *Mal.*—Homam, Ayamódkam. *Cing.*—Assamódagam. *Burm.*—Samhún. *Malay.*—Lavinju-larmisi.

Habitat.—This plant is largely cultivated in Eastern India.

Properties and Uses.—The omum seeds have stimulant, carminative, tonic and antispasmodic properties, useful in flatulence, colic, atonic dyspepsia, diarrhoea, cholera, hysteria and spasmodic affections of the bowels. The seeds yield an oil on distillation with water which is used in cholera, colic and indigestion. The dose is from 1 to 3 drops on sugar or made into an emulsion with gum arabic. Externally it is applied to relieve rheumatic pains. The oil has also powerful antiseptic properties and, therefore, it and the omum water which is the distilled water (prepared by distilling 3 lbs. of the bruised seeds in six quart bottles of water and distilled over four) are useful in cholera, especially in the early stages to check the vomiting and purging and to stimulate the system. The dose of the omum water is from 1 to 2 ounces repeated as often as necessary; the dose for a child ranges from a teaspoonful to a tablespoonful according to age. The essential oil prepared from the seeds is identical with *Thymol.* The oil of thymus or thymol is obtained by exposing oil of distillation to spontaneous evaporation at a low temperature or by exposing the oil first rectified from chloride of calcium to a temperature of O° Centigrade when the oil deposits about 36% of thymol in superb tabular crystals. The seeds are also employed as stomachic and cardiac; with astringents they are used as a topical remedy in relaxed sore-throats; they form an ingredient in cough mixture; they have further the virtue of disguising the taste of disagreeable drugs and obviating their tendency to cause nausea and griping. In habitual drunkenness, dipsomania, omum is useful. On this point Mr. Wood observes:—On account of its biting or pungent, yet pleasant taste and the sensation of warmth it creates in the stomach, it has been constantly recommended, of late years, to those afflicted with the desire for alcoholic drinks. It does not of course, intoxicate, but it is no mean substitute for the ordinary stimulant, in removing almost immediately the sensation of 'gnawing' or 'sinking at the pit of the stomach' which the frequent use of spirits so invariably brings on. And I have been assured that it has been the means of rescuing many otherwise sensible and useful men from slavery to the habit of spirit-drinking."

330. PUNICA GRANATUM.

(*N. O.*—LYTHRACEÆ.)

Sans.—Dádima-phalam. *Eng.*—Pomegranate. *Hind.*, *Duk.*, and *Ben.*—Anár, Dârim. *Pers.*—Gulnâr. *Arab.*—Rumman. *Kash.*—Dhàun. *Guz.*—Dädam. *Mah.*, *Can.*, and *Kon.*—Dàlimba. *Tel.*—Dádima. *Tam.*—Mádalai. *Mal.*—Mátalam. *Cing.*—Delumgahá. *Burm.*—Salè-bin, or Talibin. *Malay.*—Dalima.

Habitat.—The Pomegranate tree is indigenous to North-Western India, being found wild in Persia, Afghanistan and Baluchistan, and cultivated chiefly for its fruit nearly all over India.

Properties and Uses.—The Pomegranate fruit has been esteemed in the East from a very remote period as food and medicine. The rind of the fruit contains tannin to the extent of 22 to 25 per cent. The root-bark contains 20 to 25 per cent of the same astringent principle, considered to be a peculiar variety and named *punico-tannic acid* which, when boiled with dilute sulphuric acid is resolvable into *Ellagic acid* and sugar. Mannite is also obtainable from the bark which was believed to be the *Punicin* or *Granatin* of former observers. According to Mr. J. Culley, an American investigator, the properties and composition of punico-tannic acid and the gallo-tannic acid obtained from galls so closely agree that both these tannins are taken to be identical with each other. A liquid volatile alkaloid named *Pelletierine* had been isolated by Tanret in 1878 from the root-bark to which the tænifuge property of the bark has been attributed. Another alkaloid, *Isopàlletierine* was subsequently discovered by the same investigator.

The Pomegranate rind is a valuable astringent in diarrhœa and the advanced stages of dysentery, usually administered in decoction which is prepared by boiling in a covered vessel 2 ounces of the bruised dried rind and 2 drachms of bruised cloves or cinnamon in a pint of water for fifteen minutes and straining; of this, when cold the dose is 1 to 2 ounces three or four times a day; in obstinate cases five drops of laudanum may be added to each dose. The powdered rind is also similarly efficacious. The root-bark, especially the *fresh* one, is a reliable remedy for the expulsion of tænia or tape-worm. It is administered in decoction which is best made by digesting two ounces of the fresh bark and a little clove or other aromatic in a pint of cold water for six hours and reducing the strained liquor by evaporation to ten ounces; or it may also be prepared by boiling 2 ounces of the sliced fresh bark in two pints of water down to one pint and straining. This quantity should be given fasting early in the morning in doses of two ounces at intervals of an hour or two, the last dose being followed by an aperient (a full dose of castor oil or compound powder of jalap with the addition of two grains of calomel), and the worm is said to be expelled within twelve hours. A fluid extract of the fresh bark in doses of half an ounce, repeated, is equally effectual. The alkaloid, *pelletierine* and its compounds have also been used as anthelmintic and tænicide; the most suitable being the tannate, which is very difficult to dissolve and therefore not readily absorbed and is administered in doses of 3 to 8 grains, fasting and then followed by a purgative.

The acid saccharine juice of the fresh fruit is much esteemed as a cooling beverage in fevers and sickness. The flowers and buds and also the juice of the leaves are used as styptic and astringent. The flower buds powdered and given in doses of 4 to 5 grains are useful in bronchitis. In relaxed sore-throat the above-described decoction with the addition of alum (in the proportion of a drachm to a pint of decoction) is a very useful gargle and it also forms a good astringent injection in vaginal discharges; in these cases the cloves or cinnamon should be omitted.

Native Indian Preparations.—*Dádimáshtaka* :— Take of pomegranate rind one seer, bamboo-manna two tolas, cardamom, cinnamon, *tejapàtra* and flowers of *Mesua ferra (nágakesara)*, each four tolas, *Ajowan*, coriander, cumin seeds, long pepper root, long pepper, black pepper and ginger, each 8 tolas, sugar one seer. Powder the ingredients and mix. Dose, about one drachm in chronic bowel-complaints.

331. QUASSIA EXCELSA.

(*N. O.*—SIMARUBACEÆ.)

Eng :—Quassia wood. *Vernaculars* :—Koshia.

Habitat.—The wood is so called after Quassi, Coissi or Quass, a negro of Surinum who first discovered its tonic and febrifuge properties and used it as a cure for the malignant fevers so prevalent in moist, tropical countries; the species which he used was *Quassia Amara*, a small branching tree growing to the height of 16 or 20 feet in the woods of Surinum, Guiana, Cayenne and Trinidad. But that which is now generally employed is a lofty tree called in the Carribee Islands, "Bitter Ash; it is the *Simaruba Excelsa* of botanists. The quassia wood is obtainable in all Indian bazaars in the form of yellowish white shavings, chips, or raspings or large dense billets.

Properties and Uses.—Quassia is a bitter tonic without astringency; and as it contains no tannin it can be ordered with iron preparations. It invigorates the digestive organs with little excitement of the circulation or increase of animal heat. It is most suitable in dyspepsia and anorexia. Its virtue is due to a bitter crystallizable principle called *Quassin*, which, when heated, melts like resin; both alkalies and acids increase its solubility in water. A strong decoction of quassia is a good poison for flies and fish; similarly it acts in various diseased conditions of the blood, destroying unhealthy organisms, and acting as a true febrifuge like quinine. When injected into the rectum a strong infusion will cause the death of thread-worms. The infusion of the Phamacopœia intended for internal administration is made by pouring a pint of boiling water on 2 scruples or 40 grains of the chips or raspings; it is given as a tonic and antiseptic, in bilious fevers, together with alkaline salts; in gout with aromatics and ginger; in hysteria with camphor and tincture of valerian; in dyspepsia with sulphate of zinc or iron or with mineral acids. The dose is from 1 to 4 ounces.

332. QUERCUS INFECTORIA.

(*N. O.*—CUPULIFERÆ.)

Sans., and *Mah.*,—Majüphala. *Eng.*—Oak Galls. *Hind.*—Müphal. *Ben.*—Majuphal. *Bom.* and *Kon.*,—Maiphala. *Pers.*—Mazu. *Tel.*—Mashikàya. *Tam.*—Màchakài.

Habitat.—The tree bearing the oak galls of commerce is a native of Greece, Asia Minor and Syria extending to Persia, whence they are imported into India.

Properties and Uses.—The galls are excrescences caused by an *Hymenopterous* insect named *Cynips Gallæ tinctoria*, which punctures the twigs or young branches of the oak and deposits its ova. The irritation produced causes a flow of the natural juices of the plant to the part, which surround the ova and develop into a gall, sometimes of considerable size. Within the gall thus formed the larva undergoes its various transformations until the winged insect bores a passage for itself from the centre to the surface and escapes. The best quality of galls are those collected before the fly has escaped. They are darker in colour and known in the bazaars as the "black" or "blue" variety, the "white" or perforated galls being lighter in colour.

Most of the above vernacular names signify "magic nuts" from the fact that galls have been much employed in India by magicians.

The principal chemical constituent of galls is *Tannin* or *Tannic acid*, usually distinguished as *Gallo-tannic acid*, which exists to the extent of 50 to 60 or 70 per cent, and about 3 per cent of *gallic acid*.

The galls constitute a powerful vegetable astringent. The powder is used to some extent in India as an astringent in diarrhœa. A more general application is in the form of an ointment or suppository usually combined with opium as a remedy for hæmorrhoids. Tannic and Gallic acids which the galls contain are valuable styptics and astringents, useful in all internal hæmorrhages, in excessive secretions from different parts of the body and for cutting short local inflammations as in various forms of sore throats, nasal catarrh and gonorrhœa. Tannic acid is used as an antidote in poisoning by the alkaloids to form tannates which are only partially soluble.

333. QUICK LIME.

Hind.—Chunna. *Bom.*, and *Mah.*—Kalichuna. *Tam.*, and *Mal.*—Chunnambu. *Tel.*—Thàlchani Sunnam. *Can.*—Sunna. *Kon.*—Chunno.

Properties and Uses.—Lime water is given mixed with milk to children in acidity of the stomach. Mixed with gamboge, quick lime is applied externally to painful and gouty joints. It is also used as a caustic in the bites of rabid dogs.

334. QUINETUM.

Syn:—CINCHONA FEBRIFUGE; MIXED CINCHONA ALKALOIDS.

(*N. O.*—CINCHONACEÆ.)

Production.—This amorphous powder is prepared from the red cinchona bark grown at the Government cinchona plantations at Darjeeling (India).

Properties and Uses.—Quinetum contains all the febrifugal alkaloids of the *Cinchona succirubra* in the proportion of quinine 25, cinchonidine 50, and cinchonine 20 in 100 parts. It is a valuable febrifuge, but takes a longer time to act and will not replace quinine in pernicious fever. Although it has the same apyretic effect as quinine, yet it is less powerful; larger doses are, therefore, required at longer intervals before the paroxysms. It has its disadvantages, however, being apt to create nausea, vomiting, with a burning sensation at the pit of the stomach, extending in some instances to the throat and occasionally diarrhœa. Like quinine, if given in sufficient doses to produce its specific effect, it gives rise to headache, singing in the ears, giddiness and other symptoms included under the term "quinism"; but all these pass away on the discontinuance of the remedy, leaving no after-ill-effects. It is, in fact, a thoroughly safe and efficacious remedy in ordinary simple intermittents, in chronic cases and as a tonic, although not so effective in the severer forms and remittent fevers as quinine. The dose is from 5 to 10 grains twice or thrice daily during the intermission or before the paroxysms. Fresh lime juice is recommended as an eligible vehicle for its popular use. Or it is administered in the form of pills with an effervescing mixture, with the object of obviating the ill effects, such as the irritability of the stomach which it frequently produces. In debility after fevers it is recommended as a tonic given in small doses. In enlargement of the spleen it is also recommended in combination with sulphate of iron. In neuralgia, face-ache, Tic Douloureux (neuralgia of the head or face) recurring periodically it should be given in full doses (10 grains) thrice daily for adults.

Quinine.—This is an alkaloid which exists in the cinchona bark, and which is extracted by a chemical process, and, being afterwards combined with sulphuric acid, forms the crystallized disulphate of quinia or quinine as it is commonly called. For internal administration this is decidedly much superior to cinchona or quinetum, as it is more active and efficacious. As a tonic and antiperiodic it stands unrivalled; in agues and intermittent fevers of all kinds it is indispensable; in neuralgic affections and those arising from debility its good effect is generally marked and decided. It has been recommended as an antipyretic remedy in typhoid, typhus, small-pox, pneumonia, and acute rheumatism. It has also been employed with marked benefit in various septic states and in pyæmia and all exhausting suppurative conditions. The theory that it acts beneficially in disease by destroying minute organisms has led to its advocacy in whooping cough, intermittent hæmaturia, hay fever, chronic suppurative bronchitis, etc. The common dose is one or two grains three times a day; it is best given in solution, combined with double the quantity of dilute sulphuric or hydrochloric acid or citric acid, as it is insoluble in water. It is often given in some bitter infusion such as gentian or calumba; sometimes in infusion of roses the acid of which readily dissolves it.

---

335. RANDIA DUMETORIUM.

(*N. O.*—RUBIACEÆ.)

Sans.—Madana. *Eng.*—Emetic Nut. *Hind.*—Mainphal, *Ben.*—Mephal, Madan. *Bom.* and *Mah.*—Gélaphala. *Pers.*—Züz-ul-Kuch. *Tel.*—Mandà, Mringa. *Tam.*—Maruk-kallan-kai. Poongàrai. *Can.*—Mangari-kai. *Mal.*—Manga-kai.

Habitat.—This small thorny tree is in waste places and jungles all over India from the Himalayas to Ceylon.

Properties and Uses.—The rind and fruit have useful emetic, diaphoretic and antispasmodic properties. The bark is a sedative and nervine calmative; it is also administered internally and applied externally in the form of a paste to relieve pain of bruises and the bone-aches during fevers. It also acts as an astringent and is useful in diarrhœa and dysentery. The rind and the pulp of the fruit are generally used to produce emesis. The pulp of one ripe fruit is usually sufficient for the purpose. The active principle of the fruit is discovered to be saponin, and valeric acid is also found to be present. The pulp may be removed, dried and powdered and kept ready for use, the dose being 15 to 60 grains as an emetic and 5 to 10 grains as a nauseant, expectorant and diaphoretic. It is a useful substitute for ipecacuanha. The contents of two nuts will produce nausea and vomiting in about 10 minutes; the emesis is promoted by the administration of warm water. It is described by Sanskrit writers as the best or safest of emetics. The ancient Hindus, in fact, depended chiefly upon this drug for causing emesis. It is also used in combination with other medicines as in the following:—

Native Indian Preparations.—*Panch Kasháya*:—Take of *Justica Adhatoda*, *Acorus Calamus*, *nim* bark, leaves of *Trichosanthes dioica (patola)* and bark of *Aglaia Roxburghiana (priyangu)*, equal parts, half a seer in all, water eight seers; boil them together till reduced to one-fourth. This decoction is given with the the addition of the pulp of *Randia dumetorum* for causing emesis.

336. RAPHANUS SATIVUS.

(*N. O.*—CRUCIFERÆ.)

Sans.—Moolaka. *Eng.*—Garden Radish. *Hind.*—Müli, Muro. *Ben.*—Müla. *Bom.* and *Mah.*—Mula, Mulàbeeja. *Tel.*, *Tam.* and *Can.*—Mullangi. *Mal.*—Kankapál.

Habitat.—This annual herb is cultivated everywhere in the plains for culinary purposes.

Properties and Uses.—The seed and root yield to distillation a fœtid essential oil allied in its nature to that of mustard and other *Cruciferous* plants and containing a certain proportion of organically combined sulphur. The seeds are considered diuretic, laxative and lithontriptic; also believed to have emmenagogue properties. In one drachm doses the seeds are useful in gonorrhoea. The root is a reputed medicine for piles and gastrodynic pains. It is also given in urinary and syphilitic complaints. The juice in 1½ to 3-ounce doses, repeated as frequently as necessary or till the desired effect is produced, is very useful in relieving dysuria and strangury. The juice of the raddish is to be pressed out through a cloth by bruising it *without* water. Eaten before a meal the radish improves appetite and increases the digestive power.

---

337. RAUWOLFIA SERPENTINA.

(*N. O.*—APOCYNACEÆ.)

Sans.—Chundrika. *Hind.*—Chota-chand. *Ben.*—Chandra. *Tel.*—Pàtala-gandhi.

Habitat.—This climbing shrub is found in the tropical Himalaya and at moderate altitudes in Sikkim, Assam, Pegu and Tenasserim.

Properties and Uses.—The root is said to have been long known to Indians as an antidote to poison and to the bites of poisonous reptiles and stings of insects. It seems to have some beneficial action as febrifuge. The root is found to contain an alkaloid allied in some respects to brucine, but weaker and slower in its action than brucine. It is named provisionally *Pseudobrucine.*

---

338. RHEUM EMODI.

(N. O.—POLYGONACEÆ.)

Eng.—Rhubarb. *Hind.*—Hindi-révand-chini. *Ben.*—Banglä-revanchini. *Bom. Mah.*, and *Guz.*—Ladaki-révanda-chini. *Tel.*—Nättu iréval-chinni. *Tam.*—Vəriyättu. *Can.*—Réval-chinni.

Habitat.—This is usually known as the Himalayan Rhubarb and found wild at altitudes of 11,000 to 12,000 feet on the Himalaya, in Kashmir and in Nepal, Sikkim and Bhutan. The rhubarb of commerce known as Chinese or East Indian is attributed to *R. Officinale* and *R. Palmatum*, growing in the adjacent territory of South-eastern Thibet and North-western China.

Properties and Uses.—The officinal part of the plants is the decorticated and dried root or root-stalk, known as "rhubarb," the Indian drug being of a darker colour, inferior aroma and coarser texture and untrimmed as contrasted with the commercial variety, while the powder is of a dull brownish-yellow colour instead of bright yellow. Rhubarb root of commerce contains a large proportion of *Chrysophanic acid*, sometimes called Chrysophan, to which is due the yellow colour and probably some part of its cathartic property, although this has been attributed to cathartic acid. An allied substance, *Emodin*, has also been isolated, and a tannin named *Rheo-*

tannic acid besides resinous and mucilaginous principles. It usually contains a large proportion of crystals of oxalate of calcium. Dr. O. Hesse has shown that rhubarb contains a series of substances related to each other in chemical composition, viz., Chrysophanic acid, emodin and *Rhëin*, and these substances probably originate from an unknown constituent by oxidation.

Rhubarb has stomachic, tonic and cathartic properties; its primary action is that of a mild purgative; but it has also astringent property, so that its secondary effect is to confine the bowels, hence it is well fitted for use in simple diarrhoea, but not in constipation or any affection in which a continuous aperient action is necessary, it is not fitted for inflammatory or febrile cases although it seldom acts as an irritant. Its stimulating combined with its aperient properties render it valuable in atonic dyspepsia. Generally speaking it suits children and aged persons best. Combined with ginger, it may be given in the form of pill in cases where the bowels are sluggish. The ordinary dose of the powder is from 5 to 20 grains. Some persons have no objection to chew the root, and to such, this is a very good way of taking it. There is a large variety of medical compounds of which Rhubarb forms an important ingredient. Mixed with Grey Powder it is an excellent remedy for the irritation of the bowels, common among children when teething. As a common aperient for the young it is best given combined with magnesia. It has the property of communicating a deep tinge to the urine; this change of colour need not occasion alarm and misconception.

339. RHINACANTHUS COMMUNIS.

(*N. O.*—ACANTHACEÆ.)

Sans.—Yuthikapurni. *Hind.*—Pàlak-juhi. *Ben.*—Jui-pana. *Bom.* and *Mah.*—Gâjakarni, Gachkaran. *Tel.*, *Tam.* and *Can.*—Nâgamalli. *Mal.*—Purukolli.

Habitat.—This small shrub is said to be indigenous to the Deccan and Ceylon, cultivated in many parts of Western and Southern India.

Properties and Uses.—The leaves and root are regarded to act as antidotes to the bites of poisonous snakes and hence the name *nagamulli* by which the plant is known in South-India. The active principle is a red resinous substance named *Rhinacanthin* which is believed to be allied to chrysophanic and frangulic acids. The root powdered and made into a paste with lime-juice is applied with much benefit in eczema and ring-worm, especially that variety which is known as *dhobie itch.*

---

340. RHUS ODINA.

(*N. O.*—ANACARDIACEÆ.)

Sans., *Hind.*, *Ben.*, *Bom.* and *Mah.*—Ajashrangi. *Tel.*—Oddimanu. *Tam.*—Odiyamaram. *Can.*—Udimara. *Mal.*—Othi, Uthi.

Habitat.—This tree is mostly found on the East and West Coasts of India and also in Bengal.

Properties and Uses.—The bark is very astringent. The decoction of the bark is useful as a local application in cutaneous eruptions and obstinate ulceration and forms an excellent astringent gargle. The bark powdered and combined with margosa oil makes a valuable application for old and obstinate ulcers. The gum of the tree beaten up with cocoanut milk is applied to sprains and bruises and the leaves boiled in oil are similarly used. It is given internally in asthma and as a cordial to women. Externally it forms the basis of many of the plasters employed for rheumatism.

---

341. RHUS SUCCEDANEA.

(N. O.—ANACARDIACEÆ.)

Sans.—Karkatashringi. *Eng.*—The Galls. *Hind.*, *Guz.* and *Mah.*—Kàkad singi. *Ben.*—Kàkràsringi.

Properties and Uses.—The galls are horn-like excrescences caused by insects on the branches of *Rhus Succedanea*. They are large, hollow, thin-walled, generally cylindrical, tapering to either extremity. They are considered tonic, expectorant and useful in cough, phthisis, asthma, fever, want of appetite and irritability of stomach. Dose is about 20 grains. This medicine is much used in combination with other drugs for the disease.

Native Indian Preparations.—Take of *Karkatashringi*, root of *Clerodendron Siphonanthus (brahmayàshti,)* raisins, ginger, long pepper and *Curcumo Zedoaria (sati)* equal parts, powder and mix. Dose is about 30 grains with treacle or honey, in dry cough.—(Chakradatta).

In catarrhal fever with difficulty of breathing a power composed of equal parts of *Karkatasringi*, bark of *Myrica sapida* (*Katphala*) and long pepper is recommended to be given in doses of about a drachm with honey—(Bhavaprakasha.)

Sringyádi Churna.—Take of *Karkatasringi*, *atis* and long pepper, equal parts; powder and make into a linctus with honey. This is much esteemed as a cough linctus for children.—(Sharnghadhara.)

342. RICINIS COMMUNIS.

(*N. O.*—EUPHORBIACEÆ.)

Sans.—Erandam. *Eng.*—Castor-oil Plant. *Hind.* and *Punj.*—Arand. *Ben.*—Bherandâ. Assam-Eri. *Bom.*, *Guz.*, and *Mah.*—Erandi (oil—Erandel; root—Erandamul). *Tel.*—Eramudapu, Amudâ. *Tam.*—Amanakkai, Chittamani, Andagam. *Can.*—Haralu. *Mal.*—Chittamanakku. *Cing.*—Endaru. *Burm.*—Kesusi. *Malay.*—Miniak-jarak.

Habitat.—This plant is common and apparently quite wild in the jungles in India. It is cultivated throughout India, chiefly in the Madras, Bengal and Bombay Presidencies and the transmission of the seeds to Calcutta and Bombay for export forms an important part of the coast-wise and inland traffic.

Properties and Uses.—Two varieties of this plant are known:—(1) A perennial bushy shrub or small tree grown usually as a hedge plant with large fruits and large red seeds which are said to yield about 40 per cent of oil used chiefly for lubricating and illumination; and (2) a much smaller annual plant grown as a distinct crop or planted in rows in betel and sugarcane and other gardens, with small grey seeds having brown spots and yielding 37 per cent of oil, the better qualities of which are used for medicinal purposes. The better and purer quality of oil is the one known as cold-drawn castor oil, and it is so termed, because it is drawn from the seeds being pressed between cold, instead of hot plates; drawn in this way the oil is clear, odourless, almost colourless and less likely to become rancid by keeping. Such oil is fit for medical purposes. It is a mild, non-irritant and safe purgative, seldom griping or causing flatulency. It is administered (plain or in emulsion with mucilage) in inflammatory conditions of the bowels, in diarrhœa of childhood and, often combined with opium, in simple diarrhœa of adults; it is also useful in irritable conditions of the system to persons suffering from debility and young children; after child-birth to the lying-in-women, in operations for lithotomy, in peritonitis, dysentery and in inflammatory disease of the urinary organs. The usual dose is, for a child, about one teaspoonful, which may be gradually increased according to age to two or three tablespoonfuls, which is the full dose for an adult. It is best given floating on milk, strong coffee or omum water. In painful affections of the rectum, in piles and in cases where it is desirable to prevent the patient straining at stool, castor oil in small doses is often of great service, softening the fæces and lubricating the passages without weakening the patient. For sore nipples castor oil is beneficial if the nipple is smeared over freely with it each time the child is removed from the breast. In constipation, it is useful as an enema; two ounces of castor oil emulsified with a pint of soap-suds and water often causes a copious evacuation of the bowels in cases where a simple warm water enema has no effect whatever. In cases where a foreign body such as a small particle of steel has become imbedded in the eye the agonising pain and irritation can be temporarily relieved by the instillation of a few drops of castor oil between the lower lid and the eyeball. This may be repeated as often as necessary until medical aid is obtained for the removal of the foreign body.

Castor oil is much praised for its efficacy in chronic rheumatic affections, in which it is used in various combinations.

The root of the plant is also said to be particularly useful in complaints such as lumbago, pleurodynia and sciatica. The root-bark and leaves have purgative properties. The leaves warmed over a fire and applied to the breasts of women act as a galactagogue, *i.e.*, increase the secretion of milk. For this purpose a decoction is also used, a large handful of the plant is boiled in 6 or 8 pints of water. With this the breasts are bathed for a quarter of an hour, and then the boiled leaves, in the form of a poultice, are spread over them. In a few hours the effects of the application are manifest. A fluid extract or the juice of the leaves given internally increases the flow of milk. Cattle are fed with the leaves with the same object. The leaves applied to the abdomen are said to promote menstrual discharge. They are also applied to painful joints with much benefit.

Native Indian Preparations:—As a purgative, castor oil is recommended to be taken with cow's urine or an infusion of ginger or a decoction of the combination called *dasamula*. In affections of the eyes, castor oil leaves and root are used in a variety of forms, and several prescriptions containing them are given by Sanskrit writers. A decoction of the bark, leaves and root of the plant in goats' milk and water is recommended for use as a wash in recent ophthalmia—(Chakradatta).

The seeds freed from impurities and rubbed into a paste, boiled in milk and water and the decoction is given in lumbago and sciatica—(Bhavaprakash).

The root enters into the composition of various preparations for rheumatic affections and diseases of the nervous system. In pleurodynia or pain in the sides, a decoction of the root is given with the addition of *yavakshàra* (impure carbonate of potash)—(Sharngdhara).

---

343. ROSA DAMASCENA.

(*N. O.*—ROSACEÆ.)

Sans.—Satapattri (hundred-leafed). *Eng.*—The Damask or Persian Rose. *Hind.*—Gulab-kephul. *Ben.*—Golap-phul. *Bom.*, and *Guz.*—Gulabnu-phul. *Mah.*—(buds) Gulab-kali. *Pers.*—Guli-surkh. *Tel.*—Roja-puvu, Gula-puvu. *Tam.*—Gulappu, Irojappu. *Can.*—Gulabi-huvu. *Mal.*—Pannirpu. *Kon.*—Gulabshevante.

Habitat.—Several species and cultivated forms of roses are grown in India. *R. Damascena* with its familiar red double flowers is a shruby plant and is the most important; and it is cultivated on large areas of ground set apart as rose gardens in several places in Bengal and the Punjab, chiefly near Patna, Ghazipur and Lahore. *R. Centifolia* or hundred-leafed rose or the cabbage rose is also cultivated in many parts of India, and several less important species occur wild throughout India.

Properties and Uses.—The petals of the flowers are employed for the production of rose water and *attar* of roses. Rose water is distilled in simple native stills, a thousand roses being reckoned to produce a pint-bottle of rosewater. The average yield of good attar from a *lakh* of roses has been estimated at one tola weight or 180 grains. Rose oil or otto or *attar* of roses varies in colour from emerald green to reddish yellow. It is freely used as a perfume by the rich classes. Its distribution with *pan supari* and the sprinkling of rosewater are essential functions during festive occasions, *durbars* and *pujas* in India. Rose water forms an agreeable vehicle much used in lotions and collyria; from the petals also a syrup is sometimes made, and a conserve named *gulkand* which have mild laxative properties. The otto is seldom used medicinally except for perfuming emollients and medicinal soaps. It is the Red or French Rose (*Rosa Gallica*) whose petals are used for making the infusion of roses, which is an elegant vehicle for many active remedies, and is given with advantage in the sweats of phthisis, and with additional acid and nitrate of potash in uterine and pulmonary hæmorrhages and used topically as a gargle in throat affections which require an astringent application. *Honey of Roses* is also prepared from the leaves or fresh buds of this species which; mixed with borax, is a good application for the mouth in aphthæ or thrush.

344. RUBIA CORDIFOLIA.

(*N. O.*—RUBIACEÆ.)

Sans.—Manjishta, Chitravalli. *Eng.*—The Indian Madder. *Hind.*, and *Ben.*—Manjit. *Bom*, *Mah.*, *Can.*—Manjishta. *Tel.*—Tàmravalli. *Tam.*—Manditta.

Habitat.—This climbing plant is growing in the North-West Himalaya, Nilgiris and other hilly districts of India.

Properties and Uses.—The roots are collected and used in India for the red dye which they yield. The chemical constituents are a red principle, *Purpurin* and a yellow colouring matter, named *Munjistin.* The plant was formerly considered emmenagogue and diuretic and was much used in dropsy, paralysis, jaundice, amenorrhœa and visceral obstructions. When administered in the form of decoction, it tinges the blood, urine and even the bones, red. The fruit is useful in hepatic obstructions, and a paste made by rubbing up the roots with honey is mentioned as a valuable application for the removal of freckles and other discolouration of the skin. It is regarded astringent and useful as an application in external inflammations, ulcers and skin diseases such as pityriasis versicolor, etc. Madder is now chiefly used as a colouring ingredient of medicinal oils.

Native Indian Preparations.—Madder and liquorice root rubbed into a paste with *Kanjika* is applied over fractures to reduce inflammation and swelling.

Manjishthádya ghrita is prepared with clarified butter and a paste composed of equal parts of madder, red sandalwood, and the root of *Sanseviera Zeylanica* (*murvâ*) and applied to ulcers from burns—(Chakradatta).

---

345. RUTA GRAVEOLENS.

(*N. O.*—RUTACEÆ.)

Sans.—Sadápaha. *Eng.*—The garden Rue. *Pers.*, *Hind.*, *Bom.*, and *Guz.*—Satàp. *Ben.*—Ispand. *Tel.*—Suddhapuaku. *Tam.*—Arvada. *Can.*—Sudàbugida. *Mal.*—Arùta, Sômaràyen.

Habitat.—This plant is commonly cultivated in Indian gardens.

Properties and Uses.—It is ordinarily stimulant and antispasmodic; in large doses it acts as a narcotic poisoning. It is useful in some kinds of hysteria and in flatulent colic administered by the mouth or as enema. It is found useful in infantile convulsions and also given as a vermifuge. Powdered and combined with aromatics, the dried leaves are given as a remedy for dyspepsia and, with the fresh leaves a tincture is made which is used as an external remedy in the first stages of paralysis. By distillation with water the fresh herb yields a small quantity of volatile oil. It is a valuable resolvent, diuretic and emmenagogue. It is found to be a powerful anaphrodisiac and abortefacient to pregnant women. Externally it acts as rubefacient. The oil is the best form of internal administration, but rue tea is a popular remedy. The dose of the powdered leaves is from 10 to 20 grains. The fresh leaves are more active and their expressed juice may be given in ½ drachm doses. The dose of the oil is from 1 to 5 minims rubbed up with sugar and water; of the confection, 20 to 60 grains; of the tincture, from ½ to 1 drachm (for adults); of the fresh juice from ½ to 1 drachm (for children).

346. SACCHARUM OFFICINARUM.

(*N. O.*—GRAMINEÆ.)

Sans.—Ikshu, Rasalah. *Eng.*—Sugar-cane. *Hind.*—Ukh, ganna. *Bom.*, and *Mah.*—Ums, Sheradi. *Tel.*—Cheruku. *Tam.* —Karumbu. *Can.*—Kabbu. *Mal.*—Karimpu.

Habitat.—The common sugar-cane is very extensively cultivated throughout India in several varieties or races. Besides these varieties of this species, several varieties of Saccharum are grown as fibre-producers.

Properties and Uses.—The root of the sugar-cane is considered demulcent and diuretic. In the hot weather the thin, tender portion of the stem is cut into small pieces and very largely consumed raw throughout the country as a sweetmeat, being simply chewed. The expressed juice is also much used as a drink. The chief constituent of the sugar-cane is cane-sugar, which is a derivative of starch, a carbo-hydrate; it is believed to be produced by the action of the sun's rays in the leaves of certain plants and stored up in aqueous solution, in the tissues as reserves in the plant economy. It occurs in several members of the vegetable kingdom besides the sugar-cane, such as the beet, which is grown in India as a culinary vegetable, in the juice of certain palms, chiefly *Cocos nucifera*, *Borassus flabelliformis* and especially the date-palm, *Phoenix sylvestris.*

Native Indian Preparations.—The products or preparations of the sugar-cane as described by Sanskrit writers are as follow:—(1) *Ikshu rasa* or sugar-cane juice. (2) *Phánita* or sugar-cane juice boiled down to one-fourth; it can be drawn out in threads. (3) *Gúd* or jaggery, also known as *ras*, which is prepared by boiling the juice down to a dark-brown thick consistence, the crude form of sugar commonly used by Indians. It consists of a considerable proportion of "molasses" or "treacle" known as *chhoa* the uncrystalizable portion, *invert* sugar, of the saccharine juice which is drained off and sold as a distinct product. When the better qualities of *gúd* have been more or less completely drained of molasses they constitute the (4) coarse brown sugar known as "country" sugar or *shakkar*, which is much used and which consists of a soft, moist, partly crystalline mass varying much in quality. From the coarser description of *gúd*, the crystalline forms of sugar are directly prepared. The molasses having been pressed out, the crystalline portion is bleached in the sun, dissolved, clarified and crystallized, the resulting product being the familiar (5) white sugar known as *chini* or *safed* shakkar. Double refined and crystallized sugar, called (6) *misri* or *khand*. is also prepared in several forms, including *kuza misri*, sugar-candy, which is made by pouring the clarified solution or syrup into vessels in which strings are suspended round which the crystals congregate. The other preparations of sugar-cane are (7) *Matsyandiká* which is made by boiling the juice down to a solid consistence, but it still exudes a little fluid on drawing; (8) *gaudi* or fermented liquor obtained from treacle; and (9) *sidhu* or fermented liquor obtained from sugar-cane juice. The properties of these preparations are mostly those of sugar. (See under "Sugar.")

347. SALIX CAPREA.

(N. O.—SALICINEÆ.)

Eng.—The Sallow. *Indian vernaculars* (the flowers)—Bed-mushk.

Habitat.—This species of willow is cultivated in Persia and in North-Western India, in Kashmir, and at Peshawar and Lahore.

Properties and Uses.—The fragrant flowers on distillation yield an essential oil or attar and a perfumed water *(ma-el-khilaf)* which is much used in Northern India, chiefly by Persians and in Western India by Parsis, and regarded as stimulant and aromatic. The bark contains the crystalline glucoside *Salicin* and tannin. Salicin is contained in the bark of several species of willow grown in India; it is not, however, extracted. The leaves of this and several other Indian willows are occasionally covered with a syrupy exudation which dries up in thin, white flakes to a sugar or manna. The bark of S. Caprea is used as a febrifuge. Salicin is used as a tonic and anti-rheumatic and is also used with benefit in influenza.

348. SALVADORA PERSICA.

(*N. O.*—SALVADORACEÆ.)

Sans.—Pilu. *Eng.*—The Tooth Brush Tree. *Hind.*, and *Ben.*—Chhota-pilu, Jhal. *Pers.*—Darakht-i-miswak. *Bom.*—Pilva, Piludi, Kakhan. *Mah.*—Pilu. *Tel.*—Varagogu. *Tam.*—Ughai-puttai, Karkol. *Can.*—Goni-mara

Habitat.—This small tree is found in the arid tracts of Sind, in the Punjab and in North-Western India and Persia.

Properties and Uses.—The pieces of the root are used as tooth brushes by the people of the regions where the plant grows. The fresh root-bark, bruised and applied to the skin acts as an active external stimulant; in some cases it acts as vesicant and raises blisters. The bark in decoction is useful in low fever and as a stimulant and tonic in amenorrhœa; the dose is half a tea-cupful twice daily. The shoots and leaves are antidote to poisons of all sorts. The juice of the leaves is given in scurvy. The leaves heated and tied up in thin cotton cloth are applied in rheumatism. The fruits (small red berries) have a strong aromatic smell and are eaten; they are described as deobstruent, carminative, and diuretic; they are administered in snake-bite, both in the fresh and in the dried state combined with borax. The fruit is also held to be purgative.

349. SANTALUM ALBUM.

(*N. O.*—SANTALACEÆ.)

Sans.—Chandana. *Eng.*—The Sandal-wood Tree. *Hind.*, *Duk.*, and *Punj.*—Chandal, Sandal. *Ben.*—Swet-chandan, Pitchandan, *Kash.*, *Bom.*, and *Mah.*—Safed chandan. *Tel.*—Gandapu-chekka. *Tam.*—Chandana kattai. *Can.*—Shrigandhada-mara. *Mal.*—Chandana-maram. *Malay.*—Miniak Chandana.

Habitat.—This small somewhat delicate evergreen tree is indigenous to and cultivated in the Mysore Province, grown also in Coimbatore and the Southern parts of Madras adjoining Mysore.

Properties and Uses.—This fragrant wood has been used in India from a very early period. It occupies an important place in Hindu ceremonials, in the worship of idols and for annointing their bodies after bathing. The use of sandalwood in carving and the elegant articles such as fancy boxes &c., made from it are well-known. The wood is much used by the Parsis in their fire temples. Rich people sometimes use sandalwood for burning their dead relatives. Rich or poor, all add at least one piece of the wood to the funeral pyre. Medicinally sandalwood has been regarded as bitter, cooling, astringent and useful in bilious fevers; applied externally in the form of a paste with water in prickly and skin eruptions; to the temples in headaches and fevers and to skin diseases to allay heat and pruritus. In cases of morbid thirst the powder of the wood is taken in cocoanut water; the powder made into pills, or in cow's milk, is administered for gonorrhœa; locally applied, the powder allays prickly heat and checks copious perspiration. The essential oil contained in the heartwood, and obtained from it by means of distillation, is a popular remedy as a demulcent, diuretic and mild stimulant in gonorrhœa and kindred affections and in chronic cystitis. It is given in five-drop doses gradually increased to 10 to 20 minims; it is good to accompany it with a drop or two of liquor potassæ; it is commonly given in capsules or in emulsion. In cases of gonorrhœa, even in obstinate gleet, it is useful, and best given in a little omum water or infusion of ginger. Externally the oil is an excellent application in scabies in every stage and form.

Native Indian Preparations.—An emulsion of the wood is used as a cooling application to the skin in erysipelas, prurigo and sudamina —(Chakradatta).

Two tolas of the watery emulsion of sandalwood, with the addition of sugar, honey and rice-water is given to check gastric irritability and dysentery and to relieve thirst and heat of body—(Bhâvaprakash).

---

350. SAPINDAS TRIFOLIATUS.

(*N. O.*—SAPINDACEÆ.)

Syn :—S. EMARGINATUS.

Sans.—Phenila. *Eng.*—Soap-nut Tree. *Hind.*, *Mah.*, and *Duk.*—Ritha. *Ben.*—Bara-Ritha. *Tel.*—Kunkudu, Kùkudu. *Tam.*—Ponàn-kottai, Púvandi. *Can.*—Aradâla, Antharale, Anthuvàla. *Mal.*—Chavakàyimaram. *Kon.*—Rintya rooku.

Habitat.—This tree is common in Southern India and cultivated in Bengal. *S. Mukorossi* (*Syn* :—*S. Detergens*) is the soap-nut tree of Northern India.

Properties and Uses.—The fruits are largely used as soap-substitutes for washing. They contain about 11·5 per cent of *saponin*. Medicinally they may be employed as emetic in doses of 1 to 2 drachms, as purgative in larger doses, nauseant and expectorant in doses of 10 to 20 grains of the pericarp or pulp and kernel of the fruit. The root has also expectorant property. A thick watery solution of the drug dropped into the nostrils is said to relieve hemicrania, hysteria and epilepsy. Fumigations with it are useful in hysteria and melancholia. Made into plaster with vinegar it is externally applied to bites of reptiles and to scrofulous swellings. Pessaries made of the kernel of the seeds are used to stimulate the uterus to child-birth and in amenorrhœa.

---

351. SARACA INDICA.

(*N. O.*—LEGUMINOSÆ.)

(*Syn* :—JONESIA ASOKA.

Sans.—Asoka, Vichitrah. *Eng.*—The Asoka Tree. *Hind.*, and *Ben.*—Asok. *Bom.*, and *Mah.*—Ashoka, Jàsùndi. *Tel.*—Asok. *Tam.*—Asogam. *Can.*—Asokada-Kenkali-mara. *Mal.*—Asokam. *Burm.*—Ṭhawgabo.

Habitat.—This tree is cultivated in gardens throughout India.

Properties and Uses.—The bark is strongly astringent, as it contains tannin. It is much used by native physicians in uterine affections, especially in menorrhagia. A decoction of the bark in milk is generally prescribed. The dose is 1 ounce three times a day commenced from the fourth day of the monthly period and continued daily till the bleeding ceases. Fresh decoction must be made every day. A decoction of the bark in water with dilute sulphuric acid is also used. The bark is useful in internal hæmorrhoids also. Flowers pounded and mixed with water are useful in hæmorrhagic dysentery. The dose of the fluid extract is from 15 to 60 minims.

Native Indian Preparations.—A decoction of the bark in milk is prepared by boiling 8 tolas or 4 ounces of the bark in 8 tolas or 4 ounces of milk and 32 tolas or 16 ounces of water till the latter is evaporated. This quantity is given in two or three divided doses during the course of the day in menorrhagia—(Chakradatta).

Asoka ghrita is prepared with a decoction of the bark and clarified butter with the addition of a number of aromatic substances in the form of a paste.

352. SAUSSUREA LAPPA.

Syn :—APLOTAXIS AURICULATA, AUCKLANDIA COSTUS.

(*N. O.*—COMPOSITÆ.)

Sans.—Kushtha. *Eng.*—The Costus. *Hind.*—Kût, Kust, Pachak. *Ben.*—Páchak. *Bom.*—Ouplate, Upalèt. *Tel.*—Kustam. *Tam.*—Gostan.

Habitat.—This herb is growing abundantly on the mountains around Kashmir. The roots are dug up in large quantities in Kashmir, cut into small pieces of two or four inches long and sent down to Calcutta and Bombay, whence it is exported very largely to China.

Properties and Uses.—In China the root is used as an incense as well as a medicine. In India the drug has been used from a very remote period as a tonic and aphrodisiac; it is regarded as an aromatic stimulant useful in cough, asthma, fever and dyspepsia and as an ointment applied to ulcers and other skin diseases. It is used as an ingredient in stimulating mixtures for cholera. The root enters also into the composition of some pastiles for fumigation.

Native Indian Preparations.—*Agnimukha Churna.*—Take of asafœtida 1 part, *Acorus Calamus* 2 parts, long-pepper 3 parts, ginger 4 parts, *Ajowan* 5 parts, Chebulic myrobalan 6 parts, plumbago root 7 parts and the root of *Aplotaxis auriculata* 8 parts. Powder the ingredients, mix and pass the powder through a cloth. Dose:—

20 to 40 grains with whey or wine in dyspepsia with loss of appetite—(Chakradatta).

A liniment composed of the root of *Aplotaxis auriculata, kanjika* and castor oil is recommended to be applied to the forehead in cephalalgia—(Sharngadhara).

The fried root mixed with mustard oil, is applied to the scalp in prurigo. Equal parts of the powdered root and of rock salt, mixed with mustard oil and fermented paddy water (*kanjika*) are rubbed on joints affected with chronic disease.—(Bhávaprakash).

353. SCHLEICHERA TRIJUGA.

(*N. O.*—SAPINDACEÆ.)

Hind.—Kosum, Kosumba. *Bom.*—Kosamb. *Tel.*—Puskû, Roatanga. *Tam.*—Pu-maram.

Habitat.—This large tree is growing in the lower Himalaya towards the North-West and also in Central and Southern India, Burma and Ceylon.

Properties and Uses.—A fine quality of lac is produced on the young branches. The seeds contained in the pulpy fruit yield to expression a fixed oil which is said to be the original "Macassar Oil" and which is recommended as a stimulating and cleansing application to the scalp, promoting the growth of the hair.

354. SCILLA INDICA.

(*N. O.*—LILIACEÆ.)

Eng.—Indian Squill. *Hind.*—Jangli-pyàs. *Ben.*—Suphaidi-khus. *Bom.* and *Mah.*—Bhuikändä. *Tel.*—Adavitella-gadda. *Tam.*—Shirunari-vengayam, Kâttu-velvangâyam. *Can.*—Kádu-belluli, Kàdirulli. *Mal.*—Kântena.

Habitat.—This plant is very common in sandy soil in the Konkan.

Properties and Uses.—The squill of the Indian bazaars consists of bulbous roots which are found to be efficient substitutes for the official squill (the sliced and dried bulbs of *Urginea Scilla*). As found in the bazaars the drug is usually in the whole or unsliced state. It is much used in medicine as a stimulant, expectorant and diuretic.

355. SCINDAPSUS OFFICINALIS.

Sans.—Kari-pippuli. *Hind.*—Badi-pipli. *Ben.*—Gaj-pipul. *Bom.* and *Mah.*—Thora-pimpali. *Tel.*—Enuga pippalu *Tam.*—Atti-tippili.

Habitat.—This large climbing plant is growing in tropical parts of India, common in the Midnapore District.

Properties and Uses.—The sliced and dried fruit of this tree is sold in the bazaars as a carminative and stimulant medicine. It is chiefly used as an aromatic adjunct to other medicines. It is useful in diarrhœa, asthma and other affections supposed to be caused by deranged phlegm.

356. SEMECARPUS ANACARDIUM.

(*N. O.*—ANACARDIACEÆ.)

Sans.—Bhallàtakä, Agnimukhi. *Eng.*—The Marking-nut Tree. *Hind.*, and *Ben.*—Bhela, Bhilâwa. *Bom.*, and *Mah.*—Bibba. *Tel.*—Jeedivittulu. *Tam.*—Shònkottai. *Can.*—Gër-kâyi. *Mal.*—Chèr-mara. *Kon.*—Bibbayi.

Habitat.—This tree is found growing on the temperate Himalaya and in the hotter parts of India; common in Eastern Bengal.

Properties and Uses.—The pericarp abounds in a black, oily, acrid juice which is used as a "marking ink" for cotton fabrics; used in combination with lime water or caustic lime, it is practically indelible, being insoluble in water; when applied to the skin the juice acts as a powerful escharotic. By boiling the bruised seeds in water a dark brown oil is extracted to the extent of 32 per cent; which is closely allied to the vesicating oil of the cashew-nut, the active principles being the same, *viz.*, anacardic acid and cardol. The juice of the pericarp is hot and dry; it is occasionally used internally in small doses (1 to 2 minims) diluted with some bland oil or melted butter, in scrofulous affections and syphilis; also in palsy, epilepsy and other diseases of the nervous system. Externally it is sometimes used in small quantities as a counter-irritant in rheumatism and sprains. It should be used with caution as otherwise it causes inflammation and swelling. The vesicant oil is similarly employed to a small extent. The marking-nuts enter into the composition of some caustic applications for warts and piles. The ripe fruits or nuts, used internally, are regarded as heating, stimulant, digestive, nervine and escharotic, they are used in dyspepsia, piles, nervous debility, skin diseases, etc.

Native Indian Preparations.—Equal parts of marking-nuts, chebulic myrobalans and sesamum seeds are made into a confection with treacle and administered in doses of 40 to 60 grains.

Amrita Bhallâtaki—Take of ripe marking-nuts divided into halves, 8 seers, boil them in 32 seers of water till the latter is reduced to one-fourth and strain. Again boil the nuts in 16 seers of milk with the addition of 4 seers of clarified butter till reduced to a thick consistence. Then add sugar two seers and set aside for seven days, when the preparation will be ready for use. Dose is about 20 to 40 grains. It is a powerful restorative tonic, which increases the appetite and promotes nutrition and strength. It is useful in hæmorrhoids and other diseases of the rectum—(Chakradatta).

357. SENNA INDICA.—See *Cassia Lanceolata.*

358. SESAMUM INDICUM.

(*N. O.*—PEDALINEÆ).

Sans.—Tila, Snèhaphala. *Eng.*—Gingeli-oil plant (seed), Gingeli seed. *Hind.*, *Kash.*, and *Ben.*—Til. *Bom.*, and *Mah.*—Tal, Chokhóta. *Tel.*—Nuvvulu, Guvvulu. *Tam.*—Ellu. *Can.*—Uru-ellu. *Mal.*—Kárùellu. *Kon.*—Tilu.

Oil.—*Hind.*, and *Punj.*—Til-ka-tel, Mithá-tel. *Guz.*—Mitho-tel. *Mah.*—Chokhòta tela. *Tel.*—Manchi-nûne. *Tam.*—Nalenney. *Can.*—Ellenna. *Mal.*—Nal-ennæ. *Cing.*—Talla-til. *Burm.*—Nahu-si. *Malay.*—Miniak-bijan.

Habitat.—This small bush 2 to 4 feet in height is indigenous to India and extensively cultivated, especially in the warmer regions, for its oil-yielding seed.

Properties and Uses.—Three varieties of sesamum seeds are found which are known as black, white and red according to the colour of the seed. The black variety is the most common and yields the best quality of oil and is also the best suited for medicinal purposes. The seeds are emollient, demulcent and laxative, specially useful in piles and constipation, taken in decoction or as sweetmeats. Or, ground to a paste with water, they are given with butter for bleeding piles. They have also emmenagogue property; if taken in large quantities, they are capable of producing abortion. In amenorrhœa and dysmenorrhœa (painful menstruation), the administration of powdered seeds in ten-grain doses three or four times daily, combined with the employment of a warm hip bath containing a handful of the bruised seeds has given very beneficial results. A poultice made of the seeds is applied to ulcers. The seeds yield to expression about 30 to 40 per cent of a clear, limpid, odourless and non-drying oil, which has been used from time immemorial for dietetic purposes throughout India. It is also much used as an illuminant. Medicinally the oil may be employed for all the purposes to which olive oil is applied, as for lime liniment as an oil-dressing for ulcers, suppurating wounds, etc. It is regarded as superior to any other simple dressing, particularly during the hot season. The leaves, which abound in mucilage, act as demulcent and are useful in bowel affections such as dysentery, etc. An emollient poultice is also made from them. The decoction made from the leaves and root is employed as a hair-wash and is supposed to blacken the hair.

---

359. SESBANIA ÆGYPTIACA.

(*N. O.*—Leguminosæ.)

Sans.—Jayantika. *Hind.*, and *Ben.*—Jayanti. *Bom.*, and *Mah.*—Janjan, Shevâri. *Tel.*—Jalugu, Somanti. *Tam.*—Champai. *Can.*—Karijeenangi-mara.

Habitat.—This small tree is found wild and cultivated in almost all parts of India.

Properties and Uses.—The seeds are described as stimulant, emmenagogue and astringent and useful in checking diarrhœa, excessive menstrual flow and to reduce enlargements of the spleen. In the form of ointment the drug is used for the cure of itch and various other cutaneous eruptions. The leaves in the form of poultices promote suppuration of boils and abscesses and absorption of hydrocele and inflammatory swellings. The root well bruised and made into a paste is an excellent application for scorpion stings.

---

360. SHOREA ROBUSTA.

(*N. O.* - DIPTEROCARPEÆ.)

Sans.—Sâla, Asvakarna. *Eng.*—The Sâl Tree. *Hind.*, and *Ben.*—Sàl (the resin), Räl, Dhùnà. *Bom.*, and *Mah.*—Sal. *Bel.*—Jalari-chettu. *Tam.*—Taloora. *Can.*—Bile-bovu, Bile-bhogi-mara. *Mal.*—Karimaruthu.

Habitat.--This timber tree is common in the sub-Himalayan regions and the forests of Western Bengal.

Properties and Uses.—The bark contains tannic principles and yields, on boiling with water, an extract similar to catechu which is used to a small extent medicinally as an astringent. The resin which exudes from incisions made in the bark of the tree is also astringent and is an ingredient of stimulating plasters and ointments. With sugar it is administered internally in dysentery; also used for weak digestion, gonorrhœa and as an aphrodisiac Twenty grains of the pulverised resin mixed with a pint of boiled milk taken every morning is considered a good aphrodisiac. The resin is also used as an incense in several Hindu households every evening and during the worship of idols. Thrown over the fire it gives out thick volumes of fragrant smoke which is useful for fumigating rooms occupied by the sick.

Native Indian Preparations.—In the dysentery of children the resin is given in doses of about 20 grains with an equal quantity of sugar or treacle—(Bhâvaprakâsh).

Ointment :—Take of *rál* (resin), rock salt, treacle, wax, honey, bdellium, red ochre and clarified butter in equal parts, boil them together and prepare an ointment (Chakradatta.).

An Aphrodisiac :—A couple of ounces of the resin is powdered and fried in cow's ghee for about 10 minutes and the whole thrown into a basin of cold water. The mixture which floats on the surface is gathered with the fingers and constantly squeezed within the water; in the course of a few minutes it assumes a white colour. Removing the water from time to time and thus continuing the above process from ½ to 1 hour it gains the consistence and colour of butter. This is collected and preserved. A quantity the size of a small nutmeg is given internally twice a day.

---

361. SIDA ACUTA.

(N. O.—MALVACEÆ.)

Sans., and *Mah.*—Pàta. *Ben.*—Kureta. *Tel.*—Visha boddi. *Tam.*—Vatha-thiruppi, Mallaidàngi. *Mal.*—Cheruparuva. *Can.*—Visha khaddi.

Properties and Uses.—The root of this plant is a bitter tonic; has stomachic, diaphoretic and antipyretic properties useful in the form of decoction in febrile affections and some forms of dyspepsia and in mild cases of debility from previous illness. In the form of infusion it is given to promote perspiration and to increase appetite. The expressed juice of the root in the form of an electuary is employed in the treatment of intestinal worms. The leaves warmed, moistened with a little gingelly oil and applied to abscesses hasten suppuration.

The drug is used as a diuretic in rheumatic affections and as a demulcent in gonorrhœa and chronic dysentery.

362. SIDA CORDIFOLIA.

(*N. O.*—MALVACEÆ.)

Sans.—Balâ, Bätyalaka. *Eng.*—Country Mallow. *Hind.*, and *Duk.*—Kanghi. *Ben.*—Barelà. *Bom.*, and *Mah.*—Chikana. *Tel.*—Chitimutti, Tutturabenda. *Tam.*—Mayir-manikham, Paniyàr-tutti. *Can.*—Kisangi, Hettuti-gida. *Mal.*—Vellùram.

Habitat.—This and several other species of the genus *sida* are common in most places all over India.

Properties and Uses.—The roots of all these species are regarded as cooling, astringent and tonic, given in infusion in nervous diseases, urinary diseases and bilious disorders. The infusion is also useful in bleeding piles, in strangury and hæmaturia, in gonorrhœa, cystitis, etc. The dose is from ½ to 2 drachms. A decoction of the root and ginger is given in intermittent fever attended with cold shivering fits. The powder of the root-bark is given with milk and sugar for the relief of frequent micturition and leucorrhœa. The leaves are mucilaginous and used as a demulcent. In infusion they are prescribed in fevers as a cooling medicine. The seeds are likewise laxative and demulcent, and used in piles. Boiled milk whisked with fibrinous twigs coagulates. The fluid on decantation is given internally in piles. The leaves are cooked and eaten in cases of bleeding piles.

Native Indian Preparations.—*Másha baládi Kvátha :*—Take of the pulse of *Phaseolus Roxburghii*, root bark of *Sida cordifolia*, root of castor oil plant and of *Mucuna prurians*, *Hygrophila polysperma*, *Vanda Roxburghii* and *Withania Somnifera* (Asvagandhá), equal parts, in all two tolas, and prepare a decoction in the usual way. It is administered in 1 to 2-ounce doses, with the addition of asafœtida and rock salt, in hemiplegia, stiff neck, facial paralysis and noise in the ears with headache (Chakradatta).

Balátaila :—Take of the root of *Sida cordifolia* 4 seers, water 32 seers, and boil down to 8 seers. To this decoction add 8 seers of milk, 4 seers of prepared sesamum oil and 1 seer of the root of *Sida cordifolia* in the form of paste and prepare an oil in the usual way. The oil is used for external application in the diseases named above.

363. SIEGESBECKIA ORIENTALIS.

(N. O.—COMPOSITÆ.)

Vern: *South Ind.*—Katampam.

Habitat.—This plant is common throughout India.

Properties and Uses.—In China it is used as a remedy for ague, rheumatism, and renal colic. It contains a bitter crystalline principle named *Darutine* which is believed to be a derivative of salicylic acid. A tincture of the drug has been recommended in doses of 1 to 2 drachms as a remedy in scrofulous and syphilitic affections; externally a mixture of equal parts of the tincture and glycerine has been tried in Europe with good effect in ringworm and some other parasitic eruptions. Antiseptic properties have been ascribed to the fresh plant, applied to unhealthy sores.

364. SINAPIS JUNCEA (*See also Brassica*).

(*N. O.*—CRUCIFERÆ.)

Sans.—Sarsapah, Siddhártha, Rajikâ. *Eng.*—Indian Mustard. *Hind.*, and *Duk.*—Ràyán. *Ben.*, and *Punj.*—Râi. *Kash.*—Asúr *Guz.*—Ràyè. *Mah.*—Shiras, Mohari. *Cing.*—Abbe. *Burm.*—Mun-niyèn-zi. *Malay.*—Biji Sa-sarvi.

Properties and Uses.—There are two varieties of mustard, *siddhartha* or white mustard and *râjika* or dark brown or black variety. The latter is more pungent and preferred for external application as a rubefacient. As an emetic English mustard is more safe and efficient; a tea-spoonful in a tumblerful of warm water generally produces free vomiting in 5 or 10 minutes. It is especially indicated in drunkenness, narcotic and other poisoning and in all cases where the stomach is overloaded with hard indigestible food or intoxicating drinks when it is desirable simply to unload the stomach without producing any depressing effect on the system. For poultices, etc., Indian mustard may be substituted, but fresh seeds should, whenever practicable, be employed, since, by long keeping, they lose much of their pungency. Mustard poultices are usually made with the flour of mustard mixed to the consistence of a poultice with *cold* water, spread on a piece of stout brown paper or rag and applied to the skin, and kept for from 5 to 10 minutes, *i.e.*, till it produces redness of the skin. For delicate persons as women and children, a piece of thin muslin must be placed between the poultice and the skin. In cases of fever and acute disease, the morning or early part of the day is preferable for applying the poultice. In apoplexy, convulsions, delirium, violent headaches occurring during fevers or small-pox, mustard poultices are applied to the feet and calves of the legs. In these cases, if the patient is able to sit up for the purpose, a mustard foot-bath (made by adding a handful of mustard to an ordinary foot-bath) is even more effectual. The water should be as hot as can be well borne and the higher the fluid reaches up the leg, the better. In some head affections, *e. g.*, the early stages of insanity and delirium tremens with determination of blood to the head, sleeplessness, restlessness and anxiety, the mustard foot-bath should be used every night before bed-time. In some cases cloths steeped in a mixture of mustard and hot water are applied so as to envelop the whole of the legs and lower part of the abdomen, a cold wet towel being at the same time applied round the head.

In cholera, colic and spasms of the bowels unattended by inflammation a mustard poultice placed over the abdomen affords considerable relief. In the vomiting of fevers and pregnancy, it is applied to the pit of the stomach. In cholera when the patient is very low the poultice may be applied over the heart or the left side of the chest. In coughs with much difficulty of breathing, mustard poultices to the chest and on the back between the shoulder blades, afford relief. Whooping cough is occasionally much relieved by mustard poultices along the spine. Tooth-ache, face-ache and neuralgic pains of the head and face are frequently relieved by the application of a mustard poultice over the seat of pain.

In dropsy mustard is administered in the form of whey made by boiling half an ounce of the bruised seed in a pint of milk and straining. This quantity is given daily in divided doses.

Mustard oil is largely used in India for culinary purposes as well as for anointing the body before bathing; it is said to keep the body cool and the skin soft, to promote the growth of hair and to remove prurigo, lice and scurf.

Native Indian Preparations.—Mustard forms an ingredient of several emetic mixtures of which the following is an example: Take of mustard seeds, *Acorus calamus* root, bark of *Symplocos racemosa* and rock salt, equal parts. Powder and mix.—(Chakradatta).

Mustard enters into the composition of several prescriptions for loss of appetite, indigestion, etc. Thus, take of mustard seeds, cumin seeds, fried asafœtida, ginger and rock salt, equal parts. Powder and mix. Dose—grains 22 with butter-milk. (See also *Brassica*, P. 64.)

---

365. SMILAX CHINA.

(N. O.—SMILACEÆ.)

Sans.—Chobachini. *Eng.*—China Root. *Hind.*, and *Ben.*—Shuk chinâ, Chob chini. *Bom.*, and *Mah.*—Chob chini. *Tel.*—Pirangi-chekka. *Tam.*—Paringay.

Habitat.—This plant is indigenous to China and Japan where it is called *Too-fuh*, not found in India; but the drug, China root is common in all the bazaars.

Properties and Uses.—China root is used in India to some extent like sarsaparilla, as a depurative, alterative, antisyphilitic and aphrodisiac in the form of decoction, which is prepared by boiling 2 ounces of the root in one pint of water till the whole is reduced to ten ounces. Dose two to four ounces. It is useful in rheumatism, epilepsy, insanity and syphilis. In Hindu medicine it is used along with *anantamul* and other drugs of reputed efficacy in syphilis and rheumatism.

366. SODII BIBORAS.

Sans.—Kankana. *Eng.*—Borax, Biborate of Sodium. *Hind.*—Tinkàl. *Ben, Duk.*, and *Punj.*—Sohagà. *Kash.*—Vàvut. *Arab.*—Buraekes-sàghah. *Pers.*—Tinkar. *Thibetan*—Chúsal. *Bom.*, and *Mah.*—Kankanakhàr, *Tel.*—Velligaram. *Tam.*—Venkäram. *Can.*—Kankana khàr, Biligára. *Mal.*—Ponkáram. *Cing.*—Puskara. *Burm.*—Lakhiya. *Malay.*—Pijar.

Habitat.—This salt is brought to India in considerable quantities from Nepal and Thibet (where it occurs in the waters of certain lakes) and from Persia.

Properties and Uses.—Indian borax, which is obtainable in all the bazaars, is largely used by native gold and silversmiths and by potters as a glaze. Medicinally, borax is given internally as a diuretic and emmenagogue. If it is dirty or impure it may be rendered fit for medical use by dissolving one pound of it with one drachm of quicklime in three pints of water, straining through cloth and evaporating by exposure to the sun in an open vessel or over a gentle fire. Dose is from 20 to 40 grains for an adult. In prolonged and tedious labours dependent apparently on want of action or power in the uterus to expel the fœtus, and in abortion under the same circumstances, 30 grains of borax with 10 grains of powdered cinnamon in a little warm *conjee* may be given every one or two hours to the extent of three or four doses. This may also be given in convulsions attendant on labours. In cases of suspension or irregularity of the menstrual discharge and in some chronic uterine affections, doses of 10 grains with 10 grains of cinnamon occasionally prove useful.

Externally as a local sedative and antiseptic it is used in lotion (two drachms dissolved in a pint of water) in gangrenous buboes and sloughing ulcers. It is applied on rags well over the whole sore and renewed frequently by night and day. For dressing Delhi sores and other forms of ulcers, and for stimulating them to healthy action a favourite application is a mixture of borax, sulphur and catechu, one drachm of each in fine powder, and an ounce of ghee. To sore nipples a solution of borax (one drachm in an ounce of water) is applied before and after suckling the infant; or it may be employed in the form of ointment made by mixing a drachm of borax in an ounce of ghee. These applications are also serviceable in inflamed and painful piles. In the distressing irritation of the genital organs both in males and females, cloths saturated with a strong solution of borax (half an ounce dissolved in eight ounces of water) kept to the parts afford much relief. In the case of women the solution should also be used in the form of vaginal injection. The solution also proves very useful in allaying the irritation of nettle rash, prickly heat and other skin diseases such as psoriasis and eczema. For ringworm, a solution of borax (one drachm) in distilled vinegar (two ounces) is said to be an effectual application. In aphthæ or thrush and soreness of mouth or throat a mixture of one drachm of powdered borax and one ounce of honey is an excellent application, especially suitable to infants and young children; for this the official *Mel Boracis* and *Glycerinum Boracis* are efficient substitutes. It should be applied by means of the finger to the spot twice or thrice daily. In fissures or cracks in the tongue in adults, which occur in the advanced stages of consumption, fever, etc., an application twice the strength of the above proves highly serviceable. In mercurial salivation a solution of borax (half an ounce in 8 ounces of water) makes an excellent gargle.

367. SODII CHLORIDUM.

Sans.—Lavana. *Eng.*—Common Salt, *Hind.*—Nimak, Lon. *Ben.*—Lavan, Nún, Lun. *Bom.*—Mithú. *Mah.*—Meetha. *Tel.*—Lavanam. *Tam.*, and *Can.*—Uppu.

In India salt has been lavishly provided by Nature; it is dissolved in a wide expanse of sea which lashes the shores of the Peninsula; is stored up in mines; is spread out in salt-impregnated lakes and marshes; and is found to effloresce at many localities in the interior and on the sea-board. In Upper and Central India there are practically inexhaustible sources, in mines in the Punjáb and in the salt lakes and marshes of Rájputána. "Some salt from Thibet is imported into the Himalayan districts of Kumaon and Gárhwal. Earth salt is made under treaty with the British Government in the feudatory States of Gwalior, Dattia and Bikanir and a little salt is also made in the Patiala State in the Punjáb."

The preparation of salt by lixiviation of saline soils or by solar evaporation of the water of brine wells is practically prohibited except in the regions named above, and the demand is met by the importation in enormous quantities of Cheshire salt, chiefly from Liverpool.

Black salt (*Bit nún*) is prepared for medicinal purposes by heating the crude common salt with myrobalans.

It is regarded as a digestive. The impure sulphate of soda known as *Khari nún* is produced at the salt works by crystallization from brine. It is used to some extent as a saline purgative for cattle.

Properties and Uses.—In addition to its being an important dietetic agent used as a condiment, common salt is a good antiseptic. Moreover it is a great digestive; it is one of the constituents of the blood and of the body generally, and we find that where it is denied the digestive powers are weakened and the general tone of the system is impaired. It has also been observed that those who do not take salt are especially liable to worms in the intestines. Hence the desirability, if not the necessity, of insisting that children should eat a certain proportion with their food. On the other hand, if taken in excess, it is productive of mischievous results as it gives rise to diseases like scurvy. As a medicinal agent salt has a tonic effect, observed especially in some cases of convalescence where there is an intense craving for it which should be satisfied to a moderate, but not to an immoderate extent. In large doses (2 to 4 drachms) in solution it is given as an emetic. In still larger doses it acts as a powerful purgative. Such a solution administered by the rectum destroys and brings away worms from the large bowels. 1 lb. of salt dissolved in 3 gallons of water makes a convenient substitute for sea water. It is used sometimes in about the same proportion (1 to 30) as a gargle in chronic throat ulcerations and is a valuable antidote in cases of poisoning with nitrate of silver or after swallowing a leech.

As an external application it exerts a tonic influence and is highly beneficial in cases of debility whether local or general. The salt-water bath braces and stimulates the system and warm saline bathing and rubbing is good for rheumatic affections, sprains, etc.; if prepared artificially the above-mentioned proportion is a proper average strength.

With regard to the preservative properties of salt on animal substances—the chemical change which it effects in the juices of the meat to which it is applied, considerably modify the nutritive properties and render it less fit to nourish and sustain life, hence fresh meat is better than that which is preserved by salting, which should never be taken as a staple article of diet if it can be avoided.

---

368. SOLANUM DULCAMARA.

(*N. O.*—SOLANACEÆ.)

Eng.—Dulcamara; Bitter-sweet. *Ind. Vern.*—Anab-es-sàlab (the berries).

Habitat.—This shrub is met with in Kashmere; but the red berries are said to be imported from Persia into Bombay.

Properties and Uses.—This plant is nearly allied to the potato, which it very closely resembles in the odour of its root. Its bright scarlet berries closely resemble those of the deadly nightshade; and children are said to have been poisoned by eating the berries as are grown persons from an overdose of the decoction of the fresh twigs. The drug contains a peculiar bitter-sweet principle (hence the popular name) which is believed to consist of a poisonous alkaloid named *solanine*, resolvable into sugar and *solanidine*. The characteristic principle is now believed to be *Dulcamarin*, a yellowish substance, not an alkaloid, which has, at first, a bitter and, subsequently, a permanent sweet taste. Solanine is common to several species of *Solanum*, including the potato in which it is, however, rendered innocuous on boiling.

Dulcamara, although neglected in European medicine, is still used by Indian physicians, being regarded as alterative, diuretic, sudorific and mildly narcotic, usually in decoction. The berries are similarly employed. It is used in skin diseases and catarrhal affections; also in scrofula, chronic rheumatism and syphilis; the dose is—of the decoction, about a wineglassful; of the powder, 20 to 60 grains; of the extract, 5 to 10 grains; of the syrup, ½ to 1 ounce. For making the decoction the twigs gathered should be dried ones and as thick as a goose-quill; one ounce of them chopped up should be boiled in 1½ ounces of water until reduced to half the quantity.

369. SOLANUM INDICUM.

(*N. O.*—SOLANACEÆ.)

Sans.—Brahati, Bhantáki. *Eng.*—Indian Nightshade. *Hind.*—Barhanta. *Ben.*—Byàkura. *Bom.*, and *Mah.*—Dolimoola. *Tel.*—Tellamoolaka, Käkamâchi. *Tam.*—Karimulli. *Can.*—Kirigullagida. *Mal.*—Cheruchunda. *Kon.*—Kallánta.

Habitat.—This plant is common all over India.

Properties and Uses.—The root forms an ingredient of the much-esteemed *Dasamula Kvatha* or decoction of ten drugs, of Hindu medicine. It is seldom used alone but is regarded as diuretic useful in dropsy, and as expectorant useful in cough and catarrhal affections. The

same properties. They are useful in worms and indigestion, and given with honey in cases of cough. The flowers are highly esteemed as alteratives, depuratives and tonics, useful in skin diseases. The bark, ground small and mixed with whey, is a valuable remedy in piles. It is also used for local application. An oil prepared from the root by steeping it in water and then boiling it in sesamum oil until all the water is expelled is said to be a valuable aphrodisiac.

---

375. SPONDIAS MANGIFERA.

(*N. O.*—ANACARDIACEÆ.)

Sans.—Amràtaka. *Eng.*—Hog-plum or Wild Mango. *Hind.*—Ambrâ. *Ben.*—Amrâ. *Duk.*—Jungli ám. *Mah.*—Ambàdà. *Tel.*—Adavi-màmidi, Ambálamu. *Tam.*—Kattumâ. *Can.*—Ambate. *Mal.*—Ambâlam.

Habitat.—This tree is met with throughout India.

Properties and Uses.—The fruit is generally eaten as a condiment, and made into chutney and pickles. The pulp of the fruit is acid and astringent, useful in bilious dyspepsia. It is also a useful antiscorbutic. The leaves and bark are aromatic and astringent and administered in dysentery. The gum is demulcent. The juice of the leaves is applied locally in earache. By some the fruit is considered to be an antidote for wounds caused by poisoned arrows, and for this purpose it is eaten either green or dry.

---

376. STERCULIA FOETIDA.

(*N. O.*—STERCULIACEÆ.)

Eng.—Poon Tree. *Tam.*—Peenäthamaram. *Can.*—Pènarimara. *Mal.*—Pottakávalam, Peenári-maram.

Habitat.—This tree is found mostly in the Ghats.

Properties and Uses.—The flowers have most offensive odour and hence the name. The seeds are oily and, if swallowed, they bring on nausea and vertigo. If roasted they are edible. The oil is extracted by boiling the seeds in water. The kernels contain about 40 per cent of this; it is a fixed oil. The bark and leaves are aperient, diuretic and diaphoretic. The decoction of the capsules is mucilaginous and astringent.

377. STRYCHNOS IGNATII.

(*N. O.*—LOGANIACEÆ.)

Eng.—St. Ignatius' Beans. *Arab.*—Papità.

Habitat.—This tree is indigenous to the Phillipine Islands; but its seeds are occasionally met with in the drug bazaars of the large cities in India.

Properties and Uses.—The seeds are said to be used in cholera. They are roundish or oval and usually about an inch in length, varying much in size, and contain the same alkaloidal constituents as contained in the nux-vomica seeds, *viz.*, *strychnine* and *brucine* in varying proportion, about 1·5 per cent of the former to 0·5 per cent of the latter. The glucoside *loganin* is also believed to be present. The seeds are sometimes utilized in Europe for preparing strychnine, which they yield in somewhat larger quantity than nux-vomica. A tincture known as *Tinctura Ignatiæ* is also prepared, 1 in 10, and administered in doses of 3 to 20 minims as a nervine tonic.

378. STRYCHNOS NUX-VOMICA.

(*N. O.*—LOGANIACEÆ.)

Sans.—Kupilu, Kulaka, Vishamusti, Kàraskarah. *Eng.*—The Nux-vomica or Strychnine Tree, Snake-wood, Vomit-nut. *Hind.*—Kuchlâ. *Ben.*—Kuchilá. *Bom.*, and *Mah.*—Kàjra, Kuchalâ. *Tel.*—Mushti-vittulu. *Tam.*—Yetti-kottai, *Can.*—Käsarkä-na mara. *Mal.*—Kânjiram. *Kon.*—Kàrya-rüku.

Habitat.—This tree is wild and plentiful throughout tropical India and is found commonly in the jungles about Manbhoom, in the Madras Presidency, Malabar and Coromendel Coasts.

Properties and Uses.—The ripe fruit, which contains the nux-vomica seeds is of the size of an apple, has a beautiful orange colour and consists of a bitter gelatinous pulp, within which the lozenge-like, flattened, round seeds are found imbedded.

Nux-vomica is a powerful nervine tonic and a stimulant to the spinal cord. In excessive doses it is a virulant poison producing tetanic convulsions. No preparation of this powerful drug should be used except under careful medical superintendence. It is employed in doses of ½ to 3 grains in powder, ¼ to 1 grain of the extract and 5 to 10 minims of the tincture. It is used as a remedy in intermittents, dyspepsia, dysentery, diarrhœa due to debility, worms, hysteria, chronic constipation from atony of the bowels, rheumatism and hydrophobia. In Bombay the wood is said to be a popular remedy in the dyspepsia of vegetarians; and the juice of the fresh bark is given in doses of a few drops in cholera and acute dysentery. The root-bark ground into a paste with lime juice and made into pills are also effectual in cholera. The bark is sometimes employed in infusion or weak decoction, as a tonic and febrifuge, and the root, which is very bitter, is used to cure intermittent fevers and the bites of venomous reptiles. The paste made by rubbing the seeds of nux-vomica is used in rat-bites. The paste of nux-vomica seeds mixed with dry ginger and the horn of the antelope rubbed on a stone is used with benefit in muscular and chronic rheumatism. The oil obtained by heating the fresh seeds is also a useful external application in chronic rheumatism, also in palsy and relaxation of the muscles and tendons. Nux-vomica is useful in the treatment of tobacco amaurosis and paralysis following on exhausting diseases such as diphtheria, gastric catarrh, etc. As a respiratory stimulant it is used in bronchitis, emphysema and phthisis. The leaves of the nux-vomica tree are applied as poultice to sloughing wounds or ulcers when maggots have formed.

Nux-vomica contains two alkaloids in varying proportions, *viz.*, *Strychnine* (0·2 to 0·5 per cent) and *Brucine* (0·12 to 1 per cent) united with *Strychnic* or *Igasuric acid* as Igasurates. A glucoside named *Loganine* is present in the pulp of the fruit and to a small extent in the seeds, both of which contain strychnine. Nux-vomica also contains mucilage and sugar (6 per cent). The bark and wood contain brucine and the leaves contain 0·3 per cent of brucine, but no strychnine.

Strychnine has the same therapeutic action as the nux-vomica, but in a more powerful degree. It is prescribed in doses of $\frac{1}{32}$ to $\frac{1}{1}$ grain in solution or in pill. It may be used in almost all the cases in which nux-vomica is used. Various spasmodic diseases as chorea, asthma and epilepsy are said to be cured by strychnine. It is antagonistic to chloral and calabar bean. It is also employed hypodermically as a remedy in narcotic poisoning and against the effects of chronic alcoholism, also as an antidote to snake-bite administered hypodermically ($\frac{1}{16}$ to $\frac{1}{10}$ grain) close to the bitten part. Brucine has been used in epilepsy in doses of $\frac{1}{8}$ to $\frac{1}{2}$ grain in solution.

Native Indian Preparations:—*Samiragaja Kesari:* —Take of nux-vomica, opium and black pepper, equal parts and make into two-grain pills. These are given, one twice a day, with the juice of betel leaves in diseases of the nervous system.

Shulaharanayoga:—Take of chebulic myrobalan, long pepper, ginger, nux-vomica, asafœtida, sulphur and rock salt, equal parts and make into four-grain pills. These are given with warm water in dyspepsia with pain after meals, and in diarrhœa—(Rasendrasârsangraha).

Sàrangadhara gives the following prescription:—Take of mercury, sulphur, aconite, *ajowan*, the three myrobalans, *sarjikâkshàra* (carbonate of soda), yavakshâra (carbonate of potash), rock salt, plumbago root, cumin seeds, *sachal* salt, sea salt, *bàberang*, black pepper, long pepper and ginger equal parts, *Vishamushti* (nux-vomica seeds) equal in weight to all the above ingredients and make into pills of the size of black pepper corns with lemon juice. These pills are given to promote appetite and increase the digestive power.

379. STRYCHNOS POTATORUM.

(*N. O.*—LOGANIACEÆ.)

Sans.—Kataka, Ambu-prasàd. *Eng.*—Clearing-nut Tree. *Hind.*, *Ben.*, *Bom.*, and *Mah.*—Nirmali. *Tel.*—Chilla Chettu. *Tam.*—Tettămaram, Tettâ-kottai. *Can.*—Chali-mara, Chittu-mara. *Mal.*—Tettà-maram. *Kon.*—Chila-beeyi.

Habitat.—This small tree belongs to Bengal, Central and Southern India and Burma.

Properties and Uses.—The button-like seeds of this tree which are contained in a black pulpy fruit are noted for their property of clearing muddy water. They are sliced and rubbed round the sides of the unglazed earthen vessels in which drinking water is stored, which has the effect of acting as a mechanical precipitant of suspended matter present in the water. The action is clearly due to albumen, which, on simple maceration of the seed in water, renders it mucilaginous, yielding a white coagulum on boiling. Medicinally half to one full seed rubbed up into a fine paste with some butter-milk and given internally for one week is effectual in the treatment of long-standing and chronic diarrhœa. The powder of the seed is given internally with milk in irritation of the urinary organs and in gonorrhœa. The seeds are used as a local application in eye-diseases. They are rubbed up with honey and a little camphor and the mixture applied to the eyes in lachrymation or copious watery discharge from them. Rubbed with water and rock salt they are applied to chemosis in the conjunctiva. The fruit in its mature state is regarded as an emetic when given as a powder in doses of half a teaspoonful. The pulp is a good substitute for ipecacuanha in the treatment of dysentery and bronchitis. It is also regarded as a remedy for diabetes.

---

380. STYRAX BENZOIN.

(*N. O.*—STYRACEÆ.)

Eng.—Benzoin Tree (the resin), Gum-Benzoin. *Ind. Vern.*—(the resin) Lubhàn.

Habitat.—This tree is a native of the Malay Peninsula (Lower Siam) and Sumatra. It yields the balsamic resin, gum Benzoin, of commerce which is largely imported into India from Penang.

Properties and Uses.—Gum Benzoin is used throughout India as an incense. It is the source of benzoic acid which is largely used in medicine. It also contains cinnamic acid. It is a good stimulant and expectorant, and when burnt its vapour is deodorant and antiseptic; it is therefore used in sick rooms and hospitals. It is also diuretic and useful in calculous disorders, especially where there are phosphatic deposits. Its combinations with alkalies, *viz.*, Ammonia, Potash and Soda, called benzoates, are more decidedly diuretic and useful in dropsy and gouty concretions. Mixed with ointments it prevents rancidity; its vapour is thought to be good in whooping cough; it is a common ingredient in cosmetic washes. Its compound tincture, popularly known as Friar's Balsam has been employed as a styptic and healing application; a piece of lint or soft rag dipped into it and wrapped round a cut finger, although it will cause smarting at first will usually stay the hæmorrhage and effect a cure without the necessity for another dressing unless the wound be very severe; it is also good for distressing coughs, the dose being 30 drops to a drachm on lump sugar or in mucilage; the dose of benzoin is from 3 to 10 grains.

---

381. SUGAR.

Sans.—Sharkara. *Hind.*, and *Duk.*—Shakar. *Ben.*—Bhûra, Chini. *Punj.*—Misri. *Bom.*, and *Mah.*—Sâkar. *Tel.*—Shakkara. *Tam.*—Sharukkarai. *Can.*—Sakkre. *Mal.*—Panjasâra. *Cing.*—Sini, Sakkere. *Burm.*—Saghia or Tagiya. *Malay.*—Gúla.

Properties and Uses.—Sugar is one of the most generally used articles of diet. It is taken into the system for the purpose of maintaining animal heat. Sugar, being readily soluble in water, is the most easily digested of all the substances which maintain animal heat; and hence the reason why it is supplied to the young of the higher forms of animals; it is secreted by the female of all the mammalia, in the milk which is furnished universally to their young during the first months of their existence. The instinctive love of sugar so well known as the characteristic of the child seems to point out its adaptation to the wants of the infant system. When taken into the system it speedily undergoes decomposition; its elements seem to enter into secondary combinations which are very injurious. This is why the quantity taken in diet should be limited. The changes, however, which the sugar so frequently undergoes in the adult system do not appear to take place in children; hence the child may eat sugar with impunity, although its parents may not. The practice of inducing children to give up sugar in their tea and other food is not commendable, since sugar is said to be evidently intended by nature to supply them especially with the materials for maintaining animal heat.

Medicinally sugar is a powerful antiseptic. In gonorrhœa and vaginal discharges a solution of sugar (one drachm in three drachms of water) is an excellent application. In gonorrhœa it may be commenced with at once, the injections being repeated frequently during the day in addition to general remedies; but in vaginal discharges other remedies may be tried first. Sugar is an excellent dressing for certain forms of foul, gangrenous-looking ulcers; the sugar in grain (white or refined) is merely sprinkled on the sore. As a drawing plaster for boils equal parts of sugar and yellow soap is an old remedy, whilst crude native sugar forms an admirable application for carbuncles. In all forms of ophthalmia (country sore eyes, etc.) a solution of sugar, of the above-mentioned strength, dropped into the eye every hour or so affords relief and. if applied, early cuts short the disease at once. At bed-time, in these cases, it is good to apply to the eyelashes a little sweet oil or grease, and in the morning to wash the eyes carefully with hot milk and water. The solution is also useful for removing small foreign substances from the eye.

In Pharmacy sugar is chiefly used to cover the nauseous taste of drugs. It is used in the formation of pills and for the preparation of medicated syrups.

---

382. SULPHUR.

Sans.—Gandhaka. *Hind.*, *Kash.*, *Punj.*, *Duk.*, *Guz.*, an *Mah.*—Gundhak. *Ben.*—Gandrok. *Tel.*, *Tam.*, *Mal.*, and *Cing.*—Gandhakam. *Can.*—Gandhaka. *Burm.*—Kân. *Malay.*—Blerang.

Origin.—Sulphur, which is one of the most abundant constituents of the globe, being a constant element in most animal as well as vegetable substances and existing in the form of metallic sulphurets and in the combination of sulphuric acid with various bases such as lime, magnesia, etc., occurs naturally in some parts of India, in Nepal, Kashmir and Afghánistan and in Burma. Several kinds of sulphur are met with in Indian bazaars. A pure variety of washed sulphur known as *Amlasa gundhak* is obtained in the bazaars of Bengal.

Properties and Uses.—Sulphur acts as a laxative and alterative when administered internally and is used both externally and internally in skin diseases, rheumatism etc. It is a reputed remedy for itch in the form of ointment—one part of finely powdered or sublimed sulphur mixed with six parts of kokum butter or any bland oil. Some other forms of chronic skin disease improve under the use of sulphur ointment or, better still, of so-called "balsam of sulphur" which is simply a solution of sulphur in warm olive or sesamum oil. A liniment composed of two ounces of powdered or sublimed sulphur and a pint of Nim oil well rubbed in twice daily is very beneficial in cases of chronic rheumatism. Relief is also obtained from dusting the affected part with flour of sulphur at bed-time, enveloping it in flannel, and covering the whole with plantain leaf to prevent the escape of the fumes. A sulphur bath is generally efficacious for skin diseases such as itch; the sulphur bath is commonly made by adding the "flower" or "milk of sulphur" to boiling water and using it when sufficiently cool.

As an alterative sulphur is given in doses of from 5 to 20 grains three times a day, and as a purgative from 1 to 3 drachms. The milk of sulphur is best given in milk and acts all the better mixed with an equal weight of magnesia; of this combination about a drachm is the maximum dose. In piles, a mixture of equal parts of sublimed sulphur and cream of tartar is taken in milk, (the dose being half to one teaspoonful once or twice daily), so as to keep the bowels gently open. It is also well adapted for habitual constipation and also acts beneficially in cases of chronic dysentery. It must be noted in all cases where sulphur is administered internally it communicates to the stools a peculiarly disagreeable odour of sulphuretted hydrogen.

Native Indian Preparations.—In skin diseases sulphur is administered internally in the shape of a sulphuretted butter prepared from milk boiled with the addition of sulphur. The butter thus obtained is called *Gandha taila,* which is taken internally and applied externally in skin diseases—(Sandehabhanjani).

Sulphur and *Yavakshàra* (an impure carbonate of potash) mixed with mustard oil is applied in pityriasis, psoriasis, etc. (Chakrah).

Adityapàka taila.—Take of sesamum oil 4 seers, madder, the three myrobalans, lac, turmeric, orpiment, realgar and sulphur equal parts, in all one seer. Mix and expose to the sun. This oil is useful in eczema and scabies, etc.

Simhanada guggulu.—Take of sulphur 8 tolas, bdellium 8 tolas, decoction of the 3 myrobalans 72 tolas, castor oil 32 tolas; mix and boil together in an iron vessel till reduced to the consistence of a confection. Dose is about one drachm twice daily. It is useful in chronic rheumatism, lameness, cough, asthma and skin diseases —(Chakrah).

383. SWERTIA CHIRATA.

(*N. O.*—GENTIANACEÆ.)

SYN: *Ophelia Chirata: Gentiana Chirayita.*

Sans.—Kiràta-tikta, Kiràta-nàmá. *Eng.*—Chirata, Chiretta. *Hind.*, and *Duk.*—Charâyatah. *Ben.*—Chirétà. *Punj.*—Kiraita. *Kash.*—Chiraiet. *Guz.*—Chirayata. *Mah.*—Kiräyitâ. *Tel.*—Nela-vému. *Tam.*—Nila-vémbu, Chiráyatu. *Can.*—Kiriyâtu. *Mal.*—Kiriyät. *Cing.*—Bincohamba. *Burm.*—Sekhägi. *Malay.*—Chrita.

Habitat.—This annual herb is indigenous to the temperate Himalaya at altitudes above 4,000 feet from Simla to Nepal and Bhutan. The drug consists of the entire dried plant including the branched stems and roots, brought down in large quantities from Nepal, and met with plentifully in the bazaars in Bengal. Numerous varieties of this drug are found in almost every part of India.

Properties and Uses.—The whole plant is intensely bitter. It is officinal in the Pharmacopœias of Great Britain and the United States. The numerous varieties met with in India, although differing more or less from the officinal chiretta in many respects, are similar in bitterness and possess, for the most part, the same medicinal properties. The principles to which the bitterness is due are *ophelic acid* and *chiratin.* Chiretta has been in use in India from a very remote period; it is used in the form of infusion (half an ounce of the bruised plant infused in one pint of hot water for twenty or thirty minutes) in all cases of debility after fevers, in indigestion, atonic dyspepsia, loss of appetite, etc., also given in mild cases of ague or intermittent fever. It is said to be especially serviceable in the dyspepsia of gouty persons, combined with acids or alkalies, preferably the former. It also possesses anthelmintic properties, besides all the stomachic, tonic, febrifuge and anti-arthritic virtues ascribed to gentian. It is antibilious and without aroma or astringency and therefore does not constipate; hence it is much esteemed as a remedy in liver disorder. Dose of the infusion is two to three ounces thrice daily.

Native Indian Preparations.—Chiretta is much used in fevers of all sorts in a variety of forms and in combination with other medicines of its class, for example:—Take of chiretta, *gulancha*, raisins, emblic myrobalan and zedoary root, equal parts and prepare a decoction in the usual way—(Bhaishajyaratnâvali).

Kirâtâdi taila, or oil of chiretta:—Take of chiretta one seer, water sixteen seers, boil together till reduced to four seers and strain. Boil this decoction of chiretta, with four seers each of prepared mustard oil, *kânjika* and whey, and two tolas each of the following substances in the form of a paste, namely, root of *Sansviera Zeylanica (murva)*, lac, turmeric, wood of *Berberis Asiatica*, madder root of *Citrullus Colocynthis*, *pâchak* root, root of *Pavonia Odorata*, of *Vanda Roxburghii (rasna)*, *Scindapsus Officinalis* (*gajapippali*), long pepper, black pepper, ginger, root of *Stephania Hernandifolia* (pâthâ), *indrajava* seeds, *sochal*, *vit* and rock salts, root of *Justicia Adhatoda* (*vâsakâ*), *Calotropis gigentea*. *Ichnocarpus frutescens* (*shyâmalata*), *Cedrus Deodara*, and the fruit of *Trichosanthes palmata* (mahâkâla). The oil thus prepared is rubbed on the body in chronic fever with emaciation and anæmia (Bhaishajyaratnavali).

---

384. SYMPLOCOS RACEMOSA.

(*N. O.*—STYRACEÆ.)

Sans.—Lodhra, Tillaka. *Eng.*—The Lodh tree. *Hind.*, *Ben.*, *Mah.*, etc.—Lodhra. *Tel.*—Ludduga-chettu. *Can.*—Balaloddu-ginamara.

Habitat.—This small tree is of the lower hills of Bengal. Assam and Burma. Lodh bark is obtainable in the Calcutta bazaar and other important bazaars in India.

Properties and Uses.—The bark of this tree which is used in dyeing red is found to contain the following alkaloids: *Loturine*, *Colloturine*, *Loturidine* and *Quinovin* or *kinovin*; but no tannin. The bark is considered cooling and mild astringent, useful in bowel complaints such as diarrhœa and other discharges, eye diseases, ulcers, etc. It has been been recommended in doses of 20 grains in powder, mixed with sugar, as a useful remedy in cases of menorrhagia due to relaxation of the uterine tissue, given two or three times a day for three or four days. A fluid extract in half-drachm doses would be a more suitable form for exhibiting the remedy in such cases.

Native Indian Preparations.—A decoction of the wood of the Lodh tree is used as a gargle for giving firmness to spongy and bleeding gums—(Sushruta). In bleeding from the gums a paste composed of *lodhra* bark, *rasot*, tubers of *cyperus rotundus*, and honey is applied to the gums—(Chakradatta).

The Amritasâgara recommends the following application for ophthalmia:—Take of *lodhra* bark, liquorice root, burnt alum and *rasot* equal parts and rub into a paste with water. This is applied round the eyes.

385. TABERNÆMONTANA CORONARIA.

(*N. O.*—APOCYNACEÆ.)

Sans. and *Ben.*—Tagara. *Hind.*—Chàndni. *Tel.*—Nandivardhanamu. *Tam.*—Nandiyâvartam. *Can.*—Maddarasagida. *Mal.*—Nandyarvattam.

Habitat.—Bengal and South India.

Properties and Uses.—The juice of the leaves dropped into the eye is said to cure ophthalmia. The juice of its flowers mixed with oil is used to relieve the burning sensation of sore eyes. The root is chewed for the relief of toothache. The root rubbed with water into a thin paste and administered, acts as vermicide; the same mixed with lime-juice makes a good application to eyes in eye-diseases.

386. TAGETES ERECTA.

(*N. O.*—COMPOSITÆ.)

Eng.—The French Marigold. *Hind.*, and *Ben.*—Genda. *Bom.*—Makhmal, Gul-jáfári. *Mah.*—Rojia-cha-phul.

Habitat.—This plant is commonly cultivated in Indian gardens for their beautiful flowers.

Properties and Uses.—The bright yellow flowers are much admired and made into garlands to hang round the neck of idols. The flowers yield a yellow dye which is occasionally employed by poor people. Medicinally the juice of the flowers is said to be occasionally used as a purifier of the blood and as a remedy in piles

387. TAMARINDUS INDICA.

(*N. O.*—LEGUMINOSÆ.)

Sans.—Tintrani, Amlavraksha. *Eng.*—The Tamarind tree. *Hind.*, *Ben.*, *Guz.*, and *Duk.*—Amli. *Punj.*—Imli. *Kash.*, and *Arab.*—Tamar-i-hind. *Mah.*—Chinch. *Tel.*—Chinta-pandu. *Tam.*—Puliyam-palam. *Can.*—Hunasehannu. *Mal.*—Puli. *Cing.*—Siyambula. *Burm.*—Magi. *Malay.*—Assam java.

Habitat.—This handsome evergreen tree which is indigenous to Southern India is cultivated throughout India and Burma.

Properties and Uses.—The pulp of the fruit is cooling, carminative and laxative. It is used as an adjunct to other laxatives as in the confection of senna, or to increase the action of sweet purgatives such as Cassia and Manna. The preserved pulp of the tamarind fruit is officinal in the *British Pharmacopœa.* The acidulous pulp contains acid tartrate of potassium (cream of tartar), tartaric, citric, acetic and a trace of malic acids.

Tamarinds are used largely in Indian dietary in curries, chutnies, and boiled in water and sweetened with sugar, as a cooling *sherbet* useful as a laxative for children suffering from fevers. One ounce of tamarind fruit with one ounce of dates boiled in a quart of milk and strained, forms an excellent laxative drink useful in febrile and inflammatory affections. Tamarind is a valuable anti-scorbutic and useful in preventing or curing scurvy, and "as such may be taken on board the ship or form a portion of daily rations in jails, etc." The pulp of the ripe fruit as well as a poultice of the leaves are recommended as applications to inflammatory swellings to relieve pain. Hakims consider the pulp useful for checking bilious vomiting and for purging the system of bile and to adjust humours.

The powdered seeds are said to be astringent and useful in dysentery, and as a poultice to boils. The leaves crushed with water and expressed yield an acid fluid useful in bilious fever and in the scalding of the urine. A poultice of the flowers is used in inflammatory affections of the conjunctiva. The juice expressed from them is given internally for bleeding piles. The tender leaves and flowers cooked and eaten are said to be cooling and anti-bilious. A decoction of the leaves used as a wash for indolent ulcers promotes healthy action. The juice of the leaves warmed by dipping a red-hot iron is given in dysentery. The red outer covering of the seeds is a mild astringent useful in chronic dysentery if administered in powder in half-drachm doses in the form of a bolus mixed with three times the quantity of cumin seeds in powder and a sufficient quantity of palmyra sugar-candy to taste. The ash of the bark is given internally as a digestive.

Native Indian Preparations.—In intoxication from spirituous liquors the following mixture is recommended by Chakradatta :—Take of dates, raisins, tamarind pulp, pomegranate seeds, fruits of *Grewia Asiatica* (*parushaka*) and ripe emblic myrobalans, each one tola, pound them together and make an emulsion with thirty-two tolas of water. Dose.—two ounces.

Ámlica pána :—Macerate some tamarind pulp in water, strain, and add black-pepper, sugar, cloves, camphor and cardamoms to taste. This preparation is prescribed as an agreeable cooling draught in loss of appetite and disinclination for food.

---

388. TAMARIX GALLICA.

(*N. O.*—TAMARISCINEÆ.)

Sans.—Jhävuka. *Eng.*—Tamarisk. *Hind.*, and *Ben.*—Jhän; (the galls)—Badimàyi. *Pers.*—Gazmàzaj, Gazangabin. *Bom.*—Magiyamàin.

Habitat.—This shrub is found throughout India, but common in Persia and Afghânistan.

Properties and Uses.—The galls produced on this shrub are somewhat smaller than oak-galls and three-angled; both varieties equal the true galls in their yield of tannic acid. They are used on account of their bitter and astringent effect. The tamarisk manna which is obtained in the bazaars of Northern India under the Persian name given above is found as a more or less solid mass liquifying on keeping to a honey-like consistence. It is used as a mild laxative.

---

389. TARAXACUM OFFICINALE.

(*N. O.*—COMPOSITÆ.)

Eng.—The Dandelion. *Hind.*—Düdal, Baran, Kânphûl.

Habitat.—This plant is found on the temperate Himalaya, common in Tibet and on the Nilgiris.

Properties and Uses.—The root is official and it is a valuable hepatic stimulant, being very beneficial in obstructions of the liver and visceral diseases. It is also a mild tonic, diaphoretic and diuretic. A popular combination is that of the fluid extract with podophyllin, which may be reckoned as a good remedy in liver congestion. The root is also given in dyspepsia, dropsy, skin diseases, and cachectic disorders generally. About an ounce of the sliced fresh root is put into a pint of water and boiled down to half a pint and strained; add to this quantity two drachms of Cream of Tartar and take a wineglassful twice or thrice a day.

390. TERMINALIA ARJUNA.

(*N. O.*—COMBRETACEÆ.)

Sans.—Arjuna. *Eng.*—The Arjuna Myrobalan. *Hind.*, and *Ben.*—Kahû, Arjun. *Bom.*—Arjuna-sadra. *Tel.*—Yermaddi. *Tam.*—Vella-marda.

Habitat.—Lower Himalaya, Bengal, Burma, Central and Southern India and Ceylon.

Properties and Uses.—The bark is astringent, containing about 15 per cent of tannin, also over 30 per cent of calcium carbonate. It is used to prepare a lotion applied to ulcers. As tonic it is given in decoction with milk in heart-diseases. The powdered bark is given with milk, treacle or water, in fractures and contusions with extensive ecchymosis.

391. TERMINALIA BELERICA.

(*N. O.*—COMBRETACEÆ.)

Sans.—Vibhitaki. *Eng.*—Beleric Myrobalans. *Hind.*, and *Ben.*—Bahera. *Bom.*, and *Mah.*—Behada. *Tel.*—Tâdi, Tândrakâya. *Tam.*—Tànrik-kay. *Can.*—Tàri, Shanti-mara. *Mal.*—Tänni. *Kon.*—Goting.

Habitat.—This tree is common in Indian forests.

Properties and Uses.—The beleric myrobalans are described as astringent and laxative and useful in coughs, hoarseness, eye-diseases, etc. It is a constituent of *triphala* or fruit triad (the chebulic, beleric and emblic myrobalans), a remedy prescribed in a large variety of cases. The kernel is used as an external application to inflamed parts. An oil expressed from it is used as a dressing for the hair. The unripe fruit is purgative. The ripe fruit is astringent and is employed in dropsy, piles and diarrhœa. The fully ripe or dried fruit, mixed with honey, is used as an application in ophthalmia.

Native Indian Preparations.—In hoarseness, beleric myrobalans, rock salt and long pepper rubbed into a paste with butter-milk are recommended to be used as a linctus—(Chakradatta).

Beleric myrobalans are fried in clarified butter, they are then covered with a paste of wheat-flour and slightly roasted on a fire. The cortical portion of the fruits thus prepared is recommended to be kept in the mouth for the relief of sore throat, cough and catarrh (Sharangadhara).

392. TERMINALIA CATAPPA.

(*N. O.*—COMBRETACEÆ.)

Eng.—The Indian Almond. *Hind.*—Jangli-Badam, *Ben.*—Banglà-Badam. *Bom.*, and *Mah.*—Badàm. *Tel.*—Ingudi, Tàpasa taruvu. *Tam.*—Amandi-maram. *Can.*—Bàdami-mara. *Mal.*—Katappa, Adamaram.

Habitat.—This tree is commonly cultivated throughout India.

Properties and Uses.—The kernel of the fruit yields to expression 50 per cent of oil which may be a good substitute for almond oil. The bark and leaves contain tannin. The juice of the young leaves is employed to prepare an ointment for scabies, leprosy and other cutaneous diseases and is believed to be useful internally for headache and colic.

393. TERMINALIA CHEBULA.

(*N. O.*—COMBRETACEÆ.)

Sans., and *Ben.*—Haritaki. *Eng.*—Chebulic Myrobalan, Ink-nut. *Hind.*, and *Duk.*—Pile-halra, Harda. *Punj.*, and *Kash.*—Zard halĕlà. *Guz.*—Pilo-harlè. *Mah.*—Hirada. *Tel.*—Kàrakkâya (the galls). *Tam.*, and *Mal.*—Kaduk-kâi. *Can.*.—Anile-kayi. *Cing.* Aralu. *Malay.*—Buah kaduka.

Habitat.—This tree is wild in the forests of Northern India, the Central Provinces and Bengal, common in Madras, Mysore and in the southern part of the Bombay Presidency.

Properties and Uses.—Two varieties are met with in the bazaars—one smaller than the other—the smaller being used in medicine and consisting probably of the young or unripe fruits; they are ovoid in shape and sink when placed in water. The larger fruits are rounder and smoother; they are chiefly used in tanning.

The better qualities of chebulic myrobalans contain about 25 per cent of gallo-tannic acid residing in the pulp surrounding the seed which is itself devoid of astringent principles. The galls produced on the leaves are rich in tannic acid and are used for tanning and as a mordant in dyeing. The dried unripe fruit, notwithstanding the astringent nature of its constituents, is commonly used as a purgative and antibilious: 1 to 2 drachms of the pulp, prepared by bruising 3 or 4 fruits into a paste, and taken with a little rock salt, is usually sufficient, and they may also be taken in decoction combined with aromatics. It is a popular domestic aperient and liver regulator and adjunct to other medicines. Take of myrobalans bruised 6, cinnamon or cloves bruised 1 drachm, water or milk 4 ounces; boil for ten minutes, strain and set aside till cold. This quantity taken at a draught generally produces in an adult 3 or 4 copious stools without griping, vomiting or other ill effects. It is well adapted for ordinary cases of constipation, and in other states where aperients are required. A conserve is made of the large, fully ripe fruit which is considered a good digestive. Equal parts of dried myrobalans in combination with emblic and beleric myrobalans and catechu, both finely powdered and rubbed into a thick paste with sufficient ghee or some bland oil, make an excellent ointment for chronic ulcerations, ulcerated wounds and many skin diseases attended with profuse discharge.

Native Indian Preparations.—The chebulic myrobalans and under the name of *triphala* or the three myrobalans, are extensively used as adjuncts to other medicines in a variety of diseases.

Pâthyadi Kvâtha :—Take of chebulic myrobalans, pulp of *cassia fistula*, root of *Picrorhiza Kurroa* (*Katuka*), root of *Ipomæa Turpethum* (*trivrit*) and emblic myrobalans equal parts, in all two tolas, and prepare a decoction in the usual way. Dose, two to four ounces as a purgative. Now-a-days senna and rhubarb are added to the above preparation.

As an alterative tonic for promoting strength and preventing the effects of age, chebulic myrobalan is regarded and used in the following way :—One fruit is taken every morning with salt in the rainy season, with sugar in autumn, with ginger in the first half of the cold season, with long pepper in the second half, with honey in spring and with treacle in the two hot months.

These adjuncts agree best with the humours that are liable to be deranged in the different seasons—(Chakradatta).

Amrita haritaki is thus prepared :—One hundred large-sized chebulic myrobalans are boiled in butter-milk and their seeds are taken out. Four tolas each of long pepper, blackpepper, ginger, cinnamon, plumbago root, root of *Piper Chaba* (*chavikà*), the five salts, *àjowan* and the seeds of *Seseli Indicum* (*vanayamàni*), *yavakshàra*, *sarjikäkshära*, borax, asafœtida and cloves are reduced to powder and soaked for three days respectively in a decoction of tamarind and in lime juice. This mixture is introduced within the seedless myrobalans, which are then exposed to the sun and dried. One of these prepared myrobalans is directed to be taken every morning for the relief of various sorts of dyspepsia and indigestion—(Bhaishajyarathnavali).

394. THALICTRUM FOLIOLOSUM.

(N. O. RANUNCULACEÆ.)

Hind.—Pinjàri, Gurbiani. *Pers.*—Asprak. *Mah.*—Trayamàna.

Habitat.—The herb is found on the temperate Himalaya and the Khasia Hills.

Properties and Uses.—The roots are very bitter and contain the alkaloid *Berberine*, so combined as to be readily soluble in water. A cold infusion of the root is used as a lotion for ophthalmia. It is also a valuable tonic and antiperiodic, useful in fevers and dyspepsia. The root also possesses aperient properties.

395. THEVATIA NERIIFOLIA.

(*N. O.*—APOCYNACEÆ.)

Eng.—The Exile or Yellow Oleander. *Hind.*—Pilá-Kanèr. *Ben.*—Kolkephul. *Mah.*—Pivalä-Kanhër. *Bom.*—Thivati. *Tel.*, and *Tam.*—Pachchai-alari.

Habitat.—This plant is commonly cultivated as an ornamental shrub in gardens in the plains.

Properties and Uses.—The bark is bitter and powerfully cathartic, and is said to be antiperiodic in small doses, 2 grains of the powdered bark being equal to an ordinary dose of cinchona; but its use is attended with considerable danger. The seeds contain a fixed oil which, when pure, is quite inert; but a highly poisonous alkaloid named *Thevetine* may be isolated from the cake left after expression of the seeds.

396. TODDALIA ACULEATA.

(*N. O.*—RUTACEÆ.)

Sans.—Kanchaná. *Hind.*—Jangli-kali-mirch. *Ben.*—Kada-todali. *Bom.*—Limri. *Tel.*—Konda-Kashinda. *Tam.*—Mila-karanai. *Can.*—Kada-hákukàre. *Mal.*—Kàr. *Kon.*—Gàlàyi.

Habitat.—This climbing shrub is found in the lower Himalaya, common in Bhutan at altitudes of about 5,000 feet and in Western and Southern India.

Properties and Uses.—The fresh root-bark and the whole plant are pungent and aromatic; the former is used in medicine and given in infusion in doses of 1 to 2 ounces or fluid extract in $\frac{1}{2}$ to 2 drachm doses. It has stimulant, tonic, carminative, diaphoretic, antiperiodic and antipyretic properties, useful in fevers, especially of that sort of remittent which is commonly called the hill-fever. It is said to be superior to quinine or Warberg's tincture as antiperiodic and antipyretic, to gentian and calumba as tonic, and as diaphoretic to pulvis Jacobi. The root-bark contains the alkaloid *berberine* which is the source of its bitterness. The fresh leaves are eaten raw for pains in the bowels. The leaves when distilled yield a yellowish-green volatile oil having an odour like that of citron and containing citronella-aldehyde. Every part of the plant is possessed of strong stimulating powers. The unripe berries are pickled and eaten. The unripe fruit and root boiled with oil make a stimulating liniment for rheumatism.

397. TRAPA BISPINOSA.

(*N. O.*—ONAGRACEÆ.)

Sans.—Sringátaka. *Eng.*—The Indian Water Chestnut. *Hind.*—Singhára. *Ben.*—Paniphal. *Bom.*, and *Mah.*—Singàda.

Habitat.—This aquatic plant is found commonly floating on the surface of lakes, tanks and pools throughout India.

Properties and Uses.—The white kernel contained within the red-brown spiny fruit is used as a food by the poorer classes in Northern India, especially in the United Provinces and Kashmir, where it is cultivated for this purpose. It abounds in starch and resembles chestnut in flavour. The nutritive value of the kernels is shown by analysis to be equal to that of rice. The kernel is found to contain small quantities of manganese, while the pericarp is very rich in that metal. Medicinally the fruits are considered useful in bilious affections with diarrhœa.

398. TRIBULUS TERRESTRIS.

(*N. O.*—ZYGOPHYLLEÆ.)

Sans.—Ikshugandha, Gokshuri. *Eng.*—Small Caltrops. *Hind.*, and *Ben.*—Gokhrù. *Mah.*—Lâhân Gokhru. *Tel.*—Pallern-mullu. *Tam.*, and *Mal.*—Nerungil. *Can.*, and *Kon.*—Negil-mullu.

Habitat.—This trailing plant is common in sandy soil throughout India, plentiful in the United Provinces and in Madras.

Properties and Uses.—The entire plant including the root and the fruit is used in medicine. The fruit is covered with stout blunt spines. The plant and more especially the dried spiny fruits have been much esteemed as cooling, diuretic, tonic and aphrodisiac, used in decoction in cases of spermatorrhœa and diseases of the genito-urinary system such as painful micturition, calculous affections; urinary disorders and impotence. Water rendered mucilaginous by the plant is drunk as a remedy for impotence and an infusion of the stem is administered for gonorrhœa.

Native Indian Preparations.—A decoction of the fruits is given with the addition of *yavakshära* (impure carbonate of potash) in painful micturition—(Chakradatta). A decoction of the entire plant is given with *silàjàtu* (a bituminous substance) and honey in the same affection. Equal parts of *gokhru* and sesamum seeds taken with goat's milk and honey is said to cure impotence arising from vicious practices.

Gokshùràdyava leha or electuary of *gokshuri* is prepared as follows:—Take of the entire plant of *Tribulus terrestris* 12½ seers, water 64 seers and boil till reduced to one-fourth. To the strained decoction add 6¼ seers of sugar and again boil till reduced to the proper consistence for an electuary; then add the following substances in fine powder:—ginger, longpepper, blackpepper, cinnamon, cardamoms, flowers of *Messua ferrea* (*nâgakesara*), leaves called *tejapatra*, nutmeg, bark of *Terminalia Arjuna* and cucumber seeds each 16 tolas, bamboo-manna ½ seer, and prepare an electuary. It is given in doses of two tolas in painful micturition, suppression of urine, bloody urine calculous affections, etc.—(Bhavaprakâsha.)

---

399. TRICHOSANTHES DIOICA.

(*N. O.*—CUCURBITACEÆ.)

Sans.—Patola. *Eng.*—Wild Snake Gourd. *Hind.*—Palwal. *Ben.* Patól. *Mah.*—Kadu-padvala. *Tel.*—Adavi-potla. *Tam.*—Peyu-padal. *Can.*—Kahi-padavala. *Mal.*—Kâttu-patolam. *Kon.*—Kàdapaddoola.

Habitat.—This climbing plant is common in Bengal and cultivated in Northern India and the Punjab.

Properties and Uses.—The unripe fruit of this plant is generally used as a culinary vegetable and is considered very wholesome and specially suited for the convalescent. The tender tops are also used as a pot-herb and are regarded as tonic and vermifuge. The tender shoots and dried capsules are very bitter and aperient and given in decoction with sugar to assist digestion. The seeds are a remedy for disorders of the stomach and act as antifebrile and anthelmintic. The juice of the leaves is said to have emetic property, and that of the root, purgative, and the stalk in decoction is a reputed expectorant. The leaf-juice is rubbed over the liver in liver congestion and over the whole body in remittent

and given in infusion or weak decoction. Made into a gruel they are given as a diet to nurses to increase the flow of milk. As an application to the head they promote the growth of hair which they also prevent from falling off. The flour of the seeds is used as a poultice and is applied to the skin as a cosmetic. A poultice of the leaves is useful in external and internal swellings and burns, on account of their cooling properties.

Native Indian Preparations.—Several confections under the names of *Methi modaka, Svalpa methi modaka* etc., are recommended for use in dyspepsia, in the diarrhœa of puerperal women and in rheumatism. The following is one of them :—

Methi Modaka :—Take of the three myrobalans, ginger, longpepper and blackpepper, tubers of *Cyperus rotundus* (*mustaka*), nigella and cummin seeds, coriander, bark of *Myrica Sapida* (*Katphala*) *páchak* root, *Rhus Succedanea* (*Karkatasringi*), *ajowan*, rock salt, black salt, leaves of *Pinus Webbiana* (*talisa*), flowers of *Mesua ferrea*, *tejapatra*, cinnamon, cardamom, nutmegs, mace, cloves, sandalwood and camphor, one part each ; fenugreek seeds, in quantity equal to all the above ingredients ; powder them all and prepare a confection with old treacle. Dose, one to two drachms to be taken in the morning with clarified butter and honey—(Bhashajyaratnavali).

---

402. TRITICUM SATIVUM (T. Vulgare).

(*N. O.*—GRAMINEÆ.)

Sans.—Godhúma. *Eng.* Wheat. *Hind.*—Gèhun. *Ben.*—Gam. *Bom.*, and *Mah.*—Gahùn. *Tel.*—Godhumulu. *Tam.*—Godumei. *Can.*—Gòdi. *Mal.*—Kótampam *Kon.* - Gavu.

Habitat.—Wheat is extensively cultivated in various forms or varieties. in the Punjab, in the United and the Central Provinces, and the Bombay Presidency.

Properties and Uses.—Wheat is the most important and the most nutritive of the food-grains; it forms the staple food of the majority of the better classes of the people in Northern and Western India. Wheaten flour is useful as a dusting powder applied over inflamed surfaces as in erysipelas, burns, scalds and various itching and burning eruptions. It is employed for making yeast poultice. A mixture of flour and water is an antidote in cases of poisoning by salts of mercury, copper, zinc, silver and tin and by iodine. The flour of wheat made into conjee is taken to check profuse menstruation. It is used for the preparation of bread and cakes; bread is used for making bread poultices; the crumb of bread is employed for the preparation of charcoal poultice; it is also used as a basis for pills containing creasote and similar medicaments. The "bran" is used in the form of a decoction or infusion as an emollient bath in skin diseases such as psoriasis; and internally as demulcent. The bran bread is slightly laxative and may be used with advantage in certain dyspeptic conditions and, owing to its freedom from starch, in diabetes. As it is soft and yielding, readily adapting itself to any part to which it may be desirable to apply it, and as it retains heat for a very long time, bran poultices and dry applications are frequently made use of in the treatment of severe local pains whether spasmodic or inflammatory, in acute inflammation of the chest or abdomen and in the premonitory symptoms of croup in children.

403. UNCARIA GAMBIER.

(*N. O.*—RUBIACEÆ.)

Eng.—Gambier, Pali Catechu. *Hind.*—Kathà. *Ben.*—Papri. *Bom.*—Chinai-Kâtha. *Mah.*- Kàth. *Mal.*—Gambir.

Properties and Uses.—Gambier is the product of a shrub or bush cultivated in Malacca, Penang and Singapore. It is extracted from the leaves and young shoots by boiling and subsequent evaporation. If is imported into India in irregular, sometimes partly agglutinated, cubes. It is closely allied to catechu of the *Pharmacopœia*. It contains the same chemical constituents, principally "tannin" (catechu-tannic acid) in equal quantity (40 to 50 per cent, reckoned as gallo-tannic acid) and the yellow colouring principle *Quercetin.* It is used in tanning, and also largely used as an ingredient in *pàn-supari* (betel-leaf). Medicinally it is used as an astringent and as an application to syphilitic sores and aphthous ulcers in the mouth.

---

404. UNONA NARUM.

(*N. O.*—ANONACEÆ.)

Can.—Unâmini-gida. *Mal.*—Narumpànal. *Mah.*, and *Kon.*—Gunàmanijhád.

Properties and Uses.—The roots are fragrant and aromatic and the leaves when bruised smell like cinnamon. A sweet-scented greenish oil is obtained from the roots by distillation. An unctuous secretion exudes from the anthers. The leaves are used in rheumatism and the root in erysipelas, biliousness and fevers.

---

405. URGINEA INDICA.

(*N. O.*—LILIACEÆ.)

Sans.—Vanapalându. *Eng.*—Indian Squill. *Hind.*, and *Ben.*—Jangli-piyâz. *Bom.*, and *Mah.*—Kol-kända, Jangli-kànda. *Tel.*—Nakka-vulli-gadda. *Tam.*—Nàri-vengäyam.

Habitat.—This plant grows throughout India in sandy places near the sea and is found in the Lower Himalaya.

Properties and Uses.—As met with in the bazaars the drug consists chiefly of the bulbs whole and unsliced. It may be regarded as equal in medicinal value to the officinal drug, 'squill. It has been used in place of the imported squill as a stimulant, expectorant and diuretic. The chemical constituents of squill are a glucoside, *Scillain*, and *Sillipicrin* and *Scillitoxin* bitter principles. Mucilage, sugar and crystals of calcium oxalate are also present.

---

406. VALERIANA WALLICHII.

(*N. O.*—VALERIANEÆ.)

Sans.—Tagara. *Eng.*—Indian Valerian. *Hind.*, and *Ben.*—Tagar, Nahâni. *Arab.*—Asàrün. *Mah.*—Tagaraganthona.

Habitat.—This is one of the several plants of the *Valerian* species indigenous to the temperate Himalaya and found in Kashmir and Bhutan. The rhizomes or root-stocks are collected in Afghanistan and exported to the plains. The true valerian, *V. Officinalis*, is said to be found in North Kashmir.

Properties aud Uses.—In chemical constitution the roots of *V. Wallichii*, and those of the officinal drug resemble very closely; but the former has a more powerful odour and yields a larger proportion of volatile oil and *valeric acid* on distillation with water, and it acts as a stimulant and antispasmodic, and is indicated in nervous and hysterical symptoms.

407. VATERIA INDICA.

(*N. O.*—DIPTEROCARPEÆ.)

Eng.—White Dammer Tree, the Piney Resin or Indian Copal Tree. *Hind.*, and *Duk.*—Suféd dàmer. *Ben.*—Kûndro. *Punj.*—Sundras. *Tel.*—Telladú maramu. *Tam.*—Vellai-Kunnrikam. *Can.*—Dhupada-mara. *Mal.*. Vella-Kùnturukkam. *Cing.*—Hal-dumlua. *Malay.*—Guttah rukam putch.

Habitat. This large evergreen tree is indigenous to South-Western India, Canara and Travancore.

Properties and Uses. A fine resin, the better qualities not unlike amber, exudes from incisions made in the trunk and is used like copal for making varnishes; it is met with in the bazaars in irregular masses varying in colour, fragrance and density, the differences being due to the mode of collection and the age of the trees producing them. This resin burns with a clear, steady light, giving off a pleasant smell, but very little smoke. Combined with wax and oil with the aid of gentle heat it forms a good substitute for officinal resin as a basis for various ointments and plasters. Five ounces of white dàmmar with eight ounces of Kokum butter and two ounces of wax, melted together with a gentle heat, stirring briskly as it cools and spread on rag or lint, forms a good stimulant dressing for carbuncles and other ulcerations. From the fruit bruised and subjected to boiling is obtained a solid fatty oil known as Piney tallow, which is a useful application in chronic rheumatism and other painful affections.

408. VERNONIA ANTHELMINTICA.

(N. O.—COMPOSITÆ.)

Sans.—Samaraja. *Eng.* –Purple Fleabane. *Hind.*, and *Ben.*—Sómráj, Bakchi. *Guz.*—Kadvo-jiri. *Mah.*—Kále-jiri. *Tel.*—Adavi Jilakara, Vishakantakálu. *Tam.*, and *Mal.*—Káttujiragam. *Can.*—Kàdu-jirige. *Cing.*—Sanni-nægam. *Malay.*—Justan hutan.

Habitat.—This plant is common in waste places near villages throughout India; the dried seeds of this plant are met with in almost every bazaar.

Properties and Uses.—The seeds of this plant are highly reputed as a vermifuge in cases of round worms, which are expelled lifeless. The dose is about two to three drachms of the bruised seeds administered in electuary with honey in two equal doses and followed by an aperient. For white leprosy (leucoderma) and other chronic skin diseases the seeds are a reputed remedy given alone or in combination with other medicines. In diseases like psoriasis and lepra the remedy is recommended to be continued daily for one year, when a complete cure is said to be effected. In these cases the seeds are given with black pepper, both powdered and mixed together. Dose is about a drachm, to be taken in the morning with tepid water. The medicine should be taken after perspiration has been induced by exercise or exposure to the sun. The diet should consist of milk and rice. In leucoderma, a decoction of emblic myrobalan and catechu is given with the addition of the powdered seeds. These seeds are also used as tonic, stomachic and diuretic in doses of 10 to 30 grains in powder.

Native Indian Preparations. Externally this drug is used in a variety of forms such as paste, oil, etc.:—Take of *vernonia* seeds, seeds of *Cassia Sophora* (*Kásamarda*) and *Cassia Tora* (*Chakramârda*), turmeric and common sea-salt equal parts; rub them together into a paste with whey and fermented paddy-water (*Kánjika*) and apply over eruptions attended with itching. *Vernonia* seeds four parts and orpiment one part are rubbed into an emulsion with cow's urine and applied to the patches of white leprosy or leucoderma—(Chakradatta).

---

409. VERNONIA CINEREA.

(*N. O.* COMPOSITÆ.)

Sans.—Ardhaprasádana. *Eng.*—Ash-coloured Flea-bane. *Tam.*—Naichitte. *Can.*—Sahadevi. *Mal.*—Pirinà, Puvànkurutala. *Mah.* and *Kon.*—Säyadevi.

Habitat.—Bengal, East and West Coasts of India.

Properties and Uses.—The whole plant with its small, round, downy, tasteless flowers is used medicinally in decoction to promote perspiration in febrile affections. The seed is employed as an alexipharmic and anthelmintic and as a constitutent of *masàlàs* for horses. The whole plant is a remedy for spasm of the bladder and strangury. The flowers are administered for blood-shot eyes (conjunctivitis).

---

410. VIOLA ODORATA.

(*N. O.*—VIOLACEÆ.)

Eng.—Wild Violet. *Hind.*, *Pers.*, *Bom.*, etc.—Banafsâ (the flowers); Guli-Banafsá.

Habitat.—This and several closely allied species are found in Kashmir and the temperate Western Himalaya above 5,000 feet.

Properties and Uses.—The violet flowers and root contain an emetic principle named *violin*, believed to resemble emetine in some of its characters; the flowers also contain in addition to traces of a volatile oil, several peculiar colouring matters and *viola-quercitrin*, a yellow principle, and sugar.

The flowers are used medicinally on account of their demulcent, diuretic and mildly laxative properties; in large doses they are emetic. The usual form of preparation is syrup, of which 1 to 2 drachms may be given to infants for coughs and tightness of the chest. Mixed with almond oil and syrup of senna it makes an excellent demulcent and aperient medicine. The root is emetic in doses of a drachm and upwards.

---

411. VITEX NEGUNDO.

(*N. O.*—VERBENACEÆ.)

Sans.—Nirgundi. *Eng.*—Five-leaved Chaste Tree. *Hind.*—Sámbhalu. *Ben.*—Nisindä. *Mah.*—Nirgunda. *Tel.*—Sindhuvàrumu. *Tam.*—Chinduvärara. *Can.*—Bile-nekki. *Mal.*—Indrani.

Habitat.—Bengal and Southern India.

Properties and Uses.—This species is similar in properties to the three-leaved chaste tree (*Vitex Trifolia*) with its pale blue flowers and called *Sindhuvâra*; but somewhat weaker. The leaves of this species (*V. Negundo*) are a powerful discutient and very efficacious in dispelling inflammatory swellings of the joints from acute rheumatism and of the testes from suppressed gonorrhœa; the fresh leaves are put into an earthen pot, heated over a fire and applied as hot as can be borne without pain. A pillow stuffed with the leaves is placed under the head for relief of headache. The juice of the leaves is said to remove fœtid discharges and worms from ulcers. An oil prepared with the juice of the leaves is applied to sinuses and scrofulous sores. A decoction of the leaves with long pepper is given in catarrhal fever with heaviness of head and dullness of hearing. The leaves are given with garlic, rice, and *gud* (jaggery) as a remedy for rheumatism. The root is considered as tonic, febrifuge and expectorant, also diuretic. A tincture of the root-bark in 1 to 2 drachm doses is recommended in cases of irritable bladder and of rheumatism. The powdered root is prescribed for piles as a demulcent, also for dysentery. The fruit, especially of the three-leaved variety, is nervine, cephalic and emmenagogue and is prescribed in powder, electuary and decoction. The flowers are used as cool astringent in diarrhœa, cholera, fever and diseases of the liver and are also recommended as a cardiac tonic. The seeds form a cooling medicine for cutaneous diseases and leprosy. The flowers and stalks reduced to powder are administered in cases of discharge of blood from the stomach and bowels.

---

412. VITIS INDICA.

(*N. O.*—AMPELIDEÆ.)

Eng.—Indian Wild Vine. *Hind.*—Panjèri. *Can.*—Sambár-balli. *Mal.*—Chemparavalli. *Kon.*—Sàvirsambár.

Habitat.—Malabar Coast and Travancore.

Properties and Uses.—Formerly the juice of the root with the kernel of the cocoanut was employed as a depurative and aperient. It is now given with the addition of sugar to produce an aperient action. It is also used as an alterative in the form of a decoction and is said to purify the blood, to act as a diuretic and render the secretions healthy. The root-juice mixed with oil is an application in eye-diseases; combined with cocoanut milk it is applied to carbuncles and other malignant ulcers.

---

413. VITIS VINIFERA.

(*N. O.*—AMPELIDEÆ.)

Sans., *Tel.*, *Tam.*, *Can.*, *Mah.*, and *Kon.*—Draksha. *Eng.*—The Grape. *Hind.*—Angür. *Pers.*—Kishmish. *Ben.*—Dràkhya.

Habitat.—Grapes are largely cultivated in North-Western India, in the Punjab, Kashmir, Beluchistan and Afghànistan.

Properties and Uses.—Grapes have been known and highly esteemed in India from a very remote period; the ripe fruits partly dried in the sun and called raisins are employed in medicine as demulcent, laxative and cooling, useful in thirst attendant on fever, cough, hoarseness and consumption, the stones or the seeds contained within being rejected. They contain grape-sugar, malic and other fruit acids, acid tartrate of potassium (cream of tartar) and mucilage. The seeds contain a dense fixed oil or fat and about 5 per cent of tannic acid, which also exists in the skin of the fruit. Raisins are used as an ingredient in laxative, demulcent and expectorant medicines and of confections as a vehicle for unpleasant medicaments. Wine is made from grapes in Kashmir, but the wines used in medicine and pharmacy in India are all imported ones.

Native Indian Preparations.—Take of raisins, emblic myrobalans, dates, long pepper and black pepper, equal parts, rub them together with honey and clarified butter so as to be administered as a demulcent and expectorant linctus (Sharngadhara).

Drâkshârishta :—Take of raisins 6¼ seers and water 128 seers, boil them together till reduced to one-fourth, and strain. To the strained decoction add 25 seers of treacle and 8 tolas each of the following substances in fine powder, namely, cinnamon, cardamoms, *tejpatra*, flowers of *Mesua ferrea* (*nâgakesara*), fruit of *Aglaia, Roxburghiana* (*priyangu*), black pepper. long pepper and *bâberang* seeds, and set aside for fermentation. This liquor is invigorating and nourishing and is used in consumption, cough, difficult breathing and hoarseness—(Sharngadhara).

---

414. WITHANIA COAGULANS.

(*N. O.*—SOLANACEÆ.)

Sans., and *Ben.*—Asvagandha. *Eng.*—Vegetable Rennet *Hind*,—Akri, Punir. *Bom.*—Kakanaj. *Pers.*—Panir-bad. *Tel.*—Pannèru-gadda. *Tam.*—Amukkira. *Can.*—Amakiregadde. *Mal.*—Amukiram.

Habitat.—This small shrub is common in the Punjab, Sindh, Afghanistan and Beluchistan.

Properties and Uses.—The round capsular fruit is used in the fresh state as an emetic and in small doses as a remedy in dyspepsia. It has the peculiar property of coagulating or curdling milk; a small portion is rubbed with a little water or milk and is added to the milk to be coagulated. The dried capsules also retain the coagulating property in an equal degree. A tablespoonful of the decoction made with one ounce of the powdered fruits to one quart of boiling water is enough to coagulate one gallon of warm milk and gives an excellent curd in about half an hour. The active principle named *withanin* which resides in the numerous small seeds contained within the capsules is a ferment closely allied to the rennet of the animal organism. It is destroyed by boiling and is precipitated by alcohol, which latter does not, however, affect its coagulating property. It can be extracted from the seeds either by glycerin or by a moderately strong solution of common salt, extracts prepared by either means having strong coagulating powers even in small amounts.

---

415. WITHANIA SOMNIFERA.

(*N. O.*—SOLANACEÆ).

(*Syn : Physalis Flexuosa, P. Somnifera.*)

Sans., *Ben.* and *Tel.*—Asvagandhà. *Eng.*—Winter Cherry. *Hind.*—Asgandh. *Bom.* and *Mah.*—Asagandha. *Tam.*—Achuva-gandi. *Can.*—Sogade-beru, Hirimaddina-gadde. *Mal.*—Pivate.

Habitat.—This shrub is common in Bombay and Western India, occasionally met with in Bengal.

Properties and Uses.— An alkaloid possessing hypnotic properties and named *Somniferine* has been isolated from the plant as grown in Southern Europe. The seeds have been found to possess the property of coagulating milk, like those of *W. Coagulans*, but they also contain poisonous properties. The leaves and root are reputed to have narcotic properties; the latter is also considered diuretic and deobstruent; tonic, alterative and aphrodisiac properties are also attributed to it, and as such it is used in consumption, emaciation of children, debility from old age, rheumatism, etc.

Native Indian Preparations.—In consumption a decoction of *Ashvagandhà* root and long pepper is given with the addition of clarified butter and honey. For improving the nutrition of weakly children, the root reduced to a paste is given with milk and clarified butter for a fortnight—(Chakradatta).

Ashvagandha Ghrita :—Take of the decoction of *Ashvagandhâ* root one part, milk 10 parts, clarified butter 1 part, boil them together and prepare a *ghrita*. It is given to promote the nutrition and strength of children—(Chakradatta).

In rheumatism a *ghrita* prepared with a decoction and paste of the root is used internally and an oil prepared with a decoction of the root and a number of aromatic substances in the form of a paste is used externally.

About half a drachm of *Ashvagandha* root taken with milk or clarified butter is said to act as an aphrodisiac and restorative to old men—(Sharngadhara).

416. WOODFORDIA FLORIBUNDA.

(*N. O.*—LYTHRACEÆ.)

Sans.—Dhâtaki. *Hind.*—Dhâi, Dhauta. *Ben.*—Dhai-phul. *Bom.*—Dhayatis. *Tel.*—Seringi. *Can.* and *Mal.*—Tâmrapushpi.

Habitat.—This large shrub is common in many parts of India.

Properties and Uses.—The bright red flowers are used as a dye in Northern India and largely used as a tanning material. They contain a large quantity—about 20 per cent—of tannic acid; they are thus used as astringent in dysentery and other bowel complaints and hæmorrhages. Two drachms of the dried flowers are given in curdled milk in dysentery and with honey in menorrhagia.

Native Indian Preparations.—In the dysentery of children the following combination is given in the form of powder or decoction with the addition of honey :—

Take of the flowers of *Woodfordia Floribunda*, *bel* fruits, bark of *Symplocos racemosa* (*lodhra*), root of *Pavonia Odorata* (*bálá*) and the fruits of *Pothos Officinalis* (*gájapipul*) in equal parts, two tolas in all, and prepare a decoction in the usual way. The powdered flower is sprinkled over ulcers for diminishing their discharge and promoting granulation—(Sharngadhara).

417. ZANTHOXYLUM ALATUM.

(*N. O.*—RUTACEÆ.)

Sans.—Trimburu. *Hind.*—Tumru. *Ben.*—Tambul, Nepali-dhania.

Habitat.—This shrub or bush is common in the temperate Himalaya, in Bhutan and in the Khasia Hills, found also in the Darjeeling District.

Properties and Uses.—The carpels of the fruits yield an essential oil which is isomeric with turpentine and is somewhat similar to eucalyptus oil in odour and properties; it is said to possess antiseptic, disinfectant and deodorant properties similar to those of eucalyptus. The bark of this and several other species of the same genus contains *berberine*.

418. ZINGIBER OFFICINALIS.

(*N. O.*—SCITAMINEÆ.)

Sans.—Srangavéra. *Eng.*—Ginger. *Hind.*, *Duk.*, *Ben.*, and *Punj.*—(dried) Sònth; (fresh.)—Adrakh. *Kash.*—Shò-ont. *Bom.*, *Guz.*, and *Mah.*—(dried) Sunt; (fresh) Alen. *Arab.*—Zanjabil. *Tel.*—(dried) Sonti; (fresh) Allam. *Tam.*—Shukku; (fresh) Inji. *Kan.*—Shunti. *Mal.*—Chukka. *Kon.*—Sünti. *Cing.*—Ingúrú. *Burm.*—Ginsi-khiàv. *Malay.*—Hulya-kring.

Habitat.—Ginger is cultivated in many parts of India; on a large scale in the warm, moist regions, chiefly in Madras, Cochin and Travancore and to a somewhat less extent in Bengal and the Punjab. Ginger is always obtainable in the fresh or dried state in all the bazaars.

Properties and Uses.—Ginger in the dried state is commonly used as a condiment and a conserve is made from the fresh younger rhizomes. It possesses stimulant, carminative and stomachic properties which render it extremely valuable in dyspepsia, flatulence, colic, vomiting, spasms and other painful affections of the stomach and the bowels unattended by fever, and as a corrective adjunct to purgatives to prevent nausea and griping. It is best given either in powder in doses of 10 to 30 grains, which may be taken with 5 grains of carbonate of soda in gout and chronic rheumatism, or in the form of infusion made by macerating 1 ounce of bruised ginger in a pint of boiling water in a covered vessel for an hour and straining; of which the dose is from 1 to 2 ounces every hour. The addition of a moderate dose of carbonate of soda increases its efficacy. For children a tablespoonful of the infusion is sufficient.

In chronic rheumatism, infusion of ginger (2 drachms to 6 ounces of boiling water and strained) taken warm just before going to bed, the body being covered with blankets so as to produce copious perspiration, is often attended with the best results. The same treatment has also been found beneficial in colds or catarrhal attacks and during the cold stage of intermittent fever. In headache ginger paint or plaster made by rubbing ginger (dried) with a little water, applied to the forehead affords relief. Tooth-ache and face-ache are sometimes relieved by the same application to the face. In the collapse stage of cholera powdered ginger rubbed to the extremities is found to check the cold perspiration, improve the local circulation, and so tends to relieve the agonising cramps of that terrible disease.

Ginger with salt taken before meals is praised as a carminative; said to clean the tongue and throat, increase the appetite and produce an agreeable sensation. Relaxed sore throat, hoarseness and loss of voice are sometimes benefited by chewing a piece of ginger so as to produce a copious flow of saliva.

Native Indian Preparations.—*Samasarkara churna*: Take of cardamoms 1 part, cinnamon 2 parts, flowers of *Messua ferrea (nágakesara)* 3 parts, black pepper 4 parts, long pepper 5 parts, dried ginger 6 parts, sugar in quantity equal to all the other ingredients; powder and mix. Dose—about a drachm in dyspepsia, loss of appetite and piles—(Bhavaprakash).

Saubhagya Sunti:—Take of clarified butter 16 tolas, milk 4 seers, sugar 6¼ seers, dry ginger 1 seer; boil them together so as to make an electuary. Then add coriander 24 tolas, fennel seeds 40 tolas, *báberang* seeds, cumin seeds, nigella seeds, long pepper, black pepper, ginger, tubers of *cyperus rotundas*, leaves called *tejapatra*, flowers of *Mesua ferrea*, cinnamon and cardamoms each 8 tolas in fine powder and stir with a ladle till cold. This confection is much used as a carminative tonic in dyspepsia and in disorders of the alimentary canal in females after confinement—(Bhavaprakash).

Saindhavàdya taila:—Take of dry ginger 40 tolas, rock salt, long pepper root and plumbago root 16 tolas each, marking nuts 20 in number, fermented rice water 16 seers, sesamum oil 4 seers, boil them together and prepare an oil in the usual way. The oil is rubbed externally in sciatica and other forms of rheumatism—(Chakradatta).

---

419. ZIZYPHUS JUJUBA.

(*N. O.*—RHAMNEÆ).

Sans.—Badari, Kola. *Eng.*—Jujube Fruit. *Hind.*—Baer. *Ben.*—Kul. *Pers.*—Kunâr. *Bom.* and *Mah.*—Bor. *Tel.* Règu. *Tam.*—Elandai. *Can.*—Bogari, Ilichi. *Mal.*—Ilantha.

Habitat.—This moderate sized tree is found wild and cultivated in many parts of India and Burma.

Properties and Uses.—The fruit of the wild variety is not unlike a crab-apple in appearance and taste, very acid and astringent. It is eaten raw and also preserved by drying. The fruits of the cultivated varieties are more palatable and less acid. The fruit contains mucilage and sugar in addition to fruit acids. It is believed to purify the blood and assist digestion. The bark contains much tannin and a crystallizable principle, *Ziziphic acid*, has been isolated from a watery extract of the wood. The bark is a simple remedy in diarrhœa, in the form of powder or decoction. The powdered bark is a domestic dressing to old wounds and ulcers. The root is useful as a decoction in fever and delirium. The tender leaves and twigs are used in the form of paste as an application to boils, abscesses and carbuncles; they promote suppuration.

Index of Diseases and their Remedies.

Those in italics deserve special attention.

(N. I. P.--Native Indian Preparations.)

1. **Abscess.**—Artocarpus, Careya, Datura (to relieve pain, in the form of tincture and poultice), Hydrocotyle, (mammary) Jasminum P. and S., Jatropha, Moringa N. I. P., *Oryza S.* (poultice, as anodyne), *Papaver S.* (pp. 281 and 284), Plumbago Z. and N. I. P., Pterocarpus, S., Zizyphus.
2. **Acidity** of the stomach.—*Quicklime.*
3. **Acme.**—Citrus Bergamia or Citrus Acida.
4. **Ague.**—*See* Fever, intermittent.
5. **Ague-cake.**—*See* Spleen, enlargement of.
6. **Alcohol poisoning.**—Coffea Arabica.
7. **Alopecia.**—*See* Baldness.
8. **Amaurosis.**--Euphorbia Antiquorum.
9. **Amenorrhœa.**—Aloe B., Balsamodendron Myrrha, Boswellia, Cinnamomum Z., Hydrocotyle, *Sinapis* (for hip-bath).
10. **Anæmia.**—(*See also* Chlorosis) *Boerhavia, Citrus Medica N. I. P.*, Emblica O. and N. I. P., Musa (root), Swertia Chirata N. I. P.
11. **Anasarca.**—(*See also* Ascites and Dropsy), *Boerhavia N. I. P., Citrus Medica N. I. P.*, Croton, Cynodon, Euphorbia N., Hygrophila, Plumbago Z., Solanum J., Trichosanthes Dioica N. I. P.
12. **Anorexia.**—(*See also* Appetite, loss of), Quassia.
13. **Aphthæ.**—Bauhinia T. and V., Calotropis, Coriandrum, Emblica O., Ficus G., (for children) Indigofera, *Lawsonia*, Myrtus, Pedalium, *Rosa*, Uncaria.
14. **Apoplexy.**—*Brassica A.* and J., Camphora O., Croton.
15. **Appetite,** loss of.—Cannabis N. I. P., *Coccules C. and N. I. P.*, Nigella and N. I. P., *Quassia*, Swertia Chirata.

30. **Buboes.**—Arum, Boswellia, Erythrina, Oryza.

31. **Burns and scalds.** Acacia Arabica, Basella, Gossypium, Honey (ceromel), Lawsonia, *Linum*, *Sesamum*, (the oil for lime liniment), Trigonella, Triticum.

32. **Burning of the feet.**—Lawsonia, Mesua.

33. **Calculus.**—Cynodon, Dolichos, Lawsonia, Moringa and N. I. P., Pedalium, Styrax Benzoin (phosphatic), Tribulus.

34. **Carbuncle.**—Borassus, Coriandrum, Papaver, Sugar, Vateria Indica.

35. **Catarrh and Cold.**—Aconitum Ferox N. I. P., Agati, Allium Cepa (children), Barleria, Crocus, *Curcuma Longa* (as inhalation), Mussaenda, Myrica and Nigella (nasal), Ocimum Sanctum, Solanum J., Potassii nitras, Quercus, Zingiber.

36. **Centipedes,** bites of.—Cucurbita Maxima.

37. **Cephalalgia.**—Coriandrum, Hydrargyrum N. I. P., Nelumbium and N. I. P.

38. **Chancre.**—Adansonia, Nerium.

39. **Chest, affections** of children.—Brassica Juncea, Camphora.

40. **Chlorosis.**—Balsamodendron Myrrha.

41. **Cholera.**—*Acorus*, Andropogon C., Brassica A (plaster), *Capsicum*, Carum, Coffea (infantum), Ferula Asafœtida, Mucuna, Myrica, Myristica F., Piper Nigrum, *Ptychotis*, Strychnos Nux Vomica, *Sinapis* (plaster).

42. **Chorea.**—*Nardostachys Jatamansi*, *Strychnos Nux-vomica.*

43. **Colic.**—Acorus, Altingia, Andrographis (children), Andropogon C., and Andropogon S., Anisomeles (children), *Caesalpinia*, *Cannabis*, Carum, Cassia (for children as application), Cinnamomum Z. (cramps of the stomach), Ferula Asafœtida (flatulent), Myristica F., *Peucedanum*, Pimpinella Anisum and Ptychotis (flatulent), Trigonella, Zingiber (flatulent).

44. **Conjunctivitis.**—Acacia, Aloe L., Cassia Auriculata, (chronic) *Coriandrum*, Erythrina, *Luffa A* (granular), Nicotiana (purulent), Tamarindus, Vernonia C.

45. **Constipation**, habitual.—Aloe B. (for hysterical females), *Carica Papaya*, Cassia F., Croton N. I. P., Mimusops

58. **Diabetes.**—Acacia Arabica, Beninkasa, Borassus (toddy), Cassia Auriculata, fistula and Sophora, Citrus B., *Eugenia Jambolana, Ficus* B. and G., Musa (unripe fruit) and N. I. P., Orchis Mascula, *Papaver* and N. I. P., Pearls N. I. P., *Prunus Amygdalus, Strychnos nux vomica and Potatorum*, Triticum.

59. **Diarrhœa.**—*Acacia* A. C. and S., Aconitum H., (children) *Acorus, Aegle* and N. I. P., (chronic) *Alstonia*, Andrographis, *Areca Catechu*, (chronic) Asparagus, *Butea* (children and delicate females), Cæsalpinia Sappan, (chronic) *Cannabis* and N. I. P., Carica Papaya, *Cedrus Deodara* (atonic), also Cinnamomum M. and Z., Coffea (chronic), Eugenia Jambolana (children), also Ferona and N. I. P., Flacourtia, (chronic) *Garcinia Mangostana*, Hydrargyrum N. I. P., Mangifera, Myristica, Nigella, Oxalis N. I. P., *Papaver* N. I. P., *Plantago Ispagula*, Pterocarpus M., *Ptychotis Ajowan, Punica Granatum, Rheum Emodi* (for children during teething), Soymida, *Strychnos nux vomica* and N. I. P. (chronic), Strychnos Potatorum (for puerperal women), Trapa, Terminalia B., Trigonella, Zizyphus J.

60. **Diphtheria.**—Carica Papaya, Cuprum.

61. **Dropsy** (renal).—Achyranthes, *Boerhavia*, Cassia (incipient), *Citrullus Colocynthis*, Clitoria, *Croton*, Cynodon, Garcinia, Juniperus, Moringa, Nigella, (renal) Pavetta, Pedalium, *Scilla*, Solanum I., J. and N., Styrax Benzoin, Taraxacum, Terminalia B., Trigonella.

62. **Dysentery.**—Acacia Arabica (bloody), Adhatoda, (children) Aegle and N. I. P., Ailanthus M. (bloody), Aloe L., Alstonia, Asparagus, Bauhinia T., Bergera, Bombax and N. I. P., Butea (for children and delicate females), *Calotropis*, Cannabis, Cinnamomum, Citrus M., *Curcuma Angustifolia*, Diospyros, *Eucalyptus*, Ferona and N. I. P., Ficus B., Garcinia Mangostana (chronic), Hibiscus E., *Holarrhena*, (acute) Ixora Coccinea, Luffa P., Mangifera and Musa (chronic), Naregamia (acute), Ocimum B., Oxalis and N. I. P., *Plantago Ispagula, Punica Granatum, Ricinis*, Santalum A., and N. I. P., Saraca, Sesamum, Shorea

N.I.P., Spondias, Sulphur (chronic), Tamarindus, Toddalia, Trigonella, Tylophora, Vitex Negundo, Woodfordia.

63. Dysmenorrhœa.—Andropogon C., *Cannabis*, *Datura* (poultice or liniment), Gossypium, Musa, Nigella, *Petroselinum*, Sesamum, *Papaver*.

64. Dyspepsia.—Aconitum Ferox N. I. P., *Acorus* and N. I. P., Aegle, Ailanthus E. and M., Andrographis, Aristolochia, Asparagus (bilious), *Caesalpinia B.*, *Capsicum*, *Carica Papaya*, Cinnamomum Z., Citrus A., *Cocculus*, Coriandrum, Cuminum, Emblica and N. I. P., Ferula Asafœtida N. I. P., *Gentiana*, *Kariyat*, Melia Azadirachta, Momordica C., Myristica F., Nigella, Pearls N. I. P., Piper Nigrum N. I. P., *Ptychotis*, Quassia (atonic), Rheum, Rhus S., Semecarpus A. (bilious), Spondias M., Strychnos nux vomica and N. I. P. (with pain after meals), Swertia Chirata (gouty), Tamarindus N. I. P., Taraxacum, Terminalia chebula N. I. P., Thalictrum, Toddalia, Trigonella, Withania C., Zingiber N. I. P.

65. Dysuria.—Cannabis, Cucumis Melo, Curcuma Angustifolia, Hibiscus, Oryza, Oxalis N. I. P., Pedalium, Raphanus S., Solanum I. and J., Tribulus N. I. P.

66. Ear-ache.—Acalypha, *Allium Cepa and Sativum*, *Cannabis*, Cleome, Datura, Myristica M., Ocimum S., Pandanus, Papaver, piper betle, Trichosanthes P.

67. Eczema—(chronic). Carica Papaya, Cucumis Melo, *Curcuma longa N. I. P.*, Eclipta, Hydrocotyle, Jatropha, *Melia Azadirachta*.

68. Elephantiasis.—Calotropis, Carica Papaya, Eclipta, Hydrocotyle, Hemidesmus N. I. P., Ichnocarpus N. I. P.

69. Epilepsy.—Acorus N. I. P., Beninkasa and N. I. P., Citrullus, Cocculus (nocturnal), Datura, *Herpestis* and N. I. P., Moringa, *Moschus*, *Nardostachys Jatamansi*, Semecarpus A., *Strychnos nux vomica*.

70. Epistaxis.—Cynodon, Mangefera I.

71. Erysipelas.—Butea, Cannabis, *Melia Azadirachta*, Nelumbium and N. I. P., Oryza, Triticum S., Unona Narum.

72. **Eye-complaints** (dimness).—Agati, (photophobia) Cannabis, Jasminum S., Nelumbium, Piper betle, Pterocarpus S., (impaction of steel, etc.) Ricinis C., (lachrymation) Strychnos P., Vitis Indica.

73. **Fainting.**—Ferula Asafœtida, Ptychotis.

74. **Face-ache.**—Brassica Alba, Quinetum, Zingiberis (as poultice).

75. **Fevers.**—Aconitum F. and H. and N. I. P., Acorus, and N. I. P., Adhatoda N. I. P., Allium Sativa (intermittent), Alstonia and N. I. P. (malaria), Andropogon C. (typhoid), Andropogon M., *Berberis* (remittent), *Cæsalpinia B.* (infectious) Camphora, Croton N. I. P. (inflammatory and rheumatic) Cassia S., (bilious) Cedrus deodara, *Cinchona*, Citrullus N. I. P., Citrus Medica N. I. P., *Cocculus*, curcuma longa (intermittent), Cyperus Rotundus N. I. P., Flacourtia, Gendarusssa, Gmelina, Gossypium (intermittent), Hemidesmus N. I. P., Hydrargyrum N. I. P. (remittent), *Melia Azadirachta*, Moringa (low and remittent), Moschus and N. I. P., Myristica, Nelumbium, Nigella N. I. P. (intermittent and puerperal), Nyctanthus (bilious and intermittent), Ocimum S. Oryza, Piper nigrum and longum N. I. P. (intermittent), *Potassii Nitras* (bilious), *Quassia*, *Quinetum* (intermittent), Soymida, Strychnos nux vomica, Swertia chirata (intermittent), *Tamarindus*, Thalictrum (intermittent), Thevatia (intermittent), (remittent and hill fever) Toddalia and Trichosanthes N. I. P., Vernonia, Vitex Negundo (intermittent), Vitis Vinifera, Zingiber.

76. **Flatulence.**—Acorus, Allium Sativum and N. I. P., *Andrographis*, *Andropogon Citratis*, Butea, Capsicum, Carum C., Cicer Arictinum, Cinnamon Z., Curcuma Z., *Ferula Asafœtida* and N. I. P., Nardostachys Jatamansi, *Peucedanum*, *Pimpinella Anisum*, Piper Nigrum, Plumbago Zealanica N. I. P., *Ptychotis*, *Zingiber*.

77. **Genito-Urinary Diseases.**—*Hemidesmus*, *Hibiscus*, *R.* (female), Hydrargyrum N. I. P. *Linum*, Phœnix D. and S., *Prunus A.*, Raphanus, Rosa Strychnos P.

121. **Orchitis.**—Bassia, Butea, Cæsalpinia B., Cannabis, Gossypium, Nicotiana, Vitex Negundo.

122. **Otalgia.**—Gynandropsis, Moringa.

123. **Otorrhœa.**—Allium S., Arum, Cleome, *Curcuma longa*, *Helicteres*, Jasminum G., Oroxylum and N. I. P.

124. **Ozœna.**—Hydrocotyle, Ocimum S. and N. I. P.

125. **Palpitation of the Heart.**—Camphora, (hysterical) Citrus B., Coffea, Ferula Asafœtida, *Nardostachys Jatamansi*.

126. **Palsy.**—Cæsalpinia, Ferula Asafœtida N. I. P., (facial), Moringa, Piper longum (facial), Semecarpus.

127. **Paralysis.**—Allium S. and N. I P., *Croton* (of the tongue) Hydrargyrum N. I. P., Mucuna, Orchis, Piper longum, Rubia, (facial) Sida Cordifolia, N. I. P.

128. **Paraplegia.**—Abrus N. I. P , Allium Sativa N. I. P., Piper longum N I. P.

129. **Parotitis.**—Brassica Nigra, Datura (*See also* Mumps).

130. **Phthisis.**—*Adhatoda N. I. P.*, Beninkasa and N. I. P., *Cocculus C. and S* , Corton, Flacourtia, Herpestis N. I. P., Hydrargyrum N. I. P., Pistacia, (night-sweats) Rosa.

131. **Piles.**—(bleeding) *Acacia S.* Aloe B., Arum, Cannabis, (bleeding) Carica Papaya and Coriandrum. Curculigo, (bleeding) Cynodon, Euphorbia N., Messua N. I. P., (bleeding), Nelumbium N. I. P., *Nymphæa L.*, Ocimum B., Oxalis Corniculata N. I. P., *Papaver*, Phaseolus R., Piper Nigrum and N. I. P., *Plantago Ispagula*, Pterocarpus S., Quercus, Vitex Negundo, *Raphanus.*, Ricinis, Semecarpus N. I P., Sesamum, Sida C., (bleeding), Sodii biboras, Sphæranthus H , Sulphur, Tagetes and Tamarindus (bleeding), Terminalia B., Vitex Negundo.

132. **Pityriasis.**—Cassia S., Pongamia G., Rubia.

133. **Pleurodynia.**—Citrus Medica and N.I.P., Ricinis and N I.P..

134. **Pneumonia.**—(infants) Aloe B., Quinetum.

135. **Prickly heat.**—Camphora, Oryza S., (dusting with rice flour), Santalum album (powder).

136. **Prurigo.**—Abrus N. I. P., Acacia Catechu N. I. P., Aconitum Ferox N. I. P., Curcuma A., Curcuma longa N. I. P., Hydrargyrum N. I P., Santalum A

137. Psora.—Momordica, Naregamia, Sodii biboras.

138. Psoriasis.—Aconitum Ferox N. I. P., Carica Papaya, Cassia S. and T., Dipterocarpus, Hydrargyrum and N I. P., Pongamia, Sodii Biboras, *Sulphur* N. I. P., Triticum, Vernonia A.

139. Puerperal Diseases.—(fever) Nigella Sativa, Pedalium.

140. Rheumatism.—(chronic) Acorus, Adansonia, Alangium (acute), Allium C and S., *Andropogon Citratis* (chronic), Anisomeles, Asparagus N. I. P., Balsamodendron Mukul N. I. P., *Bryonia*, *Calophyllum*, *Calotropis*, Cannabis, Cinnamomum Z., Citrus Aurantium and Medica N. I. P., *Cocculus* (chronic), *Croton* (acute), Gaultheria, Gynocardia (chronic), *Hemidesmus*, Hydrargyrum, Hydrocotyle, Jatropha, *Melaleuca*, Michelia, *Myristica* F. and M., Papaver, (acute) Paederia Fœtida N. I. P., Phaseolus Roxburghii N. I. P., Piper longum, Plantago Ispagula, Pongamia, *Potassii Nitras* (acute), Ptychotis, Quinetum, Semecarpus, Sodii chloridum, Solanum D., Strychnos nux vomica (muscular), Sulphur, Toddalia, Trigonella N. I. P., Unona Narum, Vateria Indica, Vitex Negundo (acute), Withania Somnifera and N. I. P., Zingiber (chronic).

141. Ringworm.—Butea seeds, Calotropis, Carica Papaya, *Cassia Alata, Fistula and Sophora*, Cocos N., (of the scalp) Curcuma L., Embelia N. I. P., Hydrargyrum N. I. P., Jasminum A., *Ocimium A. and S.*, Pistia S., *Rhinacanthus*, Siegesbeckia, Sodii biboras, *Toddalia*.

142. Salivation.—Acacia Catechu, Alumen, Sodii biboras.

143. Scabies.—(Itch) Acalypha, *Cassia Occidentialis*, Sophora and tora, Jatropha, Momordica, Plumeria, Pongamia, Santalum, *Sulphur* Sesbania, Terminalia.

144. Scarletina, Scarlet Fever.—Calotropis, Tylophora.

145. Sciatica.—Allium Sativum N. I. P., Brassica N., *Citrus Medica N. I. P.*, Ferula Asafœtida N. I. P., Gaultheria, *Nyctanthes*, Piper longum N. I. P., Ricinis N. I. P., Zingiber N. I. P.

146. **Scorpion Stings.**—Allium Cepa, Argemone, *Aristolochia*, Carica Papaya, Citrullus, Cuminum, Curcuma longa, *Eclipta*, Euphorbia T., Sesbania.

147. **Scrofula.**--Acacia S., Bauhinia Variegata N. I. P., Boswellia, Caesalpinia B., *Datura* (tincture to relieve pain), *Gynocardia*, *Hydrocotyle*, *Melia Azadirachta*, Semecarpus, Siegesbeckia, Smilax, Solanum D., Vitex Negundo.

148. **Scurvy.**—Aegle, *Agave*, Allium Cepa, *Anacardium*, *Ananas*, Averrhoa Carambola, *Citrus A. B. and M.*, Hibiscus S., Opuntia, *Mangifera*, Spondias, *Tamarindus*.

149. **Skin diseases.**—Abrus N. I. P., Acacia Catechu N. I. P., Aconitum Ferox N. I. P., Balsamadendron Mukul, Bauhinia Variegata N. I. P., Boswellia, *Cassia Alata and tora*, *Cocculus*, Curcuma A. L. and Z. Embelia N. I. P., Gynocardia, *Hemidesmus*, Hydrargyrum and N. I. P., Lawsonia, *Melia Azadirachta*, Sulphur and N. I. P., Terminalia Catappa and chebula, Vitex Negundo.

150. **Small-pox.**—Curcuma L., Oryza (*Conjee*), *Potassii Nitras*, Quinetum.

151. **Snake-bites.**—Aristolochia, Bryonia, Butea, Cassia S., Gymnema, Nelumbium, Ocimum S. *Ophiorrhiza*, *Pericampylus*, Rhinacanthus, Trichosanthes Dioica N. I. P., Vernonia A.

152. **Sore Eyes.**—Mussaenda, Pterocarpus S.

153. **Sore Nipples.**—Acacia catechu, Ricinis, Tabernamontana.

154. **Sore-throat.**—*Allium Cepa*, Balsamodendron M., *Glycerrhiza*, Moringa, Piper B., and N., Punica Granatum, Quercus, *Rosa*.

155. **Spermatorrhoea.**—*Camphor*, Hibiscus E., Lawsonia, Mucuna, Pedalium, Pearls N. I. P., Tribulus, Zingiber.

156. **Spleen, enlargement of.**—Aloe L., Borassus F., *Carica Papaya*, Citrus B., *Cocculus and N. I. P.* Lawsonia, Momordica, Moringa and N. I. P., Piper L., Quinetum, Solanum J.

157. **Sprains.**—Andropogon C., Cicer, Curcuma Aromatica and Longa, Gynandropsis, Melia Azadirachta, Semecarpus A., Sodii chloridum.

Index of Therapeutic Agents, with their Definitions.

Alexipharmic.—A medicine neutralising a poisoning.

Alterative.—A medicine that alters the processes of nutrition and excretion, restoring, in some unknown way, the normal functions of an organ or of the system without producing any obvious impression on any of the organs of the body.

Anaesthetic.—A substance that produces loss of sensation and consciousness from its effects upon the brain and spinal centres.

Anodyne.—A medicine that gives relief from pain.

Anthelmintic.—An agent or medicine either killing or rendering powerless intestinal worms. A vermicide.

Antiarthritic.—A remedy against gout.

Antilithic.—An agent preventing the deposit of urinary calculi or sediment.

Antiperiodic.—A remedy which antagonises the poison of periodic disorders like ague.

Antiphlogistic.—An agent subduing or reducing inflammations.

Antipyretic.—An agent reducing the temperature of fever.

Antiscorbutic.—A remedy for, or preventive, of scurvy.

Antiseptic.—A remedy that prevents or destroys putrefaction or, what is the same thing, the bacteria upon which putrefaction depends.

Antispasmodic.—An agent allaying or relieving convulsions or spasmodic pains.

Aperient.—A mild purgative or laxative.

Aphrodisiac.—An agent stimulating the sexual passion.

Astringent.—An agent producing contraction of organic tissues or arresting haemorrhages, diarrhoeas, etc.

Attenuant.—An agent increasing the fluidity or thinness of the blood or other secretion.

Carminative.—A calming or soothing medicine, chiefly for children, that acts by relieving pain from flatulence.

Cathartic.—A medicine producing evacuations from the bowels.

Cholagogue.—A remedy promoting the secretion or excretion of bile.

Cordial.—Pertaining to the heart; exhilarant or stimulant.

Demulcent.—A substance soothing or protecting the mucous membranes.

Deobstruent.—A medicine that removes functional obstructions of the body.

Deodorant.—That which destoys, removes or corrects offensive odours.

Depurative.—A medicine that purifies or cleanses.

Detergent.—A drug purifying, cleansing wounds, ulcers, etc.

Diaphoretic.—A medicine causing an increase of perspiration.

Disinfectant.—An agent that destroys disease germs and noxious properties of fermentation and putrefaction.

Diuretic.—A medicine that increases the flow or secretion of urine.

Ecbolic.—That which produces abortion or facilitates parturition.

Emetic.—An agent that has the power of inducing vomiting.

Emmenagogue.—A medicine that stimulates the menstrual flow.

Emollient.—A substance which by external application softens the skin or internally soothes an irritated or inflamed surface.

Escharotic.—A substance that, applied to the skin, produces an eschar.

Expectorant.—A remedy that promotes expectoration.

Febrifuge.—An agent that lessens fever.

Galactagogue or **lactagogue.**—An agent that increases the secretion of milk in the breast.

Haemostatic.—An agent that arrests or restrains bleeding.

Hydragogue.—A medicine which causes free secretion from the intestinal glands and removes much serum from the blood-vessels, producing fluid or watery motions.

Hypnotic.—A remedy that causes sleep.

Lactifuge.—A drug that causes a lessening in the secretion of milk.

Lithontriptic.—A medicine supposed to possess the power of dissolving various concretions in the body, as the acids for phosphatic and the alkalies for uric acid calculi.

Masticatory.—An agent which when chewed increases the flow of saliva.

Mydriatic.—A medicine that causes dilatation of the pupil.

Narcotic.—A drug that produces narcosis or stupour.

Nervine.—A remedy that calms nervous excitement or acts favourably on nervous diseases.

Refrigerant.—A medicine having cooling properties or lowering bodily temperature.

Resolvent.—That which causes the absorption of inflammatory or other swellings.

Rubefacient.—A remedy that, by irritation of the ends of the nerves of the skin, causes distention of the capillaries and reddening of the skin.

Sedative.—An agent that exerts a soothing effect by lowering functional activity.

Sialagogue.—A drug producing the flow of saliva.

Soporific.—An agent which induces sleep.

Styptic.—A medicine that causes vascular contraction of the bloodvessels and checks hæmorrhage.

Sudorific.—A medicine inducing profuse sweating.

Vermifuge.—A medicine or agent that expels intestinal worms.

Vesicant.—A blistering agent or application.

Vulnerary.—A remedy or agent useful in healing wounds.

Index of Important Dietetic Articles used in India.

Articles of Food.	Average Percentage Composition.				Comparative Value yielded by 1 lb (in ors).	
	Proteids or Flesh-formers.	Fats and Starch or Heat-givers.	Mineral Matters or Salts.	Watery Matters.	Warmth.	Strength.
Arrow-root	4	82	1	13	...	...
Bajri	10	73	2	15	...	...
Barley, Pearl	11	72	2	15	...	90
Barley-meal	12	74	3	11	2780	...
Beet-root	1·5	10·5	1	87	...	...
Biscuits (average) ...	15·6	74·7	1·7	8	...	...
Bread, average, wheaten ...	8	50·7	1·3	40	1990	90
Breast-milk	2·4	10·2	·4	87	...	...
Butter, English, average ...	1·5	87·5	1	10	...	...
Butter, clarified	0	100	0	0	4706	...
Cabbage	3	9·5	1·5	86	...	...
Caltrops, Water *(Paniphul)*	4	82	1	13	...	...
Carrots	1	10·2	1	87·8	390	...
Chouli (Barbati Dal) ...	24	59	3	14	...	...
Coffee	3	28	10	12	...	...
Cream	2·7	29·5	1·8	66	...	...
Earthnut—*see* Ground-nut..	...	...	...	...	...	...
Eggs	13·5	11·6	1·4	73·5	...	...
Fish, average	22	14	1	63	980	129
Fish, Herrings, fresh ...	10	8	2	80	1455	...
Fish, Salmon	15	7	2	76	...	·
Flour, average	11	73	1	15	...	...
Flour, fine	13	70	0·7	16·3	2700	120
Ghee—*see* Butter, clarified..	...	...	...	...	...	...
Gram, Bengal	22·8	66·7	2·5	10	...	...
,, Black (Phaseol) ...	22	62	3	13	...	...
,, Green *(Mung Dal)* ...	24	60	3	13	...	14

Articles of Food.	Average Percentage Composition.				Comparative Value yielded by 1 lb (in grs.)	
	Proteids or Flesh-formers.	Fat and Starch or Heat-givers.	Mineral Matters or Salts.	Watery Matters.	Warmth.	Strength.
Gram, Horse	23·3	61	3·7	12	...	...
Ground-nut	31	56	4	9	...	...
Lentils *(Musur Dal)* ...	24	59	2	15	...	...
Maize	10	74	2	14	...	...
Meat	22	14	1	63	...	...
Milk, average, cow's ...	5	8	1	86	378	35
Milk, breast, *see* Breast-milk	...	...	...	...	...	...
,, tinned, Swiss condensed	12	61	2	25	...	...
Millet, Great *(Jaware)* ...	9	74	1	16	...	...
Millet, Little *(Kangni)* ...	12	70	1	17	...	...
Millet, Spiked—*see* Bajri ...	...	...	...	...	...	...
Mutton	18	5	1	76	150	140
Oats	11	69	3	17	...	...
Oatmeal	13	69	3	15	...	140
Parsnips	1	15	1	83	425	12
Peas, Common *(Matar Dal)*	25	58	2	15	...	...
,, Green	7	36	2	55	...	...
Pigeon Peas *(Arahar Dal)*..	21	61	3	16	...	...
Potato	2	23	1	74	770	24
Raddish *(Múli)*	1·2	4	0·8	94	...	...
Ragi	9	75	2	14	...	...
Rice	5	84	1	10	2750	70
Sago	0·8	86	0·2	13	...	...
Sugar	0	100	0	0	2900	...
Turnips	1	7	1	91	238	12
Varagu	12·6	73	2·4	12	...	...
Vetch *(Khesari Dal)* ...	28	56	3	13	...	...
Wheat	13	72	2	13	...	...

INDEX.

(English and Hindi Synonyms.)

C

D

E

F

Supplemental Vernacular Index.

A = Arabic, B = Bengali, C = Canerese, D = Dukni, G = Guzerati, H = Hindi, K = Konkani, M = Malayalam, Mh. = Mahrati, P = Persian, Pj. = Punjabi, S = Sanskrit, T = Tamil, Tl. = Telugu, Bom. = Bombay, Cing. = Cinghalese, Kash. = Kashmere.

A

* These figures refer to the numbers of the Drug treated in the book.

B

C

D

N

O